Homemaker/ Home Health Aide

Student Workbook to accompany
Homemaker/Home Health Aide,
H. Huber/A. Spatz
Order No. 0-8273-3438-9

If this workbook is not available
in your bookstore, ask your Bookstore
Manager to order it for you.

Homemaker/ Home Health Aide

third edition

Helen Huber, BA
Audree Spatz, MEd, BS, RN

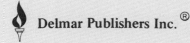
Delmar Publishers Inc.®

NOTICE TO THE READER

Delmar Staff

Executive Editor: Leslie F. Boyer
Associate Editor: Marjorie A. Bruce
Editing Manager: Barbara A. Christie
Project Editor: Ruth East
Publications Coordinator: Karen Seebald

Cover photos by Jeff Greenberg

For information, address Delmar Publishers Inc.
2 Computer Drive West, Box 15-015
Albany, New York 12212

Printed in the United States of America
Published simultaneously in Canada
by Nelson Canada,
a division of International Thomson Limited

10 9 8 7 6 5 4 3

Library of Congress Cataloging in Publication Data

Huber, Helen.
    Homemaker/home health aide / Helen Huber, Audree Spatz.—3rd ed.
        p.   cm.
    Includes index.
    ISBN 0-8273-3436-2 (pbk.).   ISBN 0-8273-3437-0 (instructor's guide)
        1. Home health aides.   2. Visiting housekeepers.   3. Home nursing.
    I. Spatz, Audree.   II. Title.
    RA645.3.H8 1989
    649'.8—dc19
                                                    88-20412
                                                        CIP

contents

part 1   Basic Principles

section 4 Promoting Health and Understanding Illness

part 2   Practical Applications

Homemaker/Home Health Aide, 3rd edition, is a comprehensive, competency-based guide to the principles and practices that home health care providers need to know to ensure quality care to the major consumers of such services—the elderly, infirm, and chronically ill.

The health care delivery system in the United States is changing rapidly. Patients who ten years ago would have spent long periods of time in a hospital convalescing from a serious illness, injury, or surgery are now released much earlier. For many of these patients, continued supportive care is required while convalescence continues. These people require care at home from trained health care providers. As the population of the United States ages, there are more elderly who can be maintained at home through the services of homemaker/home health aides. Chronically ill people of any age can be cared for at home with supportive services. Home care relieves strain on the delivery of care by means of acute care and long-term care facilities and helps maintain the independence of the individual.

In this edition of *Homemaker/Home Health Aide,* the authors continue to offer maximum exposure to the essential information and procedures that form the core of training for aides—at a level that learners can readily understand. High school students who become certified as home health aides can go immediately from high school into the job market. High school students may require additional practice for homemaking skills to compensate for the probable lack of extensive experience in this area. The text may be used effectively by adults reentering the job market. Even though such persons may have experience as homemakers, they can still benefit from a review of homemaking procedures. They may, indeed, learn new and better techniques. In addition, they will become proficient in performing technical procedures and understanding the principles underlying these procedures.

A broad scope of information is offered in this text, but due to differing state laws, each instructor will have to assume responsibility for adding or deleting procedures to meet local laws and practices. Emphasis should be placed upon the need for graduates of home health aide programs to attend in-service programs to increase and upgrade their skills.

Homemaker/Home Health Aide is divided into two major parts. Part I on basic principles offers background information and theory on which the learner builds a strong foundation prior to hands-on client care. Part I includes topics such as the vocation of home health aide, ethics and liability, communication skills development, observation and reporting skills, cultural differences, basic anatomy and physiology, human development, age-related physical and emotional problems, the relationship between health and illness, and care given to clients with specific problems.

Part II on practical applications details the procedures that most home health aides perform, including homemaking responsibilities. A step-by-step description of each major client care procedure performed by a home health aide is provided. These procedures should first be demonstrated by the instructor, practiced by the student, and then a return demonstration should be scheduled. No individual should be certified as a home health aide until these procedures can be correctly and accurately performed. The text concludes with guidance on finding employment.

It is recommended that one-half of the class time be devoted to learning the underlying theory and the second half be spent in a classroom laboratory where students can observe demonstrations of the procedures and then practice with each other before giving a return demonstration to the instructor.

In many areas of the country, a minimum training period of 90 hours is required before certification as a home health aide. Of this time, 60 hours are devoted to classroom/laboratory time and 30 hours are mandated as hands-on in the home under the supervision of a registered nurse. The necessity of a thorough understanding of both theory and practical learning cannot be overemphasized. Ultimately, the home health aide will be alone in the home setting with the client. Thus, the home health aide must be able to offer safe and medically proper care to the client and know when and how to call for assistance in an emergency.

Individual instructors will develop their own teaching plans and may choose to add new procedures to their curriculum (to the extent permitted by state laws). This text concentrates on preparing homemaker/home health aides for entry level employment. En-richment can and should be provided by each instructor. Most voluntary and proprietary agencies are or soon will be required by law to offer remedial and advanced inservice training for all practicing home health aides.

the third edition

The text was revised to reflect current issues, expanded job responsibilities, and newer or added procedures. The major changes for this edition are as follows:

- New content promoting the self-image of the homemaker/home health aide as a valued member of the health care team.
- New content emphasizing the role of the aide in relation to the nursing care plan.
- New content stressing the right of all clients to respect, courtesy, proper and safe care and confidentiality.
- New section on developing good observation skills.
- New section on how to report what has been observed about the client and his environment as they affect the care plan for the client; stresses timely reporting and documenting of accurate information.
- Added discussion of liability and what actions constitute liability on the part of the home health aide.
- Added information on ethical questions facing health care providers with guidelines on appropriate responses by home health aides.
- Added content on changes which occur in body systems as a result of aging; increased coverage of the physical and emotional effects of aging with case histories illustrating multiple problems facing the aged.
- Expanded coverage of safety in the home for the client, including the use of devices to make the environment safer and practices promoting safe living; also room-by-room guidelines for eliminating safety hazards.

- New unit on caring for the client with an infectious disease; includes extensive discussion of AIDS, with coverage of Universal Barrier Precautions to prevent the spread of the virus; a sample care plan for an AIDS client is provided.
- New unit on caring for clients with arthritis includes range of motion exercises.
- Added discussion of Diagnostic Related Grouping (DRGs) as a cost containment measure and their effect on the home health care industry.
- Expanded discussion of basic human needs.
- Added discussion of the value of humor in promoting well-being and health.
- Expanded content on cultural diversity; stresses that home health aides must keep an open mind and not judge clients because of practices unique to their cultures.
- Expanded coverage of mentally impaired clients (mental illness and retardation).
- Updated CPR information to reflect latest guidelines from The American Heart Association.

The trend continues toward certification of homemaker/home health aides. The third edition of this text meets state-mandated requirements for instruction leading to certification. In addition, the text was reviewed to ensure compliance with the *Model Curriculum and Teaching Guide for the Instruction of the Homemaker-Home Health Aide* published by the National HomeCaring Council.

supplements

The text is accompanied by a *Student Workbook* and an *Instructor's Guide*. The *Student Workbook* contains additional review questions and student projects. A Performance Evaluation Checklist is provided for each client care procedure covered in the text. The *Instructor's Guide* provides answers to the text questions, additional review questions and testing materials.

about the authors

Helen Huber received a BA in psychology from DePauw University in Indiana. She taught remedial reading and assisted in the Bureau of Testing and Research at DePauw University. Ms. Huber was coordinator and administrator for many years for federally funded adult training programs. Therefore, she is familiar with educational requirements and community needs as they relate to preparation of home health aides. Ms. Huber now serves on the Educational Committee for Social Services of the City of New Rochelle, New York, and is on the Advisory Council for Occupational Education for the City School District of New Rochelle. She also serves in a similar capacity for two proprietorial health care agencies in Westchester County.

Audree M. Spatz is a registered nurse with a BS in nursing from Ohio State University and a MEd in nursing education from Teachers College, Columbia University. She also received certification in Administration and Supervision from New York University. As Coordinator of Health Occupation of the Comprehensive Employment and Training Act (CETA) and Job Training Partnership Act (JTPA), Ms. Spatz is actively involved with the education of homemaker/home health aides. Currently she is Administrative Director of the nursing programs at Elizabeth Seton College, Yonkers, New York, including NLN-approved programs in Practical Nursing and Associate Degree Nursing. In addition, Ms. Spatz is a site accreditor for the National League of Nursing and is on the executive board of the New York State Association of Junior Colleges. Ms. Spatz serves as a member of the Burke Rehabilitation Advisory Council—Homemaker/Home Health Aide.

acknowledgments

The authors wish to express appreciation to their families who made valuable contributions and gave moral support during the writing and subsequent revisions of this text. The authors also wish to express appreciation to Alice Pagan of Any-Time Health Care, Inc. whose expertise and first-hand knowledge of the health care industry added a further dimension to this training text. The authors also wish to thank the following individuals and organizations for their assistance:

The American Heart Association

The American Cancer Society

The American Diabetes Association

Home Care Association for New York State

NLN Council of Home Health Agencies and Community Health Services

St. Joseph's Medical Center, Yonkers, NY

Everest and Jennings Inc.

Barbara Bienenstock, Mark Spatz, B. Blair Brooks, Mike Huber, and Bryan Conn who did illustrations

Marjorie Casswell, Home Aide Service of Eastern New York

Clement DeFelice, Coordinator of Physical Medicine, New Rochelle Hospital Medical Center

Registered Physical Therapists Richard Foley, Lucille Gnerre, and Adrienne Randall

Health Instructors Marguerite E. Jasper, Margery Wechsler, and Wendy Bechtold

Each person who agreed to be a subject in the illustrations

Special thanks to Leslie Boyer, Executive Editor for Health Sciences for Delmar Publishers, Inc.

Appreciation is also expressed to the following reviewers for their helpful comments:

Sylvia Watkins, PhD, RN
Assistant Administrator, The Burke Rehabilitation Center, White Plains, NY

Linda Y. Armstrong, RN
Brewster Campus/EVTC, Valrico, FL

Dorethea Y. Carter
Harding Business College, Maple Heights, OH

Phyllis Lane, RN, MS
Director, Home Health Aide Program, Queensborough Community College, Bayside, NY

M. Demeter Lyons
Director of Clinical Systems, LifePlans, Inc., Waltham, MA

Joan Schuyler
Director of Education, Watterson Skill Center, Philadelphia, PA

Carol Arledge, RN
Maringo County AVC, Linden, AL

Glenns A. Scott, RN, MA, BA
Nursing Supervisor, Watterson Skills Center, Philadelphia, PA

Jeanette Sidman, RN
Barton County Community College, Great Bend, KS

Portions of this text were evaluated by students, staff members, and instructors in various agencies, including social services, visiting nurse associations, proprietary and nonproprietary agencies, hospital home-referral departments, nursing homes and private homemaker/home health aide agencies. Evaluations served to verify technical content and compare administrative policies.

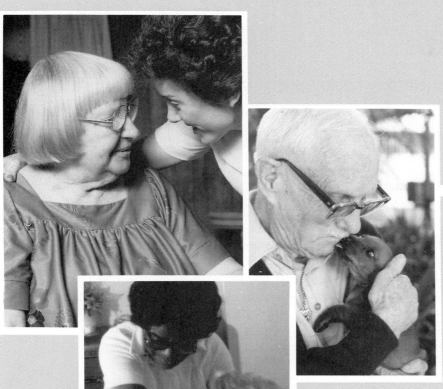

part **1**

Basic
Principles

1

Becoming a Homemaker/Home Health Aide

Unit 1
Home Health Services

key terms

chronic illness	RN	extended care facility
acute illness	LPN	

learning objectives

After studying this unit, you should be able to:
- Name three reasons why the trend toward home care has returned.
- Name the two services provided by the home health aide.
- Identify five members of the health team.
- Identify the subject areas of physician specialties.
- Explain the difference between acute and chronic illness.

Illness has always been a part of the human condition. Care has been given according to the folkways and beliefs of society. Care also depends on the knowledge and kinds of treatments available. In many early societies, home remedies using herbs and plants found in the woods were used as medicine. Attending to the personal needs of the ill was most often performed by members of the family. Even then there was often one special person who was called to help with medical emergencies. In some communities there was a midwife who came to the home during the birth of a child. For labor or delivery problems the midwife was the only trained person available. In remote areas of the country, doctors were not easy to reach. There were fewer hospitals and nursing homes than there are today. Each family had to assume the task of nursing its own family members within the home. When the mother was ill, activities in the home were usually disrupted and home services were needed to provide families with help.

the beginning of home health services

The first homemaker service was established by a social service agency in New York in 1903. Its main purpose was to provide child care. In the early 1920s employment agencies advertised for mature, practical women, experienced in child care and household management. During the 1930s the Works Projects Administration (WPA) funded a program to train "housekeeping aides." They received preservice training and some on-the-job training as well. Later, in 1959 the National Conference on Homemaker Service met in Chicago. It was decided that homemaker service should be given to families with children, chronically ill persons or aged members. It was advised that these individuals should receive care in the home whenever possible, without regard to family income. In 1960, at another conference, personal and health care was seen as an added duty of a homemaker's job; the term **home health aide** came into use. Home health aides were expected to work only under direct nursing supervision. In 1976, laws were finally passed in some states setting the standards of training for this new health career. Now the terms **home health aide** and **homemaker-home health aide** are both used.

reviving a trend toward home health care

Answering a need, home health aides practiced both homemaking and home nursing services. They provided care in the home because it was not available elsewhere. Now with well-equipped hospitals and nursing homes throughout the country, some people may be surprised to learn that there is a new trend back to home care. There are several reasons for this. One is the high cost of hospital care. In some areas the cost of hospital care may run to more than $1500 a day. That amount does not include surgeons' fees, private duty nurses, medications, and other related costs. For the average person, even with medical insurance, a long stay in a hospital could cause heavy financial burdens.

A second reason for the increase in home care is the lack of attention persons may receive in nursing homes, rehabilitation centers, or hospitals. Many facilities have cut back on the number of nurses, aides, and technicians. This means that less personal attention can be given. In hospitals, health workers are often kept busy with emergencies and acutely ill patients. The continuing but less urgent needs of the chronically ill are often neglected. A **chronic illness** is usually a long-term problem such as muscular dystrophy or diabetes. An **acute illness** refers to one which arises suddenly and requires immediate care.

A third reason for the trend toward providing home care is the vastly increased number of aged persons. Modern health care and advanced technology have resulted in a longer average life span for most people. The need for quality care and assistance for those elderly persons whose health has failed has placed strong demands on the nursing homes and **extended care facilities** that already exist. As a result, many of these facilities are filled to capacity, and there are often long waiting lists for admission. Since the needs of these elderly people cannot be put off until an opening arises, many people have turned to home health care as a satisfactory alternative.

The increase in home care is also largely due to a fourth reason: persons are usually happier and emotionally more secure in the home. A favorable mental outlook is important for improvement of a physical disorder. It is often better for a person to stay in familiar surroundings than to be moved, figure 1-1. This means being near loved ones, friends, and relatives. Try to imagine how anyone—especially the

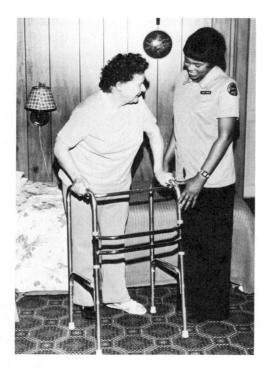

Figure 1-1 Clients are usually happier in the familiar surroundings of their own home.

older person—must feel about being taken from home, not knowing if he or she will ever return.

Elderly people often need help in meeting their personal care or health needs. Some of them live in boarding houses, in their own homes or apartments, or with their grown children. When such elderly people are disabled or in need of care, family members and health personnel must decide how to provide for them. The family may try to give the care themselves or may bring a specially trained person into the home to give the needed care. The home health aide may be the person hired to help both the person in need of care and the family to cope with illness.

DRGs

In the interest of lowering medical costs to Medicaid and private carriers, a system was devised called **Diagnostic Related Groupings (DRGs).** Under this system, careful studies were made of the number of days of hospitalization required for various medical conditions. Each specific ailment was then allocated a fixed reimbursement amount based on statistics compiled by hospitals throughout the country. The purpose was to lower medical costs to the insurance carrier and to get patients out of the hospital as soon as possible. This made hospital beds available and returned patients to their normal environments where it was expected that recovery would be hastened.

Anyone who has spent time in a hospital will realize that this plan has a great deal of merit. Hospitals must maintain a rather rigid schedule. Aides and nurses start very early with the morning routine of waking patients, bathing, changing linens, giving medications, taking blood and urine samples, bringing bedpans and feeding. Although everyone is wakened at an early hour, there are a limited number of aides and nurses. Thus, some patients are not given their baths and do not have their beds changed until late in the afternoon. Such patients feel that they have had their rest disturbed for no good reason.

It is also true that most people are happier in familiar surroundings and it is reasonable to expect that being at home would speed recovery. There is not the regimentation of a hospital and tasks may be done at the client's own pace. This allows the patient to feel more relaxed, more comfortable, and less fearful. After all, if the doctor sends you home, it must mean that you are getting better!

You can see that DRGs have some very positive benefits. However, there are also negative aspects that must be mentioned. Some people heal faster than others. Some do not want to leave the safe environment of a hospital. There have been cases where the patient left the hospital too soon and complications developed. For that reason, hospitals and doctors have been very cautious and conservative with the DRGs and if they feel there is any chance of complications, they will reassess the patient and change the grouping to allow for more days in the hospital. This reassessment is very important because a patient that is released too soon and has a severe setback might sue the hospital, doctors, and nurses for malpractice.

Before a DRG patient is released from the hospital, a detailed patient care plan is prepared by the medical team and a discharge planner. One reason for making such a careful plan is to make sure that the home care team will have full information as to how to deal with normal recovery, will know how to recognize a problem and will know what to do if one occurs. This is for the welfare of the patient as well as for the protection of the hospital and medical team. Included in the release plan should be schedules for physical therapy, occupational therapy, any special or unusual treatment plans, and medication schedules as well as a complete dietary plan prepared by a dietician or nutritional therapist.

A good discharge plan simplifies the job of a home health aide because there will be no doubts about what care is required for the client. The release plan will be discussed with the health care agency so that the aide's supervisor will be fully aware of all aspects of the care plan. Thus, if an aide on the job does have questions, he or she will be able to contact the agency supervisor for advice.

role of the home health aide

The duties of the home health aide fall into two categories. One is to perform homemaking duties and the other to provide limited health care in the home. Homemaking duties involve helping with upkeep of the home and with running the household. Doing the client's laundry, preparing meals, and going to the market are all part of an aide's duties. A home health aide is not expected to do heavy cleaning such as washing windows, waxing furniture and floors, or moving heavy furniture. However, the home must be kept clean and neat. Guidelines will be presented throughout the text to help the students know what they are expected to do.

The other main duty is to provide safe and proper health care within the home. This is only done under the supervision of other health team members. Usually, the community health nurse guides the health services given. The community health nurse may be a member of the public health department, Visiting Nurse Association, or a home referral service. The home health aide will be informed as to what should and what should not be done. Preparing for emergencies is included in the education of the home health aide.

As a home health aide, you will be pursuing a career that can bring satisfaction and fulfillment if you are willing to learn and use necessary skills. As an aide you must understand how important it is to give compassionate and competent client care. You will also be expected to clean and maintain the home efficiently.

In most cases, you will move from one assignment to another as clients become well enough to care for themselves. Therefore, you must learn to adjust to different circumstances quickly and easily. In the space of one week's time, you may be called upon to deal with the problems of a dying elderly person in one home, and also care for a newborn infant in another home. However, certain client care factors are consistently applied regardless of the type of home or medical situation.

Each person in your care has his or her own set of special problems, but every one needs understanding, kindness, and the best of care, figure 1.2. You must be aware of the

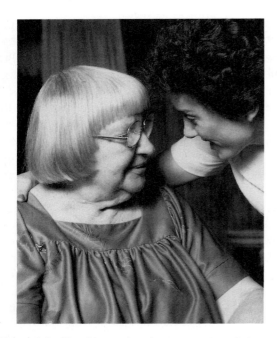

Figure 1-2 Touching and caring are good medicine.

physical needs, diet requirements, and psychological support necessary for each client. You must try to create the best atmosphere for recovery and comfort. Each case demands standards of cleanliness and neatness of the home. In addition, each case requires a client care plan which is well organized.

It will be necessary for you to adjust to many life-styles as you move from case to case. People have different religions and cultures. You should respect the ethnic and religious differences of all families. Sensitivity to the needs of all the family members is very important, figure 1-3.

Your main duties focus around caring for the client and keeping the home clean. You will be taught the basics of nutrition. This knowledge is used to plan, shop and prepare attractive meals for your clients. You will also learn the fundamentals of body structure and function. By learning to recognize what is considered to be normal, you will be more alert

to the abnormal condition. Knowing the difference is helpful in recognizing what is a crisis and what is not when unexpected situations come up. You will be expected to assume responsibilities as you become a member of the health team.

In each unit of this text you will find new words to master and new techniques to learn. As your knowledge grows, so does your confidence as an individual. In becoming a home health aide you can be proud of your newly acquired skills. Satisfaction comes in being able to serve those who need your skills.

the health care team

The home health aide is one member of the larger health care team. Even though working in the home creates physical distance between the aide and other members, the team still exists. In order for the aide to work best within the team, the duties of other members should be clearly understood.

Specially trained health care personnel who are part of the health team may include:

Nurses and Nursing Assistants
Dentists and Dental Surgeons
Occupational Therapists
Speech Therapists
Radiation Therapists
Paramedics
Dietitians
Physical Therapists
Social Workers
Pharmacists (druggists)
Physicians
Laboratory Technicians
Mental Health Consultants

The physician usually directs the care a client receives. A client who has many health problems may also have many doctors. The client usually has a family doctor, also called a

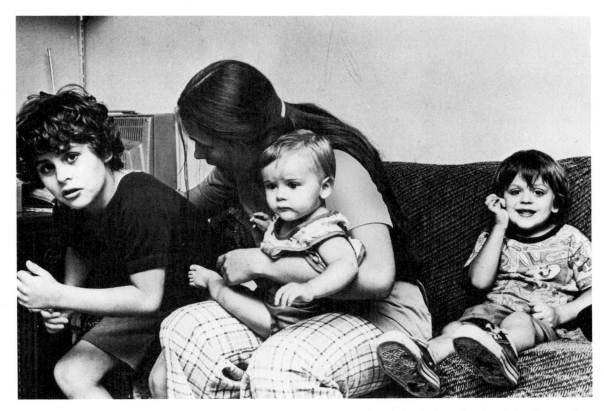

Figure 1-3 The home health aide should be sensitive to the emotional and physical needs of each family member.

general practitioner. For specific problems, however, the client may have a specialist. The home health aide should learn the medical specialties which exist, figure 1-4. The home health aide works most closely with the agency supervisors and reports directly to them.

Registered nurses (**RN**s) may take a two-, three-, or four-year educational program. At all levels of nursing a state examination must be passed before one may practice nursing. A public health nurse usually supervises the home health aide. This nurse is an RN and usually has a four-year college degree, or has taken a special course in public health nursing. Licensed practical nurses (**LPN**s) study for 10 to 18 months and must pass a state

licensing examination. In some states they are called licensed vocational nurses (**LVN**s).

A home health aide, as a member of the health team, has a responsibility to the client. Because the aide spends a large amount of time with the client, the role is important. From day to day the home health aide provides for the client's safety and comfort.

It is most important to remember that the aide may be the first to observe any changes in the client's condition. Such changes must be reported immediately to the supervisor. Most often the nursing supervisor will contact the doctor and a family member if it is necessary. Each client and each home situation is different. The home health aide must understand assignments clearly. Giving a full report

CHART OF MEDICAL SPECIALISTS

TITLE	AREA OF SPECIALIZATION
Pediatrician	Infancy through teenage years
Gerontologist	Diseases and disorders of the aged
Psychiatrist	Mental and emotional disorders
Internist	Internal organ disorders
General Surgeon	Emergency and routine surgery
Obstetrician/Gynecologist	Prenatal and postnatal care
	Female sex organ disorders
Plastic Surgeon	Skin grafting—burn care
	Cosmetic surgery—reconstructive surgery
Dermatologist	Skin disorders—allergies, warts
Ophthalmologist—Oculist	Eye disorders
Orthopedic Surgeon	Bone disorders—fractures, arthritis
Otolaryngologist (or ENT specialist)	Ear, nose and throat
Cardiovascular Surgeon	Heart and circulatory diseases
Hematologist	Blood disorders
Pathologist	Laboratory study of cellular disease
Endocrinologist	Glandular system disorders, diabetes, dwarfism, etc.
Oncologist	Cancer
Gastroenterologist	Stomach and intestinal disorders
Proctologist	Lower bowel disorders
Radiologist	X-ray diagnosis and therapy
Anesthesiologist	Anesthesia for surgical patients
Urologist	Urinary tract diseases

Figure 1-4 These are only some of the medical specialists who may be members of the health team.

to the correct person is also an important part of the job. Each aide must know who should be called and when they should be called for instructions.

A caring and dedicated home health aide will continue to learn new skills and be ready to face the challenges of medical advances as more is learned about illness and its effects on the client, family and health team. For that reason, home health aides should seek out opportunities to attend in-service programs at the local hospitals and health care facilities. The more an aide knows, the better care he/she can provide.

summary

- The need for educated, dedicated home health aides has grown. Many factors show that the need for home care will become even greater.
- The home health aide is expected to give safe and proper care to the client. The aide should be able to provide skilled care.
- To observe and report accurately is important to the other members of the health team.
- The aide should cooperate with other family members as well as the client.

review

1. What are the two main services provided by the home health aide?
2. List three reasons for the returning trend toward home care.
3. What is the difference between *acute* and *chronic* illness?
4. List five members of the health team.

Unit 2
Developing Good Habits and Practices

key terms

theory
practice
interaction
child abuse
interpersonal
  relationships

oral hygiene
evaluation
components
hygiene

confined
offensive
procedure

learning objectives

After studying this unit, you should be able to:
- List three good study tips.
- Define interpersonal relationships and interaction.
- Give an example of self-understanding.
- Identify the need for evaluation.
- State the difference between theory and practice.
- Give four examples of good personal hygiene.

At first glance, the role of a home health aide may appear to be quite simple. It is made up of everyday tasks: keeping a house in order, preparing and cleaning up after meals, and providing for the comfort and safety of a client. Students may feel that they already know how to take care of a house. Most people have been doing housekeeping tasks since early childhood. Often it is thought that there is nothing new to learn about familiar jobs. The student may ask, "Why don't we get to the important things? After all, I want to care for the sick. Why should I waste time learning homemaking skills?"

Everyone can benefit by learning new ways to do certain jobs. Once the new method is learned, the aide can compare it with the old way and may discover a more efficient technique.

By learning to focus on the components of a task, the aide will find understanding comes more easily. **Components** are the separate parts that make up a whole. Learning how to do something, when to do it, and what should be done first will add up to a more complete understanding. Students must learn how and when to do all the tasks that need to be done. They also learn what tasks are most important. In

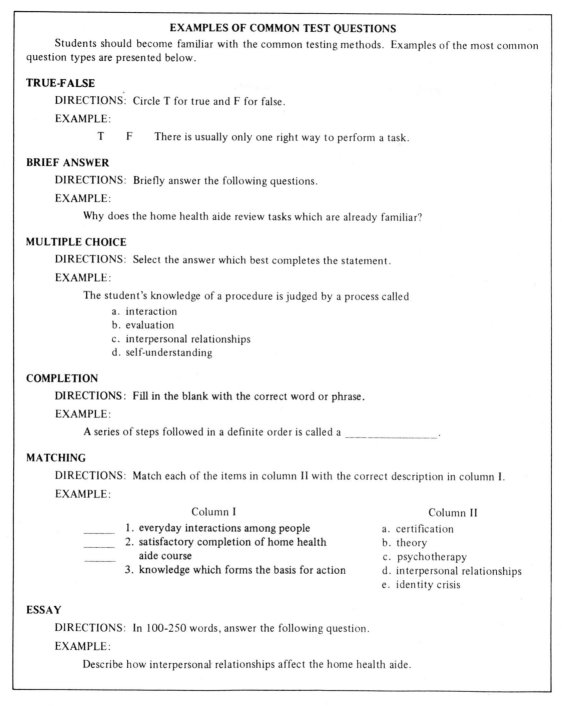

EXAMPLES OF COMMON TEST QUESTIONS

Students should become familiar with the common testing methods. Examples of the most common question types are presented below.

TRUE-FALSE

DIRECTIONS: Circle T for true and F for false.

EXAMPLE:

      T   F   There is usually only one right way to perform a task.

BRIEF ANSWER

DIRECTIONS: Briefly answer the following questions.

EXAMPLE:

Why does the home health aide review tasks which are already familiar?

MULTIPLE CHOICE

DIRECTIONS: Select the answer which best completes the statement.

EXAMPLE:

The student's knowledge of a procedure is judged by a process called
    a. interaction
    b. evaluation
    c. interpersonal relationships
    d. self-understanding

COMPLETION

DIRECTIONS: Fill in the blank with the correct word or phrase.

EXAMPLE:

A series of steps followed in a definite order is called a _____.

MATCHING

DIRECTIONS: Match each of the items in column II with the correct description in column I.

EXAMPLE:

                      Column I   Column II

_____ 1. everyday interactions among people   a. certification
_____ 2. satisfactory completion of home health   b. theory
        aide course   c. psychotherapy
_____ 3. knowledge which forms the basis for action   d. interpersonal relationships
                                                    e. identity crisis

ESSAY

DIRECTIONS: In 100-250 words, answer the following question.

EXAMPLE:

Describe how interpersonal relationships affect the home health aide.

Figure 2-1 Instructors, certification officials, and employers may use different kinds of tests to evaluate the aide's knowledge.

this way, the student completing the course will become a useful and successful home health aide.

learning procedures

There are many ways to perform household tasks and care procedures. However, in most procedures there are only two ways, the right way and the wrong way. A **procedure** is best described as the steps used to complete a particular task. A procedure can be either a specific nursing procedure or a homemaking procedure. Each student will be required to demonstrate full understanding and acceptable performance of all the procedures taught during the course. In order to become certified as a home health aide the student will be judged on the performance of the skills taught. The judging process is known as an **evaluation**. After each procedure is studied and practiced, the student will be graded on performance. Written examinations are also given for evaluation purposes, figure 2-1. Evaluation helps the student know which areas require extra study or practice.

There are usually two parts to the instruction given to the home health aide. The first is called theory. **Theory** is the information which forms a basis for action. In classroom lectures and in the assigned readings, the student learns theory. The second component is devoted to practice. **Practice** is the actual performance of the procedures. Practice is combined with the theory, figure 2-2. This allows the student to build skills in both areas at the same time. The home health aide learns client care procedures and homemaking procedures, figure 2-3.

forming study habits

Study habits differ from person to person. Some people need more time for study than others. Some are able to perform certain tasks more easily than others. Students must recognize their own needs in forming study habits. Study tips and other learning practices are listed in the workbook.

I HEAR AND I FORGET

I SEE AND I REMEMBER

I DO AND I UNDERSTAND

Chinese Proverb

Figure 2-2 Listening is not enough. Study and practice are necessary in order to learn.

READING ASSIGNMENTS

1. Set aside a time for daily study. When possible, it should be the same time each day/evening.

2. Choose a quiet, well-lighted place. Use that place regularly.

3. Identify the objectives of each assignment. Student objectives are presented before reading material, study these first.

4. Build a larger vocabulary by looking up words which are not familiar. Keep a dictionary nearby; a thesaurus is also helpful. Vocabulary lists are presented, use them as a guide.

GUIDELINES FOR GOOD HABIT DEVELOPMENT

1. How long is your attention span? Check yourself by looking at a watch at the beginning of your study time. Check yourself when you are finished, or you will lose the information you have studied. This give you a starting point.

Figure 2-3 Guidelines and study tips for the homemaker home health aide (*continued*)

2. Plan for definite study periods. Learning to increase your attention span must take place on a regular basis. This does not mean the night before a test. In other words, you must put yourself on a steady daily schedule or nightly schedule if you have an evening class.

3. To make it worthwhile, you must give yourself a REWARD for developing new study habits. You have achieved something new and good. You may do this in the following manner:

   a. Short-term: After one period of studying, give yourself a pep talk saying, "I am proud of myself. I have done something I never thought I could do!" In other words, pat yourself on the back.

   b. Long-term: After many periods of studying, that is, for a hour or more, give yourself a break. A suggestion for you: study one hour before/after dinner and then watch a television program or call a friend. Do not spend a long time on the phone! If need be, you may return to the books for a long period of studying.

4. You can build your time and attention span slowly but steadily. Once you have increased your attention span, the results will show in your classroom work. Your classroom participation will increase and your test grades will be higher. All this work will make you a happier person and your family will be proud of you.

Your instructor may give you a worksheet to help you organize your work/study period. Complete it for one week and then discuss it with your instructor. This may help you to better manage your activities of daily living.

Figure 2-3 (Continued)

ATTENDING CLASS

1. Come to class prepared.

2. If the lecture or discussion is not clear, ask questions. Do not fear looking foolish. Other students may have the same questions.

   Caution: Remember it is not safe to practice procedures which you do not fully understand.

3. Take notes during lectures and after a film has been shown.

PRACTICING PROCEDURES

1. At home, practice the homemaking procedures taught in class. If possible, practice nursing skills with family members.

2. Before going to the home to which you have been assigned, plan the day's activities: (1) Note the tasks that should be done, (2) the time it should take to do them and (3) the most important tasks to finish that day.

Figure 2-3 (Concluded)

working with others

Nurses and home health aides are employed in the service of giving care to ill persons. Delivering this service makes it necessary for the home health aide to work closely with family members. Conflicts and arguments among family members sometimes occur. Everyone has probably observed or been a part of a family dispute. What happens when an outsider enters into a family argument? In most cases, the family will band together and turn against the outsider. The family could turn away or show anger if the aide interfered in a family matter. Consider, for instance, the following situation:

You are assigned to a home by the agency for whom you work. There are two children (ages 4 and 6) and a new baby. Your job is to keep the house in order, prepare meals, and give care to the children and the mother. The mother is sitting in the kitchen having coffee; you are at the stove making formula for the baby. The two children burst into the room, fighting over a toy. One child falls against you, the aide; the baby's bottle of formula drops. Formula and broken glass cover the floor.

What would be your reaction? What reaction is likely to bring the best results? Concern for the safety of the children should be the first response of the home health aide. The children should be told that you are glad that no one was hurt. Then take them from the kitchen and clean up the broken glass and spilled formula.

In most instances, discipline must be left to the mother or other adult family member. If you should come up against special problems about child behavior, you should call your supervisor for advice. Nearly everyone today is aware of the fact that some children are disciplined too severely. This is called **child abuse.** If you have cause to think that a child is being beaten or otherwise mistreated, you should report to your supervisor immediately. Do not try to interfere, but report such information at once.

interpersonal relationships

When people live, work or play together, one person acts and the other reacts or responds to the act. This process is called an *interaction.* Figure 2-4 shows that several persons may be involved in a situation—the arrows point to all the possible interactions.

People are expected to handle interactions as a part of everyday life. The feeling and understanding which results from the interactions between two or more persons is

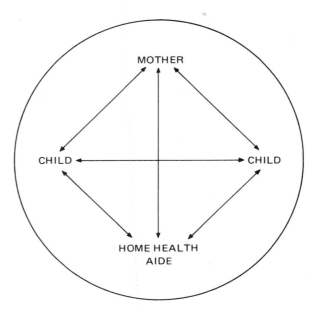

Figure 2-4 Many interactions may take place between the home health aide and family members.

called **interpersonal relationships.** To the person entering a service occupation, interpersonal relationships can determine success or failure. Each of the persons who are involved in these relationships is entitled to be treated with dignity. Everyone should follow the golden rule—treat others as you would like to be treated. This helps to establish good interpersonal relationships.

In figure 2-5, look at the combinations of relationships which may develop for the home health aide. The home health aide must remember that he/she is entering a home where an illness or a problem already exists. An illness or problem may cause the family members to be unhappy or disorganized. Anger, fear and other emotional reactions may be present. The client may be in pain, cranky, sad or depressed. The home health aide who is aware of the source of the problem often finds it easier to accept the family's behavior. As a result, awkward interpersonal relationships can often be avoided.

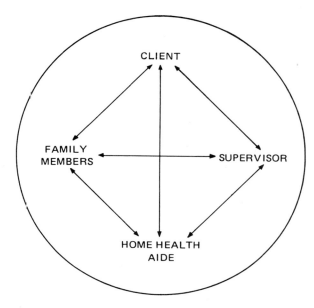

Figure 2-5 Learning to handle relationships is part of the home health aide's job.

developing self-understanding

The secret of understanding others begins with self-understanding. You know what makes you feel good. When others are kind to you, compliment you on a job well-done, tell you how well you look, don't you suddenly feel terrific? Think how you have felt when you have been criticized or when you have had a really "bad" day. Everyone shares those feelings. All individuals have the same basic needs, figure 2-6. The physical needs are food, shelter, clothing, sleep and, of course, good health.

All people have psychological needs as well. These include the need for love, having a feeling of belonging, and a feeling of well-being, to name a few. When these needs are not met, an individual may not function at his or her highest level. This can lead to stress and even illness. The person who is sensitive to his or her own needs and desires is better able to relate to others. This can be an asset to someone entering the health care field. All people must be treated with respect!

Some people have a very low opinion of themselves. They always "put themselves down." They say such things as, "I'm so dumb," "I'm so fat," "Nobody likes me," or "I know I'll fail." At the other extreme are those who brag about where they have been, who they know, and how important they are. Most people are comfortable around those individuals who are secure but modest about their success. Unfortunately, it is often much easier to judge others than to judge oneself.

PHYSIOLOGICAL	PSYCHOLOGICAL
1. Hygiene	1. Sexual
2. Comfort	2. Spiritual
3. Safety	3. Cultural
4. Body Alignment	4. Self-esteem
5. Mobility	5. Belonging
6. Rest and Sleep	6. Stimulation
7. Nutrition	7. Loss and Death
8. Elimination	8. Knowledge
9. Respiration and Circulation	9. Coping Mechanisms
10. Fluid Balance	10. Growth and Development
11. Growth and Development	11. Intellectual Achievement

Figure 2-6 Basic human needs

Self-understanding is a growth process that continues throughout life. People who have found a goal and get pleasure from their work probably feel good about themselves. As a result, they develop feelings of self-esteem. This usually makes them less critical of others and they are better able to understand others. Part of self-understanding is accepting one's own failures and weakness. Accepting others becomes easier after admitting that no one is perfect.

personal health and hygiene

A home health aide must observe the personal **hygiene** standards expected of any health team member, figure 2-7. When working in other people's homes, the aide should reflect the highest standards. This means being clean and well groomed each workday. The person who goes on a job unbathed, with dirty hair and nails, and wearing wrinkled, spotted clothes makes a bad impression. A sloppy appearance implies that the person also has a poor self-image and sloppy working habits.

An aide should wear a clean uniform, clean undergarments, and comfortable, polished shoes.

An aide in a proper uniform has a professional appearance and makes the client feel more secure. A recent survey of hospital and nursing home patients showed that they feel uncomfortable when nurses and aides wear street clothes. They say they are unable to dis-

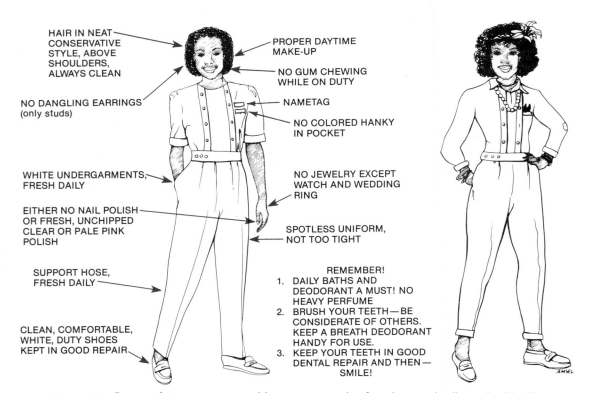

HAIR IN NEAT CONSERVATIVE STYLE, ABOVE SHOULDERS, ALWAYS CLEAN

PROPER DAYTIME MAKE-UP

NO GUM CHEWING WHILE ON DUTY

NO DANGLING EARRINGS (only studs)

NAMETAG

NO COLORED HANKY IN POCKET

WHITE UNDERGARMENTS, FRESH DAILY

NO JEWELRY EXCEPT WATCH AND WEDDING RING

EITHER NO NAIL POLISH OR FRESH, UNCHIPPED CLEAR OR PALE PINK POLISH

SPOTLESS UNIFORM, NOT TOO TIGHT

SUPPORT HOSE, FRESH DAILY

REMEMBER!
1. DAILY BATHS AND DEODORANT A MUST! NO HEAVY PERFUME
2. BRUSH YOUR TEETH—BE CONSIDERATE OF OTHERS. KEEP A BREATH DEODORANT HANDY FOR USE.
3. KEEP YOUR TEETH IN GOOD DENTAL REPAIR AND THEN— SMILE!

CLEAN, COMFORTABLE, WHITE, DUTY SHOES KEPT IN GOOD REPAIR

Figure 2-7 Contrast between proper and improper grooming for a homemaker/home health aide.

tinguish a nurse or a doctor from an aide or housekeeper. It is, then, reassuring to a client to have their home health aide properly groomed and wearing a crisp, fresh uniform. When an aide looks professional, he or she will most likely behave in a professional manner. Whether a female aide wears a skirted or pant uniform is a matter of local custom and personal preference.

There are, of course, clients who request that an aide dress in regular clothes and not be in uniform in the home. In all situations, the aide must follow the agency supervisor's directions.

It is also important for the home health aide to wear a name tag at all times. The name tag gives the name of the aide and the proper title.

Bathing, brushing the teeth, and wearing a neat hair style is also part of good grooming. Fingernails should be short, smooth and clean. Jewelry should be limited to a watch and a wedding band. Small post earrings for pierced ears are usually acceptable. Bracelets and dangling necklaces are not worn as they may catch on bedding or furniture. A ring might scratch the client, or become lost.

Good grooming is important not only for appearance but also for safety reasons. Jewelry and rough fingernails could cause scratches. The danger of infection is always present if the skin has been scratched. Dirt and germs may easily enter an opening in the skin. Infected wounds heal more slowly among clients who are **confined** to bed. The home health aide must not add pain or discomfort to the client by being careless.

Personal cleanliness is also necessary to prevent and remove body odors. A home health aide is in close contact with clients; odors can be quite **offensive.** Remember, there are clients who are allergic to perfumes. Body odors should be removed with soap and water, not covered up with perfume. A considerate home

health aide will check mouth odor as well. Brushing teeth regularly and using mouthwash helps prevent mouth odors. Eating garlic and onions, and smoking cigarettes increases the need for oral hygiene. **Oral hygiene** means keeping the mouth clean and healthy. One important way to improve oral hygiene is to have annual dental checkups. It must be emphasized that an aide should not smoke while on duty unless the client has given permission. The aide must recognize that a client with a lung disease, allergies, respiratory illness, or personal distaste for the smell of smoke has the right to refuse to allow the aide to smoke within the home.

attitude

Have you ever said, "I don't like your attitude"; or, "That one really has an attitude"? **Attitude** refers to state of mind, behavior, or conduct about some matter. A home health aide who has "a bad attitude" will not be able to do good work. Such an aide might seem angry when performing personal tasks for a client and thereby make the client uncomfortable and embarrassed. For example, when a client must use a bedside commode for a bowel movement, there will be an unpleasant smell in the room. If a home health aide is unwilling to accept dealing with such conditions, the client may be aware of the aide's attitude. This does not lead to a pleasant working relationship.

When you decide to become a home health aide, you must prepare yourself to face some tasks that are very personal and not always pleasant. Your client may be cranky and even disagreeable. As a professional home health aide, you must develop a positive attitude toward all your clients. You will have to work with a variety of clients in a variety of homes. You must take pride in helping each of them feel better. With the right attitude, your work will be satisfying to you and to your clients. A healthy attitude about yourself and your work will make you a more professional home health aide.

summary

- A practicing home health aide will be faced with many new learning situations.
- Students can learn by doing, by studying, and by observing. The person who develops good study habits now is laying a foundation for good work habits later.
- To be successful in their roles, home health aides must be sensitive to the emotional and physical needs of others.
- Student home health aides must pay special attention to the interpersonal relationships they form with their families, their classmates, the clients with whom they work, and their instructors. As these relationships develop, the student will also grow in self-understanding.
- As a member of the health care team, the home health aide must also be concerned about the image conveyed to others by his or her personal grooming.
- Personal cleanliness and a neat appearance reflect a positive self-image and also contribute to the quality of care delivered. Attention to all of these factors will make for a better life and a more successful career as a home health aide.

review

1. What is the difference between theory and practice?
2. What is an interpersonal relationship?
3. List three good study tips.
4. Why are evaluations helpful?
5. Give four examples of good personal hygiene.

Unit 3

Adjusting to Working Conditions and Meeting Ethical Standards

learning objectives

After studying this unit, you should be able to:

- Identify two vocational adjustments required of a home health aide.
- Identify three homemaking duties of the aide.
- Name two client care responsibilities.
- Define ethics and identify two examples of an ethical practice.
- Explain why accurate observation, reporting and documentation are important tasks for the homemaker/home health aide.
- Define the term "confidentiality."
- Explain what is meant by "liability" and give five examples of actions to avoid.

A **vocation** is the occupation or profession for which one has been specially educated. In every new field of employment it is necessary to make adjustments, both mentally and physically, in order to gain satisfaction from the job.

vocational adjustments

The home health aide will encounter irregular working hours and must be able to adjust to a variety of assignments, settings, and equipment. The aide must also learn to follow instructions and adhere to established policies.

Setting up a workable schedule and learning client care responsibilities and limitations are also adjustments the home health aide must make.

working hours

Working hours may be irregular. Some cases assigned to a home health aide may require the aide to work through the night. The aide may be asked to work on varying shifts or on weekends. It is common for a home health aide to be assigned several part-time cases. Three different clients might be visited in one day or on different days of the week. Due to this irregularity of assignments, a home health aide must be **flexible.** This means being able to quickly adjust from one type of situation to another.

variety of assignments

The aide must adjust to different family situations and varied health care needs of the clients. In one home, the aide might be expected to care for infants, preschool children, and teen-

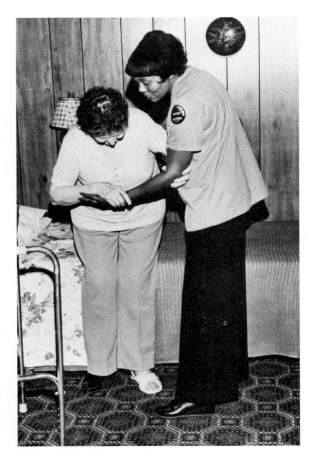

Figure 3-1 Assisting the client with medically recommended physical activities is one of the aide's duties.

agers. In another, there may be only middle-aged or elderly people. No two family situations are the same. This means the aide will have to establish new interpersonal relationships in each case. The medical conditions can range from sick infants to terminally ill clients. The aide must be prepared to give safe and medically proper care in each situation, figure 3-1.

variety of settings and equipment

The aide must also adapt to homes which are not as well equipped as others. Some homes have modern equipment and beautiful furnishings. Others offer the bare necessities of life. The home health aide must not make judgments about people based on their belongings. Some clients prefer simple living. The aide should also remember that most people who live in poverty do not do so by choice. The home health aide will be expected to treat all clients with dignity regardless of their financial position. Each human being is entitled to respectful and complete care. That is the only kind of care for which a home health aide is trained.

following instructions and policies

Another vocational adjustment is learning to carry out the assignment according to instructions. The aide must follow the doctor's orders and the directions of the supervisor. The comfort and well-being of the client should always take top priority. This means that it is the most important part of client care. In case of an emergency or any unexpected problem developing, the aide should immediately report to the agency supervisor or the employer. Before taking a case, a home health aide should be sure to ask for all vital information. In addition, the supervisor will provide a home care plan for the client, outlining the specific care to be provided and the aide's responsibilities. This includes duties, client needs, and the name and phone number of the person to be contacted in emergencies.

self-scheduling

A successful aide learns **self-scheduling.** Self-scheduling will be a necessary part of organizing the care for each client. The instructions may include: light housekeeping, laundry and ironing, meal preparation, marketing, personal care of the client and other members of the family. The aide will have to decide the best way to plan each day's activities. This will require flexibility and practical judgment. Some pitfalls to avoid are:

- gossiping with the client or family member instead of working
- watching a favorite television show
- jumping from one job to another and one room to another without organizing priorities
- putting off unpleasant tasks because they are disagreeable
- talking to friends on the phone or doing personal business.
- stopping frequently for a cup of coffee or a cigarette
- trying to do too much in one day, and doing nothing well

The best way to deal with a new set of circumstances is to look the situation over carefully and get organized. On entering a new situation, it is human nature to think about the end result. Often one is tempted to try to do everything in one day. This leads to frustration and nothing gets done well. Begin by asking where supplies are stored. Communicate with the client or family and supervisor to find out exactly what is expected. Prepare a written plan each day for the cases assigned. At the end of the working day, see what did not get done. Revise the plan for the next day. It is best to select only one big project for each day. After the routine tasks and client care procedures are done for the day, tackle the larger job. These tasks can be planned for periods when the client does not require your full attention. The household often will function better as a result of preplanning and organization.

A home health aide may be assigned to work with several clients each week. The aide should prepare a schedule for each assignment. In this way the aide's time can be used most efficiently. Each daily plan should be flexible enough to allow for the unexpected. The supervisor can make suggestions and help define the duties in each case. The aide must perform these duties in the time allotted.

When beginning a new job, the aide must adjust to the client's or family's routine. Aides should not reorganize the entire house or daily schedule to suit themselves. Major changes should be made only with the approval of the client or a responsible family member. An aide's job is to make the family comfortable and to assist them, not to change their lifestyle. A well-organized home health aide saves time and effort by planning ahead and anticipating possible problems.

knowledge of role and responsibility

Home health aides must keep in mind the purpose of their vocation. This purpose is to provide safe health care and to maintain a clean living area for the client. A client deserves the highest quality care available. An aide should be able to care for the client and the home in the time allotted. Home and health are combined in the vocational title. It is important for a home health aide to be fully aware of the extent and limitations of responsibilities in both areas. This means knowing what the aide should do and what the aide should not be expected to do, figures 3-2 through 3-6.

Clients may ask the aide to perform skills that have not been included in the instructions. How can the aide inform the client that what has been requested is not part of the assigned duties? Anger and hostility accomplish nothing. The aide should say, "This procedure

---

A. Routine home health aide functions include the following:

1. With guidance from the nurse or agency supervisor, arrange the schedule so that the client follows medical recommendations such as increased physical activity and other activities of daily living.
2. Keep an Aide Care Plan as part of the client record.
3. Take temperature, pulse, and respiration.
4. Assist the client on and off the bedpan, commode or toilet.
5. Assist with bathing of the client in bed, or in the tub, or in the shower as determined by the doctor, nurse, or agency supervisor.
6. Assist with the care of teeth and mouth.
7. Assist with grooming—care of hair, including shampooing; shaving; and the ordinary care of the nails.
8. Assist the client with dressing.
9. Assist the client with eating.
10. Assist the client in moving from bed to chair or wheelchair and assist the client in walking.
11. Accompany the client to obtain medical care (when practical).
12. Prepare and serve meals according to instructions.
13. Wash dishes as needed.
14. Make or change the bed.
15. Send soiled linen to the laundry or add to the laundry you will do.

16. Do light housekeeping; i.e., dusting and vacuuming the rooms the client uses.
17. List needed supplies.
18. Shop for the client if no other arrangement is possible.
19. Do the client's personal laundry if no family member is available or able; this may include necessary ironing and mending.
20. Notify supervisor or nurse to whom you report of any change in the client's condition.

B. Special Home Health Aide Functions:
With the permission of the supervising public health nurse, the public health nurse may teach and closely supervise the home health aide in the following procedures:

1. Reinforcing dressings and changing simple nonsterile dressings.
2. Applying prescribed ice cap or ice collar.
3. Applying ace bandages.
4. Assisting with prescribed skin care.
5. Taking the blood pressure.
6. Assisting with the change of ostomy bags.
7. Measuring intake and output as ordered.
8. Preparing modified diets, as prescribed by the physician.
9. Performing simple urine tests for sugar, acetone, or albumen and recording the results.
10. Assisting the client with prescribed exercises that have been taught by appropriate professional personnel.
11. Helping the client relearn household skills.

* In other states, aides may have different work standards and duties.

Figure 3-2 Functions approved by the New York State Department of Health which are to be performed by a home health aide.*

CLIENT CARE RESPONSIBILITIES*

Give simple emotional and psychological support to the client and other household members.

Encourage the client to become as independent as possible within the doctor's guidelines.

Make occupied or unoccupied bed.

Provide Personal Care:

    Mouth care
    Daily shave
    Nail care
    Shampoo
    Hair care
    Bed bath - complete or partial
    Shower - tub
    Bedpan - urinal as requested or scheduled
    Assistance with bathroom use
    Assistance with dressing
    Denture care

Transfer client from bed to chair and return client back to bed.

Take and Record:

Temperature	Intake
Pulse	Output
Respirations	
Blood Pressure	

Assist with oral medications which are self-administered.

Accompany client to doctor's office or to areas outside the home if permitted.

Assist client with medically recommended physical activities.

Carry out procedures assigned and demonstrated by supervisor including:

    Range of Motion
    Physical Therapy
    Urine Test - Sugar/Acetone
    Diet Preparation
    Prosthesis application
    Special skin care
    Minor dressing changes

*(Procedures listed here will be explained later in the text.)

Figure 3-3 Client care services are given under the direction of a nursing supervisor.

Do not assist with medications without permission of the supervising nurse or doctor.

Do not give injections.

Do not change sterile dressings.

Do not neglect or change the doctor's orders.

Figure 3-4 Limitations are set for the protection of the client and the home health aide.

was not included in my studies, and it would not be right for me to take unnecessary risks. Shall I call the supervisor?" If the request involves a housekeeping task, the aide might say, "There are many things I can do, and am ready to do. However, we are taught that we should not be expected to do this."

The following list summarizes the guidelines the home health aide is to observe in all assignments:

1. Follow your client's Plan of Care.
2. Work carefully.
3. Be sure you are insured if you are expected to transport your client in your car.
4. Provide only those services for which you have been trained.
5. Call your local emergency number if emergency medical care is needed.
6. Only give first aid for which you have been trained.
7. Do not provide more or less of a service.
8. Report unsafe working conditions to your supervisor.

What you do for the patient and how you do it are important. Much of the information in this book is directed toward teaching you the "what" and "how" of being a Homemaker/Home Health Aide. Your technical knowledge and skills are what the client wants and needs. An equally important part of your job responsibility involves some ac-

HOME CARE RESPONSIBILITIES

Do light housekeeping to assure that rooms are clean and in order.

Prepare shopping lists and run errands if permitted.

Purchase clothing or household items using the client's cash or check, if permitted.

Prepare and serve food that meets nutritional and dietary guidelines.

Launder, iron, mend and store clothing and linens.

Clean and operate equipment properly:
    small appliances
    washer and dryer
    refrigerator
    stove
    vacuum cleaner

Figure 3-5 Home services help maintain a safe, healthful environment.

HOME CARE LIMITATIONS

Do not do heavy housework including:

    window washing

    cleaning venetian blinds

    waxing furniture and floors

    laundering curtains

    shaking rugs or draperies

    lifting or carrying full garbage cans

    carrying firewood or containers of coal and ashes

    moving heavy furniture

DO NOT DRIVE CLIENTS OR FAMILY MEMBERS AROUND AND DO NOT RUN ERRANDS WITHOUT THE SUPERVISOR'S PERMISSION.

Figure 3-6 The aide should politely refuse to do tasks which are not within the set responsibilities.

tivities that are not seen by the client. These responsibilities include observing, reporting, documenting, following rules of ethics and confidentiality, and understanding liability.

Because the Homemaker/Home Health Aide usually spends more time with the patient than any other member of the health care team does, he or she is often able to see actions or reactions that no one else sees, or to make other unique observations. What the Homemaker/Home Health Aide does with this information is very important to the total care of the patient.

observing

All five senses (seeing, hearing, touching, smelling and tasting) should be used in the day-to-day work of the Homemaker/Home Health Aide. Let's consider each sense:

1. Seeing

Look at the patient carefully, watching for any changes since your last visit. Some of the things you might note are facial expression, posture, skin color and cleanliness, rashes, discharges, redness, swelling, evenness of facial features, way of walking (gait), steadiness, stains on clothing.

Look at the home for safety hazards (frayed electric cords, wet floors, slippery throw rugs, loose steps), cleanliness, medications sitting out, food supply, spots, stains and spills on clothing, furniture or floors.

2. Hearing

Listen to the patient: What is being said? How is it being said? Is the patient's speech clear or slurred? Is it logical or nonsensical? Are the words sad, angry, friendly, or hostile? Do you hear wheezing, coughing, or gasping for breath?

Listen to the home: Does the faucet drip? Does the refrigerator vibrate? Is the radio or TV volume too loud to permit conversation? Are the telephone and door bells loud enough for the patient to hear?

3. Touching

Does the patient's skin feel hot, cold, or moist? Is it rough, or puffy? What is the pulse rate?

Are the sheets dry? Is the diaper wet? Is the bread dried out? Are the crackers soggy? Is the bath water too hot?

4. Smelling

Does the client have bad breath or body odor? Does the odor smell like perspiration, urine, feces, alcohol, or fruit? Is there an odor from a wound or dressing?

How do the bathroom, bedroom, and kitchen smell? How does the inside of the refrigerator smell? Have items of food spoiled?

5. Tasting

Is the food too salty or too spicy?

Develop the habit of paying attention to everything you see, hear, touch, smell, and taste in the home. Ask yourself at each visit, "Is anything different today from what it was the last time I was here?" If you don't take the time to be a careful observer, you may overlook some small but important signs of change.

Changes in the client's physical or mental condition, social support system, or household environment may occur suddenly. Some examples of sudden changes to look for:

Physical: cuts, fractures, strokes, heart attacks, paling of the skin

Mental: a previously cheerful and cooperative person doesn't seem to recognize you today or appears disoriented

Social Support: a spouse dies; close friends have retired and moved away

Household: a broken water pipe floods the kitchen

These sudden changes are usually easy to observe and describe. Sudden changes are usually of a severe nature and require an immediate **intervention** (an action to improve the situation).

More often, however, changes occur gradually. These changes are not as obvious to the Homemaker/Home Health Aide who sees the patient frequently as they may be to someone else, such as the supervisor, who sees the person infrequently. You've probably heard someone say, "My goodness, you've grown so tall since I saw you last!" or "Hasn't Aunt Maude failed since her operation?" In each of these cases, the people living with the child or Aunt Maude was unaware of the changes.

It is in regard to slow changes that the Homemaker/Home Health Aide needs to use skill in observation. As you work in the home over a period of time, you will become familiar with the patient's lifestyle, habits, social activities, and place of residence. If you fail to be alert to gradual changes, you may miss them. Some examples of gradual changes to look for:

Physical: patient moves more slowly or holds onto furniture; patient doesn't watch TV as much; hair color changes and becomes dull; appetite decreases; weight loss occurs

Mental: increasing "forgetfulness"; crying; suspicion of longtime friends

Social support: family or friends visit less frequently or write less often

Household: carpet becomes frayed; refrigerator doesn't keep food as cold; electric cords fray; chair joints loosen

Asking yourself "What's different today?" and really using your senses and powers of observation can be of great help. The fact that something out of the ordinary happens one time may not mean anything at all, or it may be the first of a series of happenings that will lead to something bad or dangerous. Write the "odd thing" in your notes for later reference.

Looking, hearing, touching, smelling, and tasting will give you a lot of information. It is your responsibility to transmit the information to your supervisor.

reporting

Some important instructions that you need during your orientation to the agency is how to report information, who to report it to, and when to report it. You have a right to know these "who, what, when, and how" procedures and a responsibility to ask if you aren't told.

In most agencies, one person will be in charge of the care given to the patient. This person may be called the "supervisor," or "case manager." This is the person you will probably be instructed to contact when you have information to share about the patient.

You will need to exercise judgment in making these reports: Some things need to be reported immediately, even while you are with the patient. Some things need to be reported as soon as you leave the home. Other things can wait until a regular conference, staffing, or written report. Anything you learn that puts the patient in danger should be reported immediately. Such things usually involve physical problems (chest pain, falls, or deep cuts, for example). Other observations may leave you unsure, and you would want to talk them over with the supervisor at your first opportunity. Some observations that leave you unsure might be forgetfulness, decreased appetite, or reduced social contacts. Still other things can wait for regular contact times.

Throughout your career as a Homemaker/Home Health Aide, and especially as a beginner, you should remember that it is **always** better to report something even if you aren't sure how important it is, rather than to risk endangering the patient, the agency, and yourself by not reporting it. Good supervisors can help you learn how to sort out the "crisis" from the "unusual," and develop good judgment in reporting. You should never feel or be made to feel that the supervisor is "too busy" or that your information might be "too unimportant." Your supervisor is employed to help you give good client care, and, as you read earlier, a very important part of that care is what you observe and report. When you talk over your observations and your feelings with the supervisor, you can speak freely and voice your opinions and small details. All of these help the supervisor to make decisions; he or she can help you learn to be more concise and accurate in your oral reports as time goes by.

On the other hand, your supervisor is a busy person, so you won't want to waste her time or yours in long, dragged-out stories either. It's a good idea to practice what you're going to say so you can get the story organized in a logical sequence and make it easier for the supervisor to understand.

documenting

Writing down your observations and actions is a very important part of your job. Your agency will show you the forms they want you to use, and will tell you how often you need to document something in writing, where to do it, and where and when to turn it in.

There's a saying that "The job ain't over 'til the paperwork's done." This certainly holds true in home health care. The information you write, which may be called a "narrative," "observation," "notes," or "charting" becomes part of the client's record, or chart. The information contained in client records is of critical importance for these reasons:

1. It is a lasting record of what was done to, for, and by the patient.

2. It is a record of what was observed about the client.
3. It is a record of how the client reacted to the care that was given.
4. It contains information that can be used by other team members in evaluating the care that was given, and in deciding if changes in the care plan should be made.
5. If the patient or family is unhappy with services and decides to complain, or, in the event of legal action, the client record can be used to show that certain things were done on certain dates and times.

When you are writing these reports, it is important that you:

1. **Be factual:** Write only those things that you know to be true, not what someone told you or what you think might be true.
2. **Be objective:** Write what you actually did, saw, heard, smelled, felt, or tasted. Don't try to interpret the cause or the feelings that went along with the observation. If you feel that you really must put something in the record that's your own interpretation, identify it as such.

Don't diagnose. If the client complains of pains in his chest and arm, don't write "Mr. Peterson had a heart attack and I called the ambulance." Instead, write "Mr. Peterson complained of severe grabbing pains in his chest and upper left arm. His face was pale and moist. I called the ambulance. . . ."

If you observed a large discolored area on the client's arm, write a description of it. Don't write "Mrs. Jones has a big bruise on her arm where I think her husband grabbed her when he got mad because she wet the bed." However, if the client told you this was what had happened, you could record it as "Mrs. Jones told me that her husband was angry because she had wet the bed,

her by the arm. There is a two-inch discolored, purple area on her left forearm just below the elbow.''

3. **Be concise:** Plan your words before you write them. Use enough words to give clear information, but don't "write a book." The important facts should be obvious to another person reading your notes.

4. **Be neat:** Take care that your handwriting or printing is legible. If your writing is very small or very sprawling, try to improve it. If you make a mistake, cross it out with a single line and initial the mistake; this shows you made and corrected the error.

5. **Be accurate:** Be sure the record shows exactly what you did, and if it's appropriate, what the client's reaction was. If you weren't able to carry out some activity that was assigned, give the reason ("I couldn't do the laundry because the washer was broken"). This shows that you didn't forget the activity or purposely fail to do it. Be sure measurements (pulse, temperature, intake and output) are correct.

6. **Sign and date every entry in the record:** Most agencies will want you to sign your name and title (Mary Simmons, HHA) at the end of every entry. It's important to put the date (month, day, and year) and the time the visit began and ended.

7. **Be sure what you write relates to the goals** set for and by the client. Don't let yourself fall in the bad habit of continually writing "No change," "Client was okay today," or other meaningless phrases. If the goal is to have the client learn better housekeeping methods, you might write "Today Mrs. Kitt washed the dishes immediately after lunch."

8. **Be descriptive:** "The kitchen was a mess" doesn't give as much information as "The sink was piled full of dishes coated with dried-on food. Spilled milk had soured on the floor. Roaches were crawling across the counter."

9. **Use the correct words:** In unit 4 you can find some lists of the proper words to use in describing your observations. Try to use these words properly, instead of using slang, and learn their correct spelling. Your reports will be more respected if you learn to use the right words.

confidentiality

Maintaining confidentiality means that you don't talk about your clients or their families with anyone outside the agency. There are federal and state laws that protect the privacy of information; you should become familiar with those laws. Put in simple terms, it means **don't gossip about the client.** Don't tell your family, your friends, or anyone else any details about the client; this includes not revealing even the name or address of the client. In small towns or neighborhoods, it's hard to avoid the inquisitive friend or neighbor who wants to know about the people you work with. Sometimes another client asks questions about a friend who also receives Homemaker/Home Health Aide service. You should not even acknowledge that the person is a client. It's a good idea to practice some responses so you won't be caught offguard. Try some comments like "I'd rather not discuss my work" or "If you're interested in how Mrs. Chambers is feeling, why don't you call her? I'm sure she'd like to talk to you."

signments can be stressful and frustrating at times. It's hard to work with a dying child or to deal with your own feelings over working with an abusive family. Don't "unload" on your own family. Do your talking to the one person who can best understand your feelings, help you deal with them, and perhaps make some changes to improve the situation. That person is the supervisor in your agency. He or she is there to help you, to listen, to advise, and to understand. You need to be careful, however, in picking the time and place to do this. Don't do it in the grocery store checkout lane or the church aisle. Remember that in places like those, other people will be able and eager to overhear your conversation and pass it on as gossip to other people. Eventually, the story often gets back to the very person about whom you were talking. Your reputation, and that of your agency, will be destroyed.

Keeping client information confidential also means that if you're approached by a newspaper, television, or radio reporter and asked to give information or pose for pictures regarding your job or clients, you should refer the reporter to your supervisor for approval.

It's just as important to use good judgment in what you say about your co-workers, supervisor, or the agency. If you're unhappy or dissatisfied with working conditions or behaviors, express that discontent to someone in the agency who can do something about it. Don't do your griping to your family and friends. This would only give the agency a bad reputation, and no improvement in conditions would result.

liability

Liability refers to the degree to which you are held responsible for something that goes wrong on the job. Probably the most important protection from liability that is available to you is to **do only and exactly what your supervisor instructs you to do.** When you follow these instructions, your agency assumes responsibility for your actions. There are some pitfalls that you should recognize and avoid:

1. **Doing more than is assigned.** Practice saying "no" in a nice way, encouraging the patient to contact the supervisor if more services are wanted. When you do something that wasn't assigned, you are assuming responsibility (liability) for these acts, and your agency is no longer responsible.

2. **Doing less than is assigned.** This may put the client in danger and lead to a charge of **negligence,** which means "an action or lack of action that leads to an accident or injury."

3. **Doing hasty, careless or slipshod work.** You've received training in the proper way to carry out your work activities. It's your responsibility to work carefully. Sometimes, even with the greatest amount of care being taken, accidents happen: a valuable vase breaks while you're dusting it or a client falls. If you've been carrying out your assigned duties and exercising a normal amount of care, you are not usually held liable for the damage or injury that results; agencies carry liability insurance to cover these kinds of accidents.

4. **Using your car for work activities without notifying your insurance company.** This particularly applies to taking clients out in your car without letting your insurance agency know. If an accident occurs, you might be heavily liable for injury. It's also a good idea to be sure the agency approves of your taking clients in the car. You'll want to find out what kind of automobile insurance the agency might carry.

5. **Failing to do accurate reporting and documentation.** If you see a client doing something wrong, such as failing to take medicine properly or abusing another family member, and you don't include that in your report because you tell yourself "She doesn't like the taste of that medicine and anyway, it's so expensive" or "He's such a nice man, he couldn't possibly have

meant to bruise his wife like that,'' you're leaving yourself open to charges.

6. **Failing to act in an emergency.** You should know what the emergency plan is for each client you care for, and you should be prepared to follow it. In a life-threatening situation, call for an ambulance before calling the Supervisor. But don't try to perform First Aid or CPR if you haven't been trained to do so.

7. **Attempting to do things that are beyond your abilities.** It's okay to say ''I don't know how to do that. Let's see if we can get someone who does.'' You aren't employed as a nurse, a plumber, an electrician, or a counselor . . . don't try to be one.

8. **Injuring yourself or the client** by doing something you aren't assigned or adequately trained to do. If you have been assigned to do something you don't feel comfortable doing, ask for more training. Trying to do something without assignment and adequate training, such as moving a client with a Hoyer lift, can leave you liable for injury that results.

9. **Failing to report** unsafe working conditions that later cause injury to you or another Homemaker/Home Health Aide. Don't take unnecessary risks. Follow the agency procedures for reporting.

ethics

Ethics is a standard or code of behavior. Medical ethics is the standard of professional conduct of health team members. Doctors and nurses take an oath when they are licensed in which they promise to help and heal their clients without causing unnecessary pain or suffering. Although there is no written code for home health aides, there is a definite set of standards which they are expected to uphold as they practice their profession. A home health aide must:

- Be dependable and reliable. When accepting a job, you must be on time and prepared to fulfill all obligations.
- Maintain high standards of personal health and appearance.
- Be honest in your dealings with clients and co-workers. Stealing involves not only the taking of objects or money, it also means falsifying reports of time and activities.
- Carry out the responsibilities of the job in the best way you possibly can. This means being sure you understand the assignment and how to do it and asking when you aren't absolutely sure.
- Show respect for the client's privacy and modesty. The client must be protected from embarrassment.
- Recognize and honor the right of the client to determine his or her lifestyle, even if it's not one you would choose for yourself. Be flexible and nonjudgmental in working with clients whose lifestyle or values differ from your own.
- Never discuss the financial, emotional, family, medical, or other problems of the client with outsiders.
- Respect the cultural and religious practices of the client and the family.
- Avoid discussions with the client of **diagnosis** and **prognosis** (the medical condition and probable outcome). When a client brings up this subject, the aide should suggest that these matters be discussed with the doctor, supervisor, or members of the family.
- Keep your professional life separate from your personal life. Personal problems of the home health aide should not be discussed with the client or the client's family. Working hours should be devoted to the needs of the client.
- Control your normal reactions to severe illness or the living conditions of the client.

There may be sights and odors which could be upsetting, but the aide must conceal such reactions from the client and the client's family.

- Maintain safe conditions in the working environment. An aide should follow basic rules of safety in caring for the client and when working with equipment and supplies.
- Never walk out in the middle of an assignment. Some people may be more pleasant to work for than others. If personality conflicts or the work load are impossible to deal with, the aide should try to finish the shift, then call the agency supervisor and explain the problem. If the aide is working a private case or did not get the job through an agency, the problem should be discussed directly with the employer. Having accepted the duties as an employee, a home health aide is ethically bound to give service for the wages paid.
- End the relationship with the client when your assignment there is over. If another homemaker/home health aide is assigned to care for that person, your continued contact will make it difficult for the newly assigned worker to establish a good working relationship with the client.
- Refuse tips. Accepting tips is considered unprofessional behavior and may cause your dismissal.
- Say something good about your agency and co-workers, or say nothing.

ethical dilemmas

The homemaker/home health aide may be faced with ethical problems while caring for a client. For example, an aide may be asked in the workplace to perform tasks that are not part of the job description. Instead of getting angry or upset when asked to do such tasks, an aide may say that the agency must give permission before such work can be done. By letting the agency supervisor explain to the client what is or is not allowed, the aide keeps a good relationship with the client and the client's family.

Sometimes homemaker/home health aides find themselves in a home where the family members are abusive and hit or otherwise harm the client or each other. Aides must report such behavior to their supervisors immediately.

What can a homemaker/home health aide do if a client or member of the client's family makes a sexual advance? An aide should not tolerate this kind of behavior. A health aide should never become sexually involved with a client. The aide must firmly state that such behavior is not acceptable. If that does not solve the problem, walk away from the client and tell him/her that you are going to report this incident to the supervisor. You must not permit or put up with sexual harrassment. Try to handle the situation with diplomacy and tact, but always refuse to participate in any sexual behavior.

Sometimes a client is so grateful for the care provided or the attention given by an aide that he or she will offer extra money or gifts to the aide. Sometimes a client may be confused or under the influence of medication and offer money to the aide. Although it may be tempting, accepting a tip or gift under these circumstances is not ethical practice. If the client continues to offer extra money or gifts, report this to your supervisor.

Sometimes a client may become too attached to one particular health aide and may become very dependent or manipulative of the aide. This could lead to a variety of problems. The aide may feel that it is all right to "let down" on the job because the client likes him/her so much, or the client may avoid asking the aide to perform certain tasks. The client may wheedle the aide to "break the rules" such as by adding salt to a salt-free diet or sugar to a sugar-free diet.

When a client becomes too dependent upon an aide, the client may stop trying to improve their own ability to perform the activities of daily living. The aide's job is to help the client achieve the maximum quality of life and become as self-sufficient as possible.

For these reasons, some agencies prefer to rotate homemaker/home health aides occasionally. A particularly difficult case is another reason for rotation. Such a case would occur if the client requires a great deal of personal service, or if the environment is especially depressing, or if a client is extremely demanding. In these situations the aide may suffer "burn out." This means that the aide loses interest or enthusiasm for the job and becomes less effective or careless. Generally, a home health aide is assigned a client who has an immediate need. For example, such a need would occur if a client had just returned from the hospital or nursing home and had no one at home to help him/her until self-care could be resumed. A home health aide would also be needed during the terminal stages of a client's illness. If the client is resuming self-care, an agency will "wean" the client by slowly cutting the aide's hours to the point where the client realizes there is no longer a need for an aide.

Another ethical problem a homemaker/home health aide may face relates to the instructions given by the client to the family or physician regarding the desire of the client to die with dignity. Clients may decide, while in full control of their mental faculties, that they do not want to be kept alive by machines. For example, a client may sign a "Living Will" (see appendix H) which states that he or she is not to be placed on life support systems such as intravenous feeding, oxygen, dialysis, or other mechanical devices. There is still a great deal of controversy about such decisions. In some areas, physicians and hospitals refuse to follow such instructions. This, of course, is not a decision in which an aide would be involved. However, if a client makes his wishes known to an aide, the aide should immediately report such information to the supervisor. An aide **may not, cannot,** and **should not** attempt to advise a client in this regard.

Another choice a client may have to make is whether to die in a hospital or at home. The client and/or the client's family may ask the aide for advice. The homemaker/home health aide should reply that she is not qualified or permitted to comment. The aide can then report the request to her supervisor at the agency who can arrange for counseling for the client and/or family or for referral to an appropriate agency.

Another ethical question is what forms of address to use. A homemaker/home health aide should introduce herself or himself as "Ms., Mrs., or Mr. Smith." The client should be addressed as "Ms., Mrs., or Mr. Jones." Although our society is very informal today, calling a client by his or her first name is unprofessional and demeaning to the client unless the client requests it.

applying ethical standards at work

The home health aide who adheres to ethical standards will always be worthy of employment. Home health aide is a challenging and ever changing vocation. Every job will be different. Some jobs will be more interesting than others; some will be extremely difficult.

A pleasant, calm manner is the best asset a home health aide can develop. One can be sympathetic and understanding of the client's condition but one should not become emotionally involved with the client or family.

Sometimes, the interpersonal relationships within the family unit are poor. The home

The following situation is a common one many homemaker/home health aides meet on an assignment. Remember that information about the client's condition is not to be shared with friends and neighbors. Select the proper responses to the situation. If you select an inappropriate response, discuss the response with your classmates and/or teacher and determine why it is inappropriate:

The situation: For eight months on this assignment, you have accompanied Mr. J to the neighborhood grocery each Friday morning to assist him in doing his weekly grocery shopping. You've gotten to know the check-out clerk; you, she and Mr. J have a running joke about his fondness for very ripe bananas. This past month has been different: Mr. J has had some light strokes and is not permitted to leave his apartment, so you have been doing the shopping for him at the same store.

The problem: The clerk has noticed that Mr. J hasn't been with you. You are at the cash register now, and five people are in line behind you. The clerk comments on Mr. J's absence and asks you what's wrong with him. How would you reply without revealing any confidential information about Mr. J and without hurting the clerk's feelings?

Some possible responses are listed below. Which are acceptable and appropriate?

1. I'm not allowed to talk about my clients.
2. I shouldn't tell you this, but he's been having some strokes, and frankly, he's acting kind of strange, if you ask me.
3. I'll be sure to tell Mr. J you were asking about him. I'm sure he'll be glad to know that you missed him.
4. He had other commitments.
5. It's none of your business.
6. He just didn't come today; I hope he'll be with me next week.

Responses 3, 4 and 6 are all appropriate and reveal nothing about Mr. J while still being polite to the clerk. Response 2 is a definite breach of confidentiality as well as showing disrespect for Mr. J. Response 1 is acceptable, but not very sensitive to the clerk's concern. Response 5 is unacceptable.

health aide must learn to stay out of **intrafamily** disputes. Remaining uninvolved is not always easy. One or more family members may try to get the aide involved through manipulation. **Manipulation** is trying to control another's thoughts or actions for one's own personal gain. A mother, for example, might complain to the aide about how unkind her daughter is. The aide should simply say, "Now, Mrs. Jones, you'll have to talk about that with your daughter. If you like, I'll ask her to stop in so you can clear this up." In other situations, children may try to manipulate. For example, a child might ask the aide's permission to go out knowing that the parents would never allow this privilege.

The home health aide, as a member of the health team, must respect the rights of the client. There was a time when a sick person had to accept whatever care was given, good or bad. The person was not told what treatments were being given and often was not even told what was wrong. Today, more and more sick people are aware of their individual rights as consumers.

A client can and should ask to know the facts about his or her illness from the doctor. A client has the right to refuse any treatment, or the services of the doctor or other health team members. The client may ask that other doctors be called for consultation. Of special importance to the home health aide are the following client rights:

- The right of the client to personal privacy and confidentiality.
- The right to be treated with dignity and respect.
- The right to dismiss any health team member because of that person's unsafe care practices, uncooperative attitude and careless work habits.

summary

- The person entering the vocation of home health aide must be flexible about working hours and conditions.
- A homemaker/home health aide must be capable of working in many different situations and dealing with all age groups and must be well organized in each working environment.
- A homemaker/home health aide must combine a working knowledge of homemaking with safe client care.
- It is essential that the homemaker/home health aide adhere to ethical standards of practice and respect the client's rights. As a member of the health team, the homemaker/home health aide is expected to behave in a suitable manner.
- The needs of the client should be uppermost in the aide's planning, but the other duties must also be completed.
- The homemaker/home health aide should study the housekeeping and client care responsibilities.
- When necessary, a homemaker/home health aide should inform the client as to limitations of an aide's duties.
- The homemaker/home health aide must maintain the confidentiality of the client. Information about the client must not be shared with friends and neighbors of the client or with the family of the aide.
- Accurate observations of the client's physical and emotional states and the details of the client's environment are important components of the overall care of the client. Document all observations thoroughly and accurately as required by the agency.
- The homemaker/home health aide is required to report information to the supervisor or other personnel at the agency. Know who to report to, how to report, and when to

report. Learn the procedures and also know how and when to report emergencies.

- The homemaker/home health aide can be held liable or responsible for accidents or injury to the client or environment. Perform only those activities you have been trained to do and which have been approved for the client by your supervisor. Follow the care plan for the client. Know and avoid the actions which could result in liability.

review

1. Name two vocational adjustments a home health aide might be expected to make.
2. Define ethics.
3. Name two client care responsibilities of the home health aide.
4. List three home care responsibilities of the home health aide.
5. List six characteristics of the client's physical condition that you would observe.
6. List six actions to avoid that could lead to liability.

Unit 4
Developing Effective Communication Skills

key terms

body language	tone	suffix
nonverbal	pitch	root words
communication	medical terminology	listening
aphasia	abbreviations	illiterate
dyslexia	prefix	
dysphasia		

learning objectives

After studying this unit, you should be able to:
▬▬ Identify the sender-message-receiver process.
▬▬ Explain the difference between verbal and nonverbal communication.
▬▬ List four rules for improving aide/client communication.
▬▬ Identify two examples which apply rules of good communication.
▬▬ Identify characteristics of speech which affect communication.
▬▬ Give an example of a precise way to report an observation.

What do most people think of when they see or hear the word communication? Do they think of what they say and how they say it? Do they think of words written in a book, magazine or newspaper; or do they think of television, radio or a telephone? Communication involves all of these and more. What is communication? It is simply the sending and receiving of information.

Humans have developed many methods of communication. Cave men drew pictures. Early Egyptians developed a complicated system using symbols written on stone. Indians used smoke signals. Homing pigeons carried written messages from one area to another.

Words are one of the tools of communication. From the time a baby puts two syllables together and says "ma ma" or "da da," vocabulary begins to develop. Because vocabulary is an important part of communication, and clear communication is a necessity between the aide, agency, client, and family, home health aides should continue to add new words to their vocabulary both during and after training.

basic characteristics of communication

Communication is a two-way process. It involves a sender and a receiver as well as a message. In a conversation, the role of sender and receiver alternates from one to another. In this way there is an exchange of ideas and information. **Listening** is a very important part of communication. When the receiver is so busy thinking of how to reply to the sender, the meaning of what is being said may be lost.

meaning and use of words

Insights in dealing with others can be gained by understanding the importance of accurate communication, and by listening carefully to the words communicated. Words can be soothing, harsh, cruel, or kind. Some words have a special meaning to certain people. Such words may have a strong effect or an emotional impact because of the past experiences of the listener. For instance, widow is a word used to describe a woman whose husband has died. To a recently widowed woman, the word can be frightening. A woman who has been dependent upon her husband usually has a strong feeling of loss. She also may feel anger, rejection, worry, and terrible loneliness. To a woman who has not been widowed, the word has less personal meaning and little or no emotional impact.

Words can be simple or complex. The home health aide must make sure that the words used mean exactly what they are intended to say. Words can be used as weapons to hurt or embarrass others. They can also cheer and comfort.

vocal communication

Vocal or voice communication is using speech to give a message. When speaking with clients, the home health aide should use words that the client can understand. It is helpful to get feedback from the client to be sure the client is receiving the intended message.

Voice communication is an important part of the home health aide/client relationship. The aide should be mindful of the effect that voice communication has on clients and their families and work to improve voice quality.

voice volume and tone

Loud voices often sound harsh and can cause anger in the listener. The listener may then respond harshly, causing an argument. When the aide speaks too softly, it may be hard for the listener to understand what has been said. The home health aide must use special care in communicating with clients and their families.

Tone is the expressive quality of the voice that gives meaning. When speaking, tone is a vital part of communication. A home health aide should speak clearly to be understood and pleasantly to avoid upsetting the client. An ill person and the family has had to adjust to sickness. The family may resent the added burden of the cost of the illness and having an extra person in the home. The client may be emotionally upset and frightened, feeling at the mercy of others. A pleasant tone of voice is necessary when working with people who are emotionally upset. Sometimes it is best to remain quiet.

voice pitch

Speaking voices vary in **pitch.** This quality may be high or low. Some sounds are so low or so high that the human ear cannot perceive them. In speaking, women's voices are normally higher pitched than men's. Most adult sopranos are women and basses are men.

This is mainly due to a difference in the physical structure of the vocal chords.

Some voices are very unpleasant to listen to. They may be hoarse and harsh sounding, grating to the ear. The middle range of voice is more pleasing than the very high or very low. The person who is hard of hearing, however, may be better able to understand what is said when words are spoken slowly and in a low pitch.

regional accents and speech patterns

Regional accents vary. The southern accent is a soft, slow drawl; an eastern accent is often fast, clipped and nasal sounding. There are Boston, Chicago, Brooklyn, and Bronx accents, to name a few. There is nothing wrong with any of these accents, and most people are not aware of how they sound to others. However, they are extremely aware of accents different from their own. The speed with which people speak is another difference which may be noticed.

It is possible to change speech habits. For example, "ya know," "yeah," "like," and "um" endlessly repeated during a conversation can be very boring to the listener. During class, listen carefully when another student is speaking. Try to pick out the tone, pitch, speed, and speech patterns which are most pleasant to listen to.

content of speech

An aide is expected to avoid crude and vulgar language while on the job. Also, for the sake of the client, the aide's personal life should remain separate from his or her working life. In other words, communication with the client should be limited to shared experiences in the work situation. An aide's personal problems should not interfere with the job. The client has enough problems with which to cope without adding the aide's personal problems to them. The aide cannot do proper work if attention is focused on personal problems instead of the client's needs. Anger or hostility from another area of the aide's life should never be allowed to carry over into the relationship with clients. Contact your supervisor for advice. Do not burden your client with your problems.

nonverbal communication

Communication is not limited to words. It can also involve emotions and body language, figure 4-1. Information which is expressed without the use of words is called **nonverbal communication.** It is possible to communicate without words by using gestures such as hand movements, frowns, and smiles. Use of gestures instead of words is also called **body language.** Body language may be combined with words to reinforce the meaning of the words. This reinforcement helps to make communication clear. Body language could, however, be just the opposite, or contradict, the spoken words.

Imagine an elderly client who has no control of the bowels or bladder. Some health aides tend to be very cold and businesslike when cleaning the client and changing the bed. Instead of showing patience and understanding they may become rude or unkind by making a cruel remark or by holding their nose or making a face while cleaning the client. The home health aide has a responsibility to show compassion to all clients.

Consider the following situation. The mother has just told her child to pick up the toys and clean up the mess in the room. The

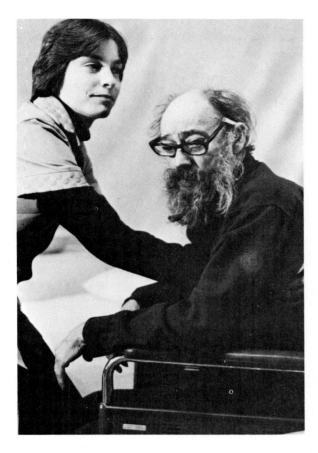

Figure 4-1 Kindness and understanding can be communicated without words.

mother is very angry because the child had not done it earlier. As the mother is walking out of the room with her back to the child, the child says, "Yes, Mama, I'm sorry." The child sticks out her tongue at the departing parent and makes a "face."

What kinds of communication are being used? This is an example of words communicating one thing, and body language another. This sort of contradiction would also be seen if a home health aide were cleaning up after a client had soiled the bed and the aide said, "Let me get this cleaned up so you will be more comfortable," and at the same time rolled the eyes and fanned away the bad odor. The aide's body language speaks louder than the words spoken to the client, and causes the client to be embarrassed. Sometimes the words lose their meaning and the body language is what is communicated. The home health aide must be careful of the message body language gives as well as the choice of words spoken.

written communication

Writing is another form of communication. However, written words have no meaning for the person who is **illiterate** (cannot read). Both reading and writing skills must be learned. As a person progresses in language skills, reading and writing skills improve and vocabulary grows.

Some people have difficulty communicating because of a learning or physical disability, such as aphasia. **Aphasia** causes a person to use words incorrectly or may totally impair a person's ability to speak. **Dyslexia** is another type of learning disability which makes it difficult for a person to read and understand the words that are seen. A person who has difficulty speaking has **dysphasia.**

medical terminology

The home health aide is usually required to keep a written record of the care given a client, and of the client's response to that care. In doing so, the aide may use special medical terminology in describing care procedures or a client's condition.

Medical terminology involves the use of special words and abbreviations that relate to medical subjects. These medical words or terms provide members of the health care team with a precise means of communicating important information about clients under their care, figure 4-2.

VAGUE REPORT	PRECISE REPORT
My client looks bluish around the lips.	Client is cyanotic.
Mrs. Jones looks as white as a sheet.	Mrs. Jones is pale.
Mr. Smith looks very red in the face.	Mr. Smith is flushed.
She feels like she's burning up.	Her temperature is elevated to 102°F.
Susan feels just like ice.	Susan's skin is cold and clammy.

Figure 4-2 Choosing precise words communicates information more clearly.

If a client under the care of a home health aide were to suddenly change color—turn pale, or red in the face, or even become blue, how could this be best described? Of course, the home health aide could say, "Mrs. Jones looks as white as a sheet" or "She looks like she's burning up" or "My client looks kind of bluish around the lips." However, by using proper medical terminology, the home health aide could communicate more clearly by saying, "My client is cyanotic (blue), the TPR (temperature, pulse, and respiration rate) is as follows," or "The client is flushed, temperature is elevated to 102° . . .," or "The client is chalky, skin is cold and clammy, TPR is. . . ." In this way, the home health aide has stated the problem in a way that communicates more facts. The supervisor does not have to waste time asking for more information and can quickly decide what should be done for the client.

prefixes and suffixes

It would be an impossible task for the aide to try to learn all of the medically related words that exist. Special dictionaries have been developed to provide members of the health care team with a reference for learning the meaning of medical words. However, most medical words can be split into distinct parts, making it possible to determine the meaning of the word from the meaning of the parts.

Medical terms are often a combination of different parts called prefixes and suffixes. A **prefix** is a syllable or word that appears at the beginning of a term. A **suffix** appears at the end of a word.

Both prefixes and suffixes have specific meanings. For example, the suffix "itis" means "inflammation of." Thus, tendonitis is an inflammation of a tendon. Another example is the word biology. The prefix "bio" means life. The suffix "ology" means "study of" or "science of." Thus, biology means the study of life, or living things. There are also **root words,** which are the main parts of a word to which a suffix or prefix may be attached. For instance, the meaning of the root word, "appendix," may be changed by adding the prefix "pseudo" which means false, and the suffix "itis" which means inflammation. The combined term, pseudoappendicitis, means a false inflammation of the appendix.

By learning some of the common prefixes, suffixes, and word roots used in medical terminology, it is possible to determine the meaning of an unfamiliar term. Figure 4-3 shows a list of some common word parts.

abbreviations

In addition to complete medical words, the home health aide should become familiar with commonly used *abbreviations* (brief, or shortened, forms of words). Some common abbreviations include Dr. (doctor), R.N. (regis-

a-, *an*-: without, not
ab-: from, away
ad-: to, toward
adeno-, *aden*-: gland, glandular
-*algia*: pain
ambi-: both
ante-, *pre*-: before
anti-, *contra*-: against
audio-: sound, hearing, dealing with the ear
auto-: self

bi-, *bis*-: twice, double
bio-: life
bronch-, *bronchi*-: air tubes in the lungs, bronchi

cardi-, *cardia*-, *cardio*-: pertaining to the heart
-*cide*: causing death
crani-, *cranio*-: pertaining to the skull
cyst-, *cysto*-, *cysti*-: bladder, bag
-*cyte*, *cyt*-: cell

derm-, *derma*-, *dermo*-, *dermat*-: pertaining to skin
dia-: through, between, apart
dorsi-, *dorso*-: to the back, back
dys-: difficult, painful

ecto-, *ex*-, *exo*-: outside of, external
-*ectomy*: surgical removal of
endo-: within, innermost
entero-: intestine, pertaining to the intestine

gastro-, *gasti*-: stomach
-*genetic*, -*genic*: origin, producing
genito-: organs of reproduction
glyco-, *gly*-: sugar
gyn-, *gyno*-: women, female

hemi-: half
hema-, *hem*-, *hemo*- *hemato*-: blood
hepato-: liver
hetero-: other, unlike, different
homo-, *homeo*-: same, like
hydro-: water

hyper-: over, increased, high
hystero-, *hyster*-: uterus
hypo-: under, decreased, low

inter-: between, among
intra-: within, into
-*itis*: inflammation, inflammation of

leuko-, *leuco*-: white
-*logy*, -*ology*: study of, science of

mal-: bad, abnormal, disordered
mast-, *masto*-: breast
micro-: small
mono-: one, single
multi-: many, much, a large amount
myo-: muscle

neph-, *nephro*-, *ren*-: kidney
neuro-, *neur*-: nerve or nervous system

-*ology*: study of a science
ophthalm-, *ophthalmo*-: eye
-*ostomy*: creation of an opening by surgery
ot-, *oto*-: ear
-*otomy*: cutting into

path-, *patho*-, -*pathy*, -*pathia*: disease, abnormal condition
ped-, *pedia*-: child
peri-: around
-*plegia*: paralysis
pneum-: lung, pertaining to the lungs
proct-, *procto*-: rectum, rectal
psuedo-: false
psych-, *psycho*-: pertaining to the mind

sep-, *septic*-: poison, rot
sub-: less, under, below
super-, *supra*-: above, upon, over

therm-, *thermo*-: heat
-*toxic*, -*tox*: poison
tracho-: trachea, windpipe

Figure 4-3 Prefixes and suffixes commonly used in medical terminology.

ā - before	P.O. - By mouth
ad lib - As desired	prep. - Prepare for
a.c. - Before meals	p.r.n. - When needed or necessary
b.i.d. - Twice a day	pt. - Patient
B.P. - Blood Pressure	P.T. - Physiotherapy, Physical Therapy
B.R.P. - Bathroom privileges	apy
c̄ - With	q.2h. - Every 2 hours
C.B.R. - Complete bedrest	q.3h. - Every 3 hours
cc - Cubic centimeter	q.4h. - Every 4 hours
H.S. - Hour of sleep	q.d. - Every day
Ht. - Height	t.i.d. - Three times a day
Lab - Laboratory	q.i.d. - Four times a day
lb. - Pound	q.o.d. - every other day
ml - milliliter	s̄ - Without
N.P.O. - Nothing by mouth	S.O.B. - Short of breath
o.d. - every day	stat - immediately
O.T. - Occupational therapy	S.S.E. - Soapsuds enema
oz. - Ounce	Temp. - (T) - Temperature
p̄ - after	T.P.R. - Temperature, Pulse, Respiration
pc - after meals	tion
	Vital signs - T.P.R. and B.P.
	Wt. - Weight

Figure 4-4 Standard medical abbreviations must be learned in order to understand medical orders and to chart correctly.

tered nurse), B.M. (bowel movement), @ (at), and ea. (each). Many other abbreviations, such as TPR (temperature, pulse, and respiration rate), will be defined throughout this text. Figure 4-4 provides a list of abbreviations that may be frequently encountered.

communication with clients

Interpersonal relationships are developed through communication. Touching, speaking, laughing and crying are all ways of communicating. The home health aide should keep in mind a few simple rules for setting up lines of communication in the work situation, figure 4-5.

Humor has been found to be so effective in healing that some health care professionals are making it a regular part of the care plan. A home health aide might ask a client what makes him or her laugh. Sometimes it might be a "corny" joke or a re-run of a com-

DO	DO NOT
Show acceptance of the client's feelings first, before explaining what can be done.	Pass judgement, argue with the client, or set blame on the client or others.
Let the client talk.	Rudely interrupt or give advice.
Show interest in what is said.	Pretend to be busy or change the subject abruptly.
Show concern for your client's condition. Ask if the client is comfortable or if you can help in any way.	Give false encouragement as to a client's prognosis.
Allow the supervisor to answer when a client wants to know about his or her medical condition.	Tell your own medical history.
Tell the client what you are going to do before you do it. Also, explain procedures as you are doing them.	Assume the client understands the steps or the purpose of a procedure.

Figure 4-5   Learning these rules helps make communication more meaningful.

edy TV show such as "I Love Lucy." Shared laughter can improve communication between a client and home health aide. However, use humor carefully and appropriately so it is not misunderstood as mocking or ignoring the seriousness of a situation. Humor can make people feel good about themselves and ease stress, figure 4-6. Some therapists prescribe "humor breaks" for families of terminally ill patients. The theory is that if you can laugh for a few moments, you may be better able to cope with illness or death.

communicating with the client's family

The more people involved in a home health care situation, the more a possibility exists for miscommunication and misunderstanding. If the client is a woman with a sick husband in the house, there may be friction when a home health aide comes on the scene. The wife may show signs of jealousy over the special attention given by a female aide to her husband. The aide may feel caught in the middle and be getting instructions or orders from all sides. The aide must keep calm and listen to the requests, questions, and advice offered. Then the aide must state that he/she is only permitted to take orders from the supervisor. If conflicting requests are made by the family, the aide must remain friendly and appear interested while going ahead with the job as assigned.

Another example would be a family that is affected by the illness of a parent. The aide should try to get the family involved in making the client comfortable. Ask family member(s) to name the client's favorite foods and to state what the client likes to talk about. Try to learn more about the client from them and then put that information to good use when caring for the client. You can be supportive of the family members by being sympathetic, by being understanding, and by listening. If you are supportive of the family, they will be able to give more support to the ailing family member.

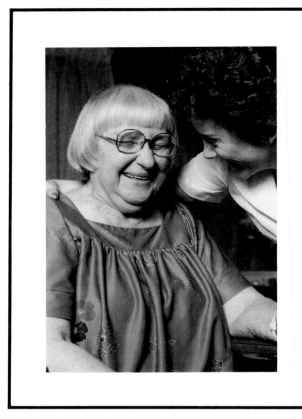

Figure 4-6 Laughter makes everyone feel better.

Sometimes family members will ask an aide to do personal work for them. This is not acceptable. The aide can say that he/she will have to get permission from the agency, or suggest that the family member call the agency to see if such a request is appropriate. It is wrong to talk back to the client or to the client's family. If an aide should find it impossible to cope with a particular client or the client's family, the agency supervisor should be advised immediately.

Stop to think about the rules in figure 4-5. Are they not based on common sense? Clients and their families are to be spoken to and treated in the same way that the home health aide would want to be spoken to and treated. Remember, too, that communication does not always need words. Sometimes a gentle pat on the arm or a smile can communicate more than any choice of words.

Communication is a combination of many skills. A home health aide must develop these skills in order to become successful. Figure 4-7 shows several examples of aide/client communication. Note how the choice of words can affect interpersonal relationships. The better responses are based on the rules shown in figure 4-5.

Guidelines for communicating with hearing- and speech-impaired clients are shown in figure 4-8, page 46.

SITUATION	POOR RESPONSE	BETTER RESPONSE
Client is in pain.	"Stop complaining; take an aspirin and you'll feel better."	"I see that you are in pain. I'll call my supervisor and see what should be done."
Client tells you all the details of her operation.	"I had a friend who had the same thing. She never got well and was in terrible pain."	"My, you've really had a rough time; you must be happy to be back home."
Client asks your advice about a personal matter.	"Well, if I were you I'd stop talking to that person. . . she's no good."	"I know that you are upset. Perhaps you should talk this over with your family."
Client complains that you did something the wrong way.	"Nobody could please you. It's no wonder you have no friends."	"The way you're used to may also be correct, but this is the way I was taught in class. I'll check with the supervisor the next time I call."
Client is restless and cranky — should be napping.	"It's your nap time and I am due for a coffee break."	"You don't seem sleepy. Would you like to talk for a while before you take your rest?"
Client on salt-free diet, says food tastes terrible.	"That's what you're to eat, so stop complaining."	"It must be hard to get used to eating your food without salt. Perhaps using the salt substitute the doctor recommended would help."
Client on sugar-free diet pleads with you to put "just a little" sugar in her tea.	"Well, just a half spoon of sugar couldn't hurt."	"I know it's not easy to give up sugar, but your health comes first. Try the sugar substitute your doctor ordered."
Client claims she needs bedpan even though she used it only 20 minutes earlier.	"It's your imagination. You know you don't need it again."	"You must be uncomfortable. I'll get it for you."
Client has soiled bed the second time in one day and is very upset.	"Why didn't you tell me you needed the bedpan. What an awful mess."	"It's hard not to feel ashamed, but it takes just a few minutes to change the linens."
It's time for lunch but the client states she is not hungry.	"Eat the soup before it gets cold."	"I can warm it up and serve it later when you feel hungry."
Aide wants to give client a bath. Client says she is too tired.	"How could you be tired? You just woke up. Anyway I have to bathe you now."	"Yes, you must be tired but I have to give you a bath before I leave this morning."

Figure 4-7 Situations can be handled more smoothly when the correct response is made.

HEARING IMPAIRMENT

1. Always be sure to get the listener's attention, verbally or by touch.
2. Position yourself so that the listener can view your face clearly.
3. Speak slowly and clearly at a full, but not excessively loud level. Form words carefully and keep sentences relatively short. Avoid unnecessary chatter that may confuse the hearing-impaired client.
4. Use facial expressions or gestures appropriately to help express yourself. Visual clues are important in helping the hearing-impaired client to understand what you say.
5. Check to make sure your client has understood what you said. If not, rephrase the message, trying to give more clues. (Example: *Message:* "The nurse will be dropping by this afternoon to check on you." *Rephrased:* "Your nurse, Ms. Anderson, will be coming here at 3:00 to check the dressing on your leg.")
5. Try to reduce distractions in the immediate environment.
6. Avoid chewing gum and placing your hands at your mouth when you speak.
7. Demonstrate your willingness to take the time and energy to communicate with your client, without losing your patience.

SPEECH IMPAIRMENT

1. Position yourself close to the client in a quiet setting in order to avoid unnecessary strain or frustration.
2. Speak to the client in a normal fashion.
3. Try to phrase questions so that they may be answered either yes or no.
4. Watch the lips of the speaker to help you pick up additional clues as to the message being communicated.
5. If you do not understand a portion of your client's message, repeat the portion of it you did understand and request clarification of the remainder. (Example: "I understand that you are hungry, but I do no understand what you would like to eat.")
6. Limit the time of your conversations so as not to tire your client.
7. Keep paper and pencil within your client's reach, if necessary.
8. Demonstrate your willingness to take the time and make the effort to communicate, without losing your patience. Provide encouragement for your client to speak.

Figure 4-8 Guidelines for communicating with hearing- and speech-impaired clients.

The following is a typical situation that may arise when caring for a client. As you read the description of the situation, consider appropriate responses. Then compare your responses with those provided and make a selection of the most appropriate ones. If inappropriate choices are made, determine why they are inappropriate.

The situation: You are the homemaker/ home health aide assigned to work with Mrs. T from 10:00 A.M. until 12:30 P.M. on Monday through Friday. One of your assigned duties is to prepare Mr. T's noon meal, with enough planned leftovers for Mrs. T to prepare a light supper for herself. Your supervisor has told you that Mrs. T has very limited money available for food purchases, so you must be careful to not waste food or plan expensive menus.

The problem: Ever since Mrs. T was a child, she has been accustomed to offering food to anyone working at her home at a mealtime. When you prepare a meal, she asks you to sit down at the table and share the meal with her. When you say that the leftovers are for her supper, she says she'll just eat cold cereal then. It looks like she's getting angry because you won't eat with her.

What are some of the responses you might make that will encourage Mrs. T to eat, but allow you to refrain from eating her food? Some possible responses are:

1. Thank you, but I'm going to eat lunch with a friend as soon as I leave here.
2. Thank you, but I have to go home and fix a meal for my family, so I'll eat with them.
3. I couldn't possibly eat your food!
4. I'm allergic to this kind of meat so I can't eat it.
5. Thank you for asking. I don't believe I'll eat a full meal right now, but if it's all right with you, I'll sit down and have a cup of tea while you eat.
6. I brought my lunch today, so I'll get it out of your refrigerator and sit with you while we both eat.
7. If I were to eat with you and then eat with my family when I get home, pretty soon I'd be too fat to fit through your door!

Responses 1, 2, 5, 6, and 7 are acceptable. If you plan to use 5 or 6, be sure your supervisor has approved your taking lunch time while in a client's home. Responses 3 and 4 won't leave Mrs. T feeling very good about herself. Can you think of some other possible responses?

- One of the skills a home health aide must develop is the art of communication.
- It is always wise to think before speaking. The tone of voice and the pitch, as well as the content of what is said, are all part of verbal communication.
- Nonverbal communication includes body language such as gestures, touching, and facial expressions.
- Communications can only be delivered when there is a sender and a receiver. This means that part of the art of communication is learning to be a good listener.
- Written communications must be very clear. This requires properly spelling words and writing clearly so that the message can be read.

- Many times a home health aide will be asked to keep a chart of the client's responses or to record certain information about the client, such as temperature, pulse, and respiration rate. Special terminology or abbreviations may be used for this purpose.
- Accuracy is an absolute must when making medical records.
- When communicating with an elderly or ill person, the home health aide should be patient and gentle.
- The aide should keep in mind that illness affects the emotions. Some clients may whine and cry. Others may appear to be angry and short-tempered.
- It is the duty of the home health aide to keep the lines of communication open. Clients and their families must be spoken to and treated in the same way that the home health aide would want to be spoken to and treated.

review

1. Give two examples each of verbal and nonverbal communication?
2. How can the home health aide give a precise report of observations made?
3. List four rules for improving communications with clients.
4. What three elements are involved in communication?

Unit 5

Understanding Differences: Individuals, Families, and Cultures

learning objectives

After completing this unit, you should be able to:
- List three ways in which families may differ.
- Identify one way illness might affect a family.
- Discuss racial and religious prejudice.
- Identify what is meant by a family unit.
- Define environment and culture.
- Describe the meaning of home.

Home is a word with a great deal of emotional impact. It has a special meaning for most people. It recalls mental images of shared family experiences and geographical locations or even of anger or sadness. One may speak of one's home as the country, state or town of birth. It may be thought of as the house where one lives. It can be a small room in a boarding house or a spacious place in the suburbs; but to the people living there, it is home. A home health aide may be assigned to many different types of homes, from modest to wealthy. The care standards provided by the home health aide are the same in all types of homes. Standards of cleanliness are to be maintained, using whatever equipment is available. An aide is expected to work with individuals and within **family units** and develop good interpersonal relationships.

The home health aide must recognize that each client is an individual who is unique in many ways from any other person. Each client has different needs, and each reacts to illness or disability in different ways. The aide must be prepared to adapt to the changing and unique needs of the client and the client's family.

the family unit—
past and present

What is a family unit? By many laws, a family unit is made up of a married couple and their natural or adopted children. A family may also include relatives such as aunts, uncles, cousins, grandparents or in-laws. In today's society, however, a family may also be made up of nonrelated members who live together under one roof. As a large or small group, they usually share some common interests and financial duties.

historical perspective

Early in this century, a majority of the population lived in rural areas. Home and family were the center of life. Farming or agriculture was the main industry or source of income. This was called an **agrarian** society. Families lived and worked together. They were self-sufficient and provided for their own needs—food, clothing, shelter. They sold grain, chickens, eggs, and cattle to bring in cash. The average farm income was often less than $900 a year. Sometimes three generations (grandparents, parents, and children) lived together, sharing responsibilities. Men and women worked side by side in the fields. Babies were cared for by the older women in the family. As the children grew up, they were given chores suited to their age. They were expected to gather eggs and feed the farm animals or milk the cows. Each member of the family unit worked to help the family survive as a whole.

Because of lack of transportation, social life was limited to the local neighborhood. It usually centered around the family, close neighbors, the school and the church. Close family and community ties provided stability and strength to the family unit.

Technological advances eventually led families away from an agrarian society. Travel became easier and industrial jobs drew families away from their rural homes. Family members became more mobile and often became separated from the main household.

current perspectives

We are now moving from being an industrial society to being a computer society. We have entered the **Age of Information** and further changes in life-style are taking place. Technology has improved the lives of family members in many ways but it has also caused new problems. Nevertheless, children still need the security of a home, figure 5-1.

Because it takes more and more income to maintain a reasonable standard of living, large numbers of husbands and wives both hold down jobs. Day care centers cannot provide adequate space for the children of these working families. For the homemaker/home health aide, this means more opportunity for work as child care providers.

As a result of cuts in federal spending, many facilities that provided child care in the past are no longer in operation. Very often, today's homemaker/home health aide is called upon to work with **special children** (children

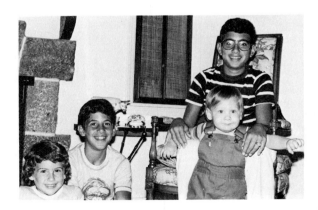

Figure 5-1 Children of today's Age of Information society still need the security of a home.

who are emotionally, mentally, or physically handicapped).

Another change within families is the increased number of **single-parent families.** It is estimated that nearly one half the marriages in the United States will end in divorce, leaving one parent with the major responsibility of child rearing. The greater independence individuals now have gives them more freedom of choice, but often leaves them in a state of loneliness. Frequent moves can be very difficult for some people. Both adults and children may find it hard to continually make new friends each time they move.

As children grow up and move away from the parental home, often moving across the country, the caregivers have become people outside the family rather than the spinster daughter or the bachelor son of yesteryear.

Changes in life-style also have altered social and moral attitudes. In some cases, these changes have weakened the family unit. Since family members cannot always rely on one another for care, they must seek help from outside the family. The trained homemaker/home health aide meets this need by giving the care formerly provided by family members.

general background about contrasts creating family differences

According to the 1988 *World Almanac,* the population of the United States is approximately 240,856,000 and the age distribution is:

0–14	21.7%
15–59	61.8%
Over 60	16.5%

As of 1986, the life expectancy at birth of males was 71.5 years and 78.5 years for females.

The total population can be divided roughly into groups according to skin color as follows:

White	80%±
Black	10%±
Other	10%±

The last category includes Native Americans (Amerinds and Eskimos), Mexicans, natives of India and Pakistan, Hispanics, Orientals, and all other nonwhite emigrants.

It is estimated that 59.3 percent of the population are members of churches, synagogues, or temples. The major religions in the United States are:

Protestant denominations (Christian, Baptist, Methodist, Episcopalian, Presbyterians, etc.). In addition, there are various *sects,* groups that are too small to be considered a denomination.
Catholic (Roman Catholic, Old Catholic, Polish National Catholic, Russian Orthodox, and American Catholic).
Jewish (Reform, Conservative and Orthodox).

There are also Muslims who follow the writings of Mohammed; Buddhists who believe in the teachings of Buddha; and athiests, who do not believe in God, to name only a few.

From reading these statistics, it is quite clear that America is truly a melting pot where people are free to practice (or not practice) religion. This is a nation which prides itself on offering the gift of freedom to all people. Freedom, however, does not mean that a person can do whatever he or she may choose. There are laws which all must follow so that we will not live in chaos.

What does all this mean to a home health aide? Prejudice grows out of ignorance and lack of knowledge about others. Prejudice is forming an opinion without knowing all the facts. Those who hold preconceived, irrational opinions often feel hatred or strong dislike for a particular group, race, or religion. Some people feel threatened by those whose skin color is different or fear practices that are unfamiliar to them. It is clear that the average individual cannot be knowledgeable about all of the differences among people. However, each individual should keep an open mind and be sensitive to the religious, cultural, or ethnic practices of others.

As home health aides go from client to client, they will meet persons of other cultures, religions, color, or nationality from their own. This can be looked upon as an opportunity to discover interesting and informative facts about others. The more a person knows, the less likely a person is to be prejudiced. An aide must always remember that there are unpleasant individuals in the world. Being unpleasant has nothing to do with one's race, color, language, or religion.

Religious practices, traditions, types of food, and manner in which food is prepared are very often determined by the culture and religion of the individual. The home health aide must (1) accept the practices of others, (2) be sensitive to the client's needs, and (3) follow the instructions given by the supervisor in meeting the needs of the client regardless of religion, color, or creed. An aide must not judge clients, but must allow them the freedom to follow their own practices and beliefs while the aide provides safe and proper health care.

Families differ in size, ages of members, likes and dislikes, customs and habits. They differ in political beliefs, financial resources, and ethnic background. Each family has its own living standards, religious practices, and standards within the community. Many normal contrasts exist. However, health or social problems can also create contrasts. Some families include children with special needs. Members of other families may have suffered emotional breakdowns. Alcoholism, psychosocial problems and addiction to drugs or gambling may cause family problems. The home health aide should be aware of these problems. They may determine how the aide plans work schedules and what work must be done.

cultural differences

Culture is the way of life which is passed down to children from generation to generation. Cultural influences include language, moral codes, customs and laws. Culture is a learned behavior. A child at birth speaks no language. A Chinese baby raised by a German family would grow up speaking German, not Chinese. Culture is the result of the social surroundings which affect the growth of an individual. The sum total of the conditions which surround an individual is called the **environment.** Examples of cultural customs which might be seen by a home health aide include:

- *When and what a family eats.* Farm families often have their main meal at noon. Those who live in cities most often have their largest meal at night when all the family members are at home. The spices and seasonings preferred by a family are often culturally determined. Greek and Italian families may use heavy garlic seasonings. Some Texans prefer hot, spicy foods because they have acquired part of the Mexican culture.
- *The accepted response to pain or grief.* American Indians have been considered a stoic people. They are taught from infancy to show no pain and not to cry. Other cultures may encourage outward expression such as screaming, crying or tearing their clothes to show grief.
- *How children are disciplined.* In Japan, children are taught from infancy not to make unnecessary noise. When a baby cries, it is picked up at once and soothed so that the cries will not disturb others. In general, American parents are more permissive than English parents. Most people discipline a

child in the way they were disciplined by their own parents.

religious practices

Whether or not one follows a religion is an individual decision. However, that personal decision is greatly influenced by one's culture. When working in a home where there are strong religious practices, the home health aide must respect the customs and practices of that family.

Most religions set aside Sunday as a day of worship and rest; exceptions to this are Judaism and Seventh Day Adventists which celebrate the Sabbath on Saturday. Special dietary laws are often observed. Some religious groups do not eat meat, limit the types of meat eaten, or restrict meat on certain days. Many nonreligious groups also do not eat meat or animal products and are referred to as **vegetarians.** Fast days (no food or drink are consumed for a certain period of time) may also be observed in varying degrees. Orthodox Jewish families may have two or more sets of dishes and utensils for cooking and eating: one set is used only for dairy foods, another set for meat dishes, and a third set is used only during the Passover celebration. Observing Jewish law in this manner is part of keeping a Kosher home. Families that practice special dietary customs will usually instruct the home health aide as to the family's special requirements. The aide must carry out such special instructions without passing judgment.

Among some religious groups, it is customary for the minister, priest or rabbi to make regular visits to the homebound members of their congregations. A telephone number of the clergy is usually given to the aide. This number should be kept near the phone so the aide can call if the need arises. To a deeply religious family, the minister, priest, or rabbi is a vital member of the health team; they give spiritual and psychological support to the client. The home health aide has a duty to respect the religious beliefs and practices of the client and family.

differences in response to illness or disability

Each family reacts to illness in a different way because no two people or two families are exactly alike. The personalities, attitudes, interests and needs differ from person to person within the family. Some differences are due to age, physical and mental condition, and the individual's place in the family unit. Illness in a family creates a special set of problems. How the family reacts might depend upon the:

- seriousness of the illness
- length of time the illness is expected to last
- probable outcome of the illness
- family member who is ill

If the head of the household is ill, there may be no money coming in to meet daily expenses and medical costs. The rest of the family may be afraid and worried. Some members may also be angry because they have to do without new clothes, or have to change their personal plans because of the illness. The person who is ill may be just as worried and upset as the rest of the family; the illness can be worsened by the added worry. When the mother of the family is ill, the household may be totally disorganized, figure 5-2. The children may fight with each other and refuse to accept any new responsibilities. A prolonged or chronic illness of the mother could cause long-term changes in the family. The children may have to take on household duties and care for each other. Family members must learn to adjust so they still have time for their own pursuits.

In the case of an acute or sudden illness, families are more able to make adjustments because they know it is only for a short time.

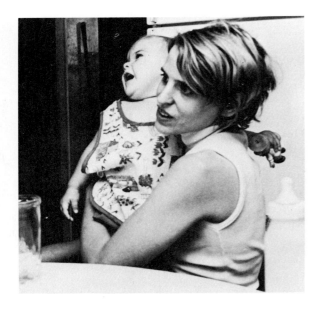

Figure 5-2 A person who is not well may find it difficult to cope with the demands of child care.

They are often cheerful and happy to be able to help out for a few days. Long-term, or chronic illness, however, can lead to sullen and uncooperative attitudes on the part of family members. They may show patience and kindness during the early days of the illness, but soon they want to get back to their own lives and may become impatient with the needs of the sick person.

A home health aide is entering a home where illness is present. A professional attitude must be developed toward the client and family. An aide should not become overly involved in the family's problems. The aide should be a sympathetic listener, but should not attempt to take charge and tell the family how to live. Each home served by a home health aide offers new challenges. Upon entering a client's home, an aide has assumed the responsibility to meet the demands of a particular medical situation and provide the needed care for the home.

An aide must be flexible enough to follow suggestions about the care of the home. Aides must also make certain that the prescribed medical needs of the client are met. A home health aide is not expected to work miracles. However, the aide who is aware of potential family problems during illness is better able to deal with them. The aide who knows how to plan, bring order out of chaos, and keep the client clean and comfortable, helps the entire family during a time of trouble.

summary

- Rich or poor, the home is usually the focus of family life. Within a home, the family unit lives by its own rules and standards.
- One of the responsibilities of the home health aide is to respect the rights of the client and the family within the home.
- When working in a home, accidents do happen. During the course of cleaning, a lamp or dish may be broken. A dark sock may get mixed in with the white laundry. An aide should be able to admit making a mistake. Most family members will understand that minor accidents do occur. However, the home health aide must make every effort to avoid making careless and possibly dangerous errors.
- Client care is always given as ordered by the doctor. A home health aide is also expected to follow the instructions of the supervisor.
- The home health aide comes into a home as a stranger to give personal care to the client and provide home care. The aide can ease some of the problems caused by illness.
- A home health aide should take pride in doing a job well.
- When helping a family in trouble, the aide should always show respect for the customs and life-styles of that family.

review

1. Name three ways that families may differ.
2. How may a family member's illness affect the entire family?
3. What is meant by environment?
4. Define culture.
5. Give two examples of prejudice.

Basic Anatomy and Physiology

Unit 6

Functions and Disorders of the Body Systems

---

key terms

epidermis	sensory deficits	oliguria
dermis	auditory	anuria
bony prominences	otosclerosis	vasoconstriction
decubitus ulcer	emphysema	vasodilation
ligaments	peristalsis	hypotension
fracture	impacted	hypertension
arthritis	incontinent	dyspnea
epilepsy	cystitis	apnea
hemophiliac	Cheyne-Stokes	tachypnea
	respirations	

---

learning objectives

After studying this unit, you should be able to:
—— Identify one function of each body system.
—— Name the five senses.
—— Identify one disorder in each body system.
—— Identify the relationship among cells, tissues, organs and systems.
—— Identify the difference between hereditary and environmental factors.

Human beings have often been compared to machines. When functioning perfectly, the body operates as smoothly as a well-oiled machine. The human body, however, is much more efficient than any machine. Unlike a machine, the human body can often repair itself, e.g., new skin can grow over a wound. When the body functions at its peak efficiency with all of its parts working like a finely tuned engine, it is in a well state.

The body is a complex organism. It is made up of millions of cells which are the smallest structural units of the body. Many cells make up a tissue and tissues make up organs, figure 6-1. Organs act together in making the total body function. All of these separate units interact within the body in systems. There are nine body systems, figure 6-2. Each body system performs a necessary function in the body.

integumentary system

The skin, which is the largest component of the integumentary system, is the body's first means of defense against germs. The skin is the largest organ of the body. It covers the entire outer surface and the inside surfaces of all the body's openings (nose, mouth, ears, vagina, etc.). Skin is made up of two layers of tissue. The outer layer is the *epidermis* and the inner layer is the *dermis,* figure 6-3. Other organs of the integumentary system are the nails, hair, oil and sweat glands, and mucous membranes.

The integumentary system protects the body from germs but also has other functions. It regulates body temperature, and works with the nervous system to sense touch, pressure, pain, heat, and cold.

The pores or natural openings in the skin surface are protected by oil glands and sweat glands. As the body perspires (sweats) through the skin pores, the air evaporates the perspiration and the body feels cooler. Secretions from these glands are helpful in keeping germs from entering the pores. When the skin is cut or there is an open sore, pathogens can enter the body easily. Once germs get beyond the skin, the other body defenses start to work. White blood cells surround the germs and try to stop them from going deeper into the body. The pus that forms on a skin wound is made up of dead white blood cells which have fought off the germs.

Hair protects the body in several ways. The eyebrows keep sweat from falling into the eyes. The tiny hairs inside the nose and ears stop small particles from entering and causing

STRUCTURAL UNIT	DESCRIPTION	EXAMPLES
Cell	Microscopic life units	Blood cells, nerve cells
Tissue	Group of specialized cells which perform a specific function	Epithelial - (skin and lined inner surfaces) Connective - (blood, tendons, ligaments, cartilage) Muscular - (heart, organ walls and muscles attached to bones) Nervous - (brain, spinal cord, and nerves)
Organ	Group of tissues which perform a particular function	Kidney, heart, liver, stomach
System	A set of organs which act together in a common purpose	Integumentary, musculoskeletal, endocrine, nervous, circulatory, respiratory, digestive, urinary, and reproductive

Figure 6-1 Cells group into larger structural units in order to perform special functions.

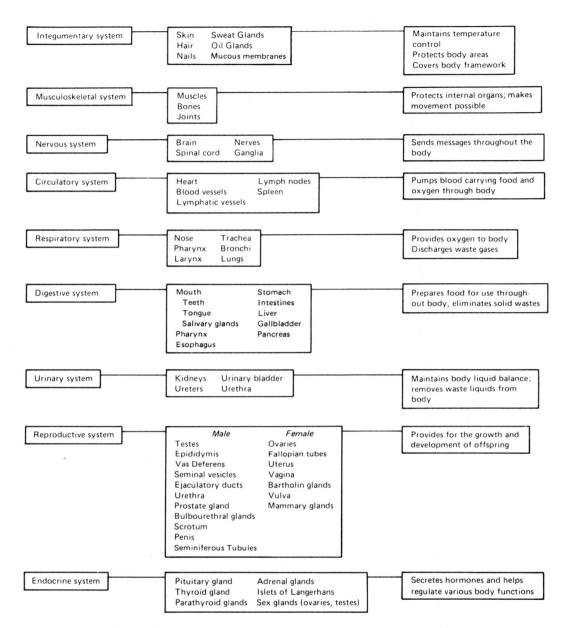

Figure 6-2 The body systems and their major organs and functions

damage. The eyelashes keep small objects from getting into the eye. These hairs all act very much like a screen door on a house in keeping out unwanted organisms. The skin itself screens out harmful rays from the sun which may cause burns and harm the body.

common disorders of the integumentary system

decubitus ulcers (bedsores). The care given to the skin of a person confined to bed or a wheelchair is extremely important. When

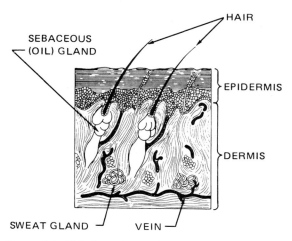

SEBACEOUS (OIL) GLAND

HAIR

EPIDERMIS

DERMIS

SWEAT GLAND — VEIN

Figure 6-3 Skin is made up of two layers of tissue—the epidermis and the dermis.

the body gets little exercise, the skin is one of the first areas to break down. The first sign of skin breakdown is the appearance of a reddened area; the ulcer may be graded as shown in figure 6-4. Breakdown most often occurs where the skin covers the bones. These places are called **bony prominences,** figure 6-5.

A **decubitus ulcer,** also called a bedsore, is a breakdown in the skin which covers a bony area. Decubitus ulcers occur most often as a result of poor blood circulation and

DEGREES	DESCRIPTION
1°	Reddened area
2°	Blistered area (which then hardens or there is a break in the skin)
3°	Tissue death
4°	Involves the muscle area
5°	Involves the muscle, tendons, bones, and maybe even the joints

Figure 6-4 Grading decubitus ulcers

constant irritation of the skin. The back of the head, elbows, knees and heels rub against bedding or clothing; these are some of the places to watch for signs of decubitus ulcers. The first sign is a warm looking red spot. Within 18 to 24 hours the red spot can become an open sore. The client's bed linens should be kept clean and dry at all times. If the client is left in a urine-saturated bed, the skin may begin to break down in seven (7) minutes. If the doctor permits, the client should be turned at least every two hours. This turning relieves the pressure on the bony prominences.

Range of motion exercises should be given as often as the doctor permits. The home health aide assists the client in arm and leg movements to increase the blood circulation near the skin's surface. Gentle massage may be given to these areas of the skin to increase circulation to these areas. There are special protective pads which may be placed on the elbows, heels and ankles, figure 6-6. The pads protect skin areas from rubbing against bedclothing, but do not take the place of good skin care.

During normal morning and evening care, the home health aide should carefully observe the danger areas. Prevention of decubiti is the first goal of the home health aide. Once a decubitus ulcer has developed it may be very difficult to clear it up.

Some other common skin disorders and their treatments are described in figure 6-7.

musculoskeletal system

The musculoskeletal system is made up of bones and muscles. It protects the internal body organs and makes body movement possible. The skull, for instance, forms a protective covering for the brain. The spinal column surrounds the spinal nerves leading from the brain. There are over 200 bones in the body, figure

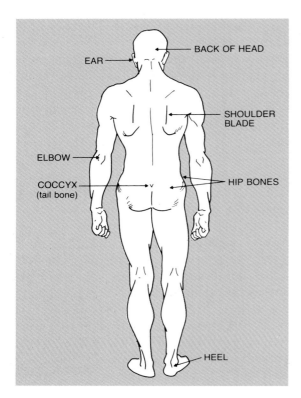

Figure 6-5 Decubitus ulcers most often form over bony prominences.

6-8 on page 63. Bones are joined together by tough elastic fibers called **ligaments.**

Joints allow the bones to be moved in certain ways, figure 6-9 on page 64. The elbows and knees have hinge joints which move in only two directions like hinges on a door. The joints at the shoulder and pelvis are ball and socket joints. They provide a circular movement. The wrist, ankles and spinal column have gliding joints connecting the various bones. These allow only a limited sliding movement.

Skeletal muscles are attached to the bones and are stretched over joints. Certain muscles produce motion by pulling on the bone when they receive messages from the nervous system. These muscles are called voluntary muscles because their movement is controlled

by the brain. For example, the eye sees a $5.00 bill on the floor. The picture is relayed to the brain. The brain, through the nervous system, tells the body to bend over and pick up the bill. This is an example of voluntary muscle action or one which the body chooses to perform.

Other muscles, called involuntary muscles, form the walls of organs. They, too, receive messages through the nervous system but they work automatically, or without any conscious effort by the individual. The heart is an example of an involuntary muscle as it pumps blood throughout the body without any conscious effort.

The musculoskeletal system constantly interacts with other systems. The interior of the bone produces new blood cells for the circulatory system. Blood vessels in the bone centers are nourished or fed by the digestive system. Muscles move in response to messages from the nervous system. It is not necessary to understand these complex interrelationships. However, it is interesting to note how one system depends on another.

common disorders of the musculoskeletal system

The musculoskeletal system can be invaded by pathogens and become diseased. However, the most common problems are fractures which are caused by falls.

fractures. A **fracture** is a break in a bone, figure 6-10 on page 65. Fractures are treated by immobilizing the bone or fixing it into position. Healing of bones may take several weeks; older people require a longer healing period.

arthritis. Another musculoskeletal problem the home health aide will probably encounter is arthritis. Although arthritis affects people

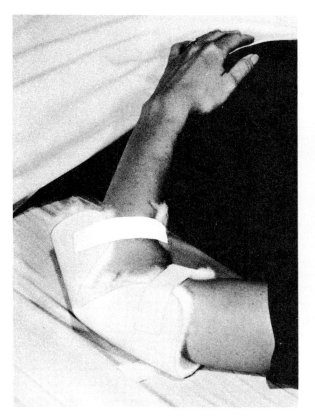

A. Elbow pad

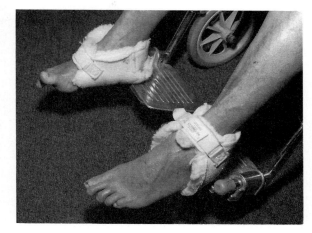

B. Heel pads

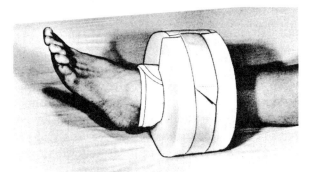

C. Ankle lift for heel protection

Figure 6-6 Pads reduce skin irritation and help prevent decubitus ulcers (courtesy of the J. T. Posey Company, Arcadia, CA).

DISORDER	DESCRIPTION	TREATMENT
Acne	Chronic inflammatory disease of the sebaceous (oil) glands and hair follicles. Characterized by eruptions, cysts, nodules, or pustules that may lead to scarring and pitting of the skin. Often appears at puberty when major body changes commence. Usually appears on the face, neck, and shoulders.	Diet modification Topical medication Cleansing of the skin Surgical skin peeling or removal
Psoriasis	Scaly, itchy skin eruptions that appear at any age	No cure, but can be controlled by topical medication to relieve itching
Dermatitis	Skin inflammation that causes itching, redness, and skin lesions (sores). May be caused by skin irritants such as poison ivy, allergies, sunburn, or adverse reaction to heat or cold	Topical medication and avoidance of causal factors
Scabies	Skin lesions caused by mites that burrow into the skin. Transmitted by direct contact, clothing, and linen. Itching may persist several days after treatment. Noticed around fingers, wrists, axilla, waist, under the breasts, abdomen, buttocks, and genitalia. Infection of the lesions is common.	(ordered by physician) Topical medication Antibiotics if infection occurs Antihistamines to relieve the itching

Figure 6-7   Common skin disorders and their treatments

of all ages, it more commonly affects the elderly. **Arthritis** is an inflammation of the joints. It is usually painful and causes the joints to swell and become enlarged. Sometimes the bones of the hands and feet curl inward and become deformed. The physician may order a splint to be applied to the affected joint in order to prevent deformities. Arthritic clients should be kept busy so that less time is available to think about the pain. The doctor may suggest some form of occupational therapy.

There is no specific cure for arthritis but there are treatments to relieve some of the symptoms. Pain, muscle spasms and cramps can be relieved by heat from hot baths, heat lamps, paraffin bath, or hot packs. Aspirin, or aspirin substitutes, are considered the safest medication for long-term use. However, the doctor should determine the amount of aspirin the client is allowed to take. Other drugs are also used in the treatment of arthritis but these drugs must be prescribed by the physician. A client with arthritis may need physical therapy or may be treated with a special diet and vitamin supplements. Complete bedrest is necessary during acute stages of the disease.

nervous system

The brain, spinal cord, nerves and ganglia make up the nervous system. This system

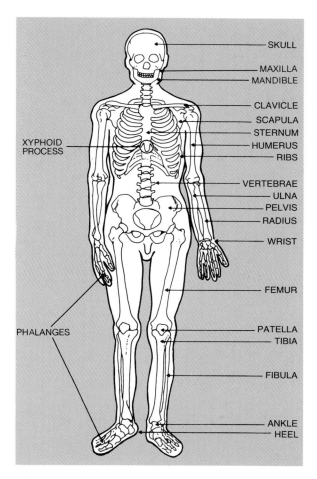

SKULL
MAXILLA
MANDIBLE
CLAVICLE
SCAPULA
STERNUM
HUMERUS
RIBS
VERTEBRAE
ULNA
PELVIS
RADIUS
WRIST
FEMUR
PATELLA
TIBIA
FIBULA
ANKLE
HEEL

XYPHOID PROCESS

PHALANGES

Figure 6-8 The framework of the body (skeleton) is made up of 206 bones.

is the communication center which sends messages to all parts of the body, figure 6-11. It is the system which allows the body to see, hear, smell, taste and touch. Sight, sound, taste, smell and touch are known as the five body senses. The brain is the master control or main switch of the nervous system. Messages are relayed to the brain from all parts of the body. The brain decides how to respond to each stimuli or message sent by the nerves. Each area of the brain performs a specialized duty. The brain alerts other control centers in the body

so that the body correctly responds to a message.

The spinal cord can be compared to the electrical wiring system in a house. All the major nerves of the body are bound together in the spinal cord and lead into the brain. The spinal cord is protected by the spinal column. If the spinal column is damaged or diseased, the spinal nerves may be affected. For example, if one suffers a broken back and the spinal cord is cut or damaged, the nerves below the cut could no longer send messages up to the brain. The parts of the body below the cut could no longer feel pain and the muscles would no longer move.

Paraplegia refers to paralysis of the lower part of the body and both legs. Quadriplegia refers to paralysis of both arms and both legs. Both paraplegia and quadriplegia are the results of tumors or injury to the spinal cord. Hemiplegia is a paralysis of one side of the body. It is frequently the result of a cerebrovascular accident (CVA or "stroke").

The nerves radiate from the spinal cord to all parts of the body forming a network. The nerve endings might be compared to the electrical outlets in the house. In the body, the nerves are usually ready to receive stimuli. For instance, the hand touches a hot surface, the nerve sends the message to the spinal cord and it goes to the brain. The brain sends back the message to move the hand. This entire process takes place in an instant so that one is only aware of the result. The time it takes to respond to a stimulus is known as reaction time. As the human body ages, reaction time often slows down a great deal. It also is affected when part of the brain has been damaged as with a stroke.

common disorders of the nervous system

epilepsy. **Epilepsy** is a condition that is characterized by various forms of recurrent

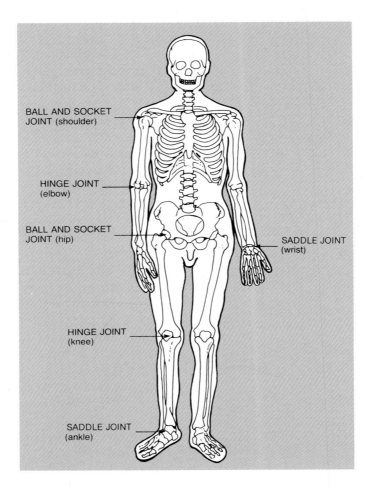

Figure 6-9   Joints allow bones to be moved in certain ways.

seizures. These seizures range in severity from momentary losses of consciousness to violent, patterned movements. Clients who have epileptic seizures are often treated with medication to control the severity and/or frequency of those episodes.

spinal cord injuries.   When a person suffers an injury to the spinal cord, loss of sensation and function in body parts below the level of that injury often results. Clients who are paralyzed as a result of a spinal cord injury are often prone to the development of decubitus ulcers and contractures.

sensory deficits.   **Sensory deficits** (decreases in sensory abilities such as hearing or vision) commonly affect elderly people, but may also affect others as a result of disease. The home health aide is likely to encounter clients whose vision or hearing is impaired. Such conditions as glaucoma (an eye disorder caused by increased pressure of the fluid within the eye) and cataracts (a cloudy area in the

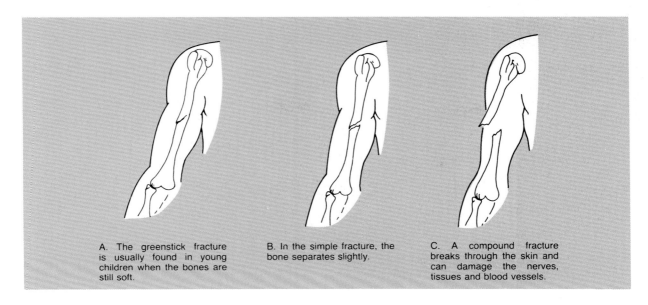

A. The greenstick fracture is usually found in young children when the bones are still soft.

B. In the simple fracture, the bone separates slightly.

C. A compound fracture breaks through the skin and can damage the nerves, tissues and blood vessels.

Figure 6-10 Three types of fractures

lens of the eye) may severely limit the vision of a client. Elderly persons who are hard of hearing may have nerve damage affecting the *auditory* (hearing) nerve, or a disorder called *otosclerosis*. This condition occurs when the tissues of the inner ear harden and sound waves are no longer carried in the usual fashion. Hearing ability gradually diminishes. Aged persons also may experience a loss of taste sensation, which may have a negative effect on their appe-

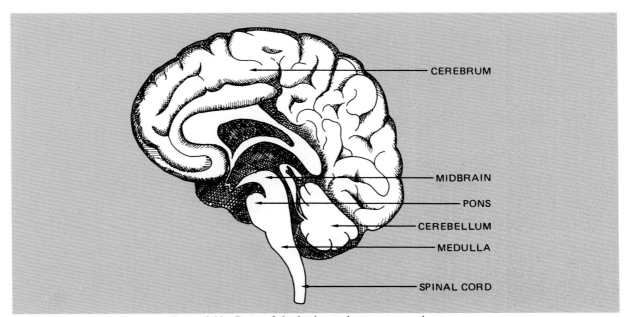

Figure 6-11 Parts of the brain send messages to the organs.

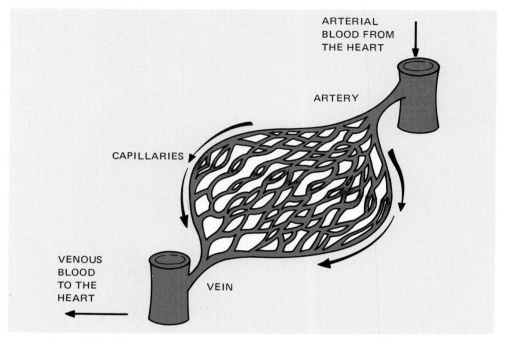

Figure 6-12 Nutrients are carried to all parts of the body by the blood vessels.

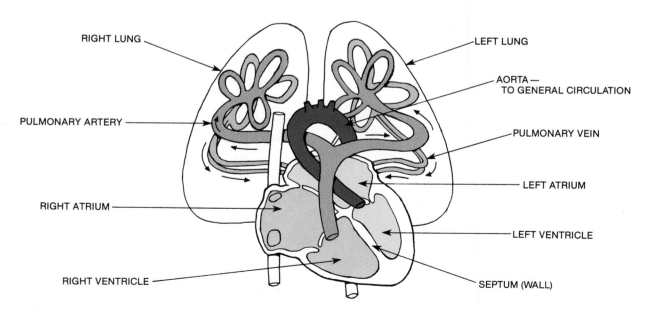

Figure 6-13 Blood is returned to the lungs in order to get rid of carbon dioxide and pick up oxygen.

tite. The home health aide should be aware of any sensory deficits a client might have, and accordingly adjust the care given.

circulatory system

The circulatory system delivers food, oxygen, and liquids to every cell of the body. It can best be described as a series of soft, flexible tubes of different sizes. These tubes are blood vessels which spread to every part of the body. Blood is carried through the vessels bringing nourishment and removing waste products, figure 6-12.

The organ which provides power to the system is the heart. The heart is a muscular organ about the size of a closed fist. Although it is one of the most important organs in the body, it has only one job. That job is to pump blood through the body. From the time the fetus is 3½ months old until death, the heart continues to pump.

The heart has four chambers. Leading into and out of these chambers are the largest blood vessels making up the circulatory system. There are three kinds of blood vessels. The arteries carry blood away from the heart to the body cells. The arteries join the tiny blood vessels called capillaries. The capillaries meet the veins. The veins carry the blood back to the heart. This blood, poor in oxygen, is then pumped into the lungs where carbon dioxide is exchanged for oxygen, figure 6-13. From the lungs, the oxygenated blood returns to the heart. The arteries carry the blood away from the heart to all parts of the body. It takes one minute for blood to leave the heart, travel through the arteries, capillaries and veins and return to the heart. This is a cycle which continues each minute of the day.

As the heart contracts (squeezes together) and expands (relaxes) it pushes the blood into the arteries. The arteries contract and expand in the same rhythm as the heart.

The pulse measured at the wrist is the expansion of the radial artery. The blood carried in the arteries is a rich, bright red color. Venous blood is a darker red because it is low in oxygen.

common disorders of the circulatory system

Circulatory disorders are very common in people over the age of fifty. These disorders may affect either the heart or the blood vessels. Circulatory conditions are the leading causes of long-term illness and death after the age of fifty. The symptoms may be so mild as to be unnoticeable. Damage may have taken place before a victim knows anything is wrong. Cardiac disorders are those which affect the heart itself. Circulatory disorders are those affecting the blood vessels carrying blood throughout the body. The parts of the body most often affected by circulatory disorders are the brain and the lower extremities (feet and legs.)

disorders of the heart

angina pectoris. Angina pectoris is a severe pain in the chest that radiates to the shoulder, neck, and left arm. It usually results from a lack of oxygen in the heart muscle. It occurs most commonly in middle-aged men.

acute coronary occlusion (myocardial infarction). Acute coronary occlusion (myocardial infarction) is commonly known as a heart attack. It occurs when a blood vessel within the heart muscle closes, or is blocked by a blood clot. The seriousness of this condition depends on the size and location of the blockage. The heart may be permanently damaged.

congestive heart failure. Congestive heart failure occurs when the heart cannot pump enough blood to meet body demands, causing congestion in the lungs and other tissues. Damage to the heart muscle is the usual cause. Acute attacks of congestive heart failure may lead to a chronic condition.

disorders of the blood vessels

arteriosclerosis. Arteriosclerosis is hardening of the arteries. **Atherosclerosis** is a type of arteriosclerosis that often occurs in the larger arteries, especially those of the heart, kidneys, and brain, figure 6-14. This condition could be compared to a piece of garden hose left lying outdoors. Dirt clogs the insides and the weather changes cause it to become hard and stiff. In the arteries, fatty deposits stop the blood from flowing through and causing loss of elasticity. Lack of blood flow causes less oxygen to reach the body cells. The body cells starve as a result.

gangrene. Gangrene is the death of body tissue caused by lack of adequate blood supply. It may be caused by disease, or by injury to a body part.

phlebitis. Phlebitis occurs when the lining of a vein becomes inflamed, causing a clot to form in the vein. This usually occurs in one leg which may become swollen and painful to touch. The area may feel warm. The physician may order anti-embolism stockings or elastic bandages (such as Ace bandages) to be applied to the affected leg or to both legs. The area should never be massaged as that may cause the clot to move to the heart or lungs, causing severe damage or death.

cerebral vascular accidents. A cerebral vascular accident (CVA) is also known as a stroke or as apoplexy. There are three main causes of a CVA.

- A small blood clot, also called a thrombus, may block a blood vessel in the brain. This prevents oxygen from reaching the brain cells.
- Arteriosclerosis (hardening of the arteries) may develop in the blood vessels of the brain.

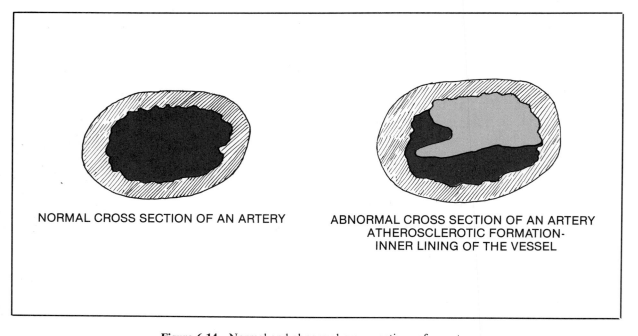

NORMAL CROSS SECTION OF AN ARTERY

ABNORMAL CROSS SECTION OF AN ARTERY
ATHEROSCLEROTIC FORMATION-
INNER LINING OF THE VESSEL

Figure 6-14 Normal and abnormal cross sections of an artery

- A small blood vessel in the brain may burst, spilling blood directly into the brain tissues.

disorders of the blood

anemia. Anemia occurs when there is a lack of adequate red blood cells. It may result from an excessive loss of blood, from malformation of blood cells, or from a lack of essential nutrients.

sickle cell anemia. In this disorder, the client's red blood cells are crescent shaped, like a sickle. The cells do not carry enough oxygen in them, causing anemia. This is an inherited disease for which there is no cure, but new drugs are helping clients. Infections, stressful situations, excessive exercise and other situations that increase the client's need for oxygen should be avoided. In the United States, this disease is usually found only in blacks.

leukemia. Leukemia is a condition in which too many white blood cells are produced. These excess white blood cells block the normal transport of oxygen to the body's tissues. They may also affect production of new red blood cells. This disease occurs most often in children and young adults.

Look up the vocabulary words related to circulatory problems: Cheyne-Stokes respirations, oliguria, anuria, vasoconstriction, vasodilation, hypotension, and hypertension. You will need to know them for the discussion in Unit 17.

respiratory system

The respiratory system consists of the nose, pharynx, larynx, trachea, bronchi, and lungs, figure 6-15. It is closely linked to the circulatory system. Blood is supplied with fresh oxygen by means of the respiratory system. Fresh air is inhaled into the body and carried to the lungs. The oxygen from the air is carried to all parts of the body by the circulatory system. As oxygen is delivered to the cells of the body, waste gases are picked up and carried back to the lungs where they are exhaled from the body. The most plentiful waste gas is carbon dioxide. In short, oxygen is inhaled and carbon dioxide is exhaled.

common disorders of the respiratory system

Diseases of the respiratory system have now been classified together as chronic obstructive pulmonary diseases (COPD).

pneumonia. Pneumonia is an infection of the lung. It is usually caused by bacteria, but there may be other causes such as a virus. It is treated with antibiotics. The client may need to be hospitalized to receive the necessary medications, intermittent positive pressure breathing (IPPB) treatments and/or oxygen.

chronic bronchitis. Chronic bronchitis often occurs in middle-aged or elderly persons. It can result from a number of acute conditions, asthma, bronchitis, cigarette smoking, air pollution.

asthma. Asthma is a condition that may be caused by an allergic reaction, although there are other causes. Often the specific substance causing the asthma cannot be determined. Symptoms may include coughing, difficult breathing, wheezing, and a feeling of tightness in the chest. The clients need much reassurance at this time.

emphysema. Emphysema is a lung condition in which the air sacs within the lung lose their elasticity. Breathing is difficult for the person affected by this disease. Medications can relieve the symptoms of emphysema, but there is no cure.

digestive system

The digestive system changes food into a form that can be used by all the cells of the body. Those parts of food which cannot be used by the body are expelled as waste products.

Food is the fuel burned by the digestive system to provide energy for the entire body. This use of food can be compared to gasoline in a car which burns to give power to the car, or oil in a furnace which produces heat. In the body, the fuel is food; the process of burning this fuel is called metabolism.

Metabolism depends on the proper functioning of each organ of digestion, figure 6-16. The digestive process begins the moment food is taken into the mouth. The teeth and tongue tear the food into small pieces and mix it with saliva so that it can be swallowed easily. In the saliva, chemical substances called enzymes start to break down the foods into products that can be used by the rest of the body. From the mouth the partially processed food is swallowed, moving into the esophagus. An involuntary wavelike muscle action called **peristalsis** moves food through the esophagus

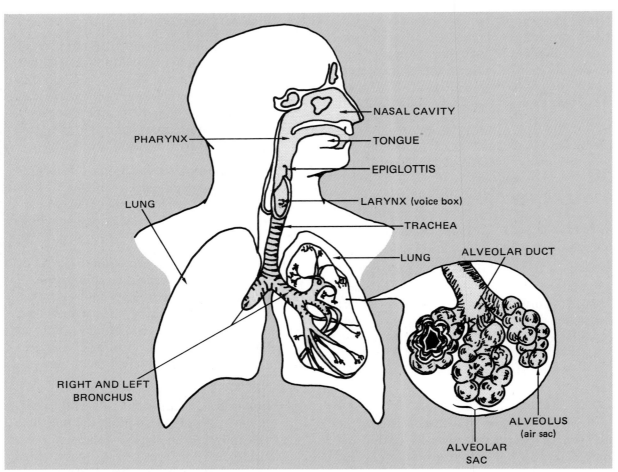

Figure 6-15 The respiratory system (from Ferris, et al, *Body Structures and Functions,* 5th edition, Delmar Publishers, 1979).

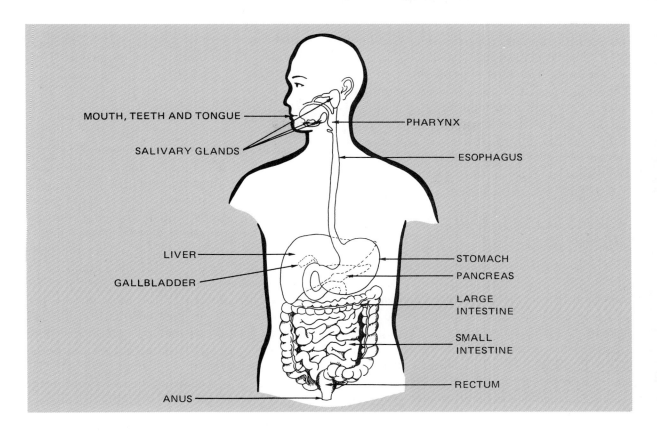

Figure 6-16 Organs of the digestive system

and then into the stomach. Sometimes the body rejects or refuses food during the digestive process. When this occurs, the voluntary and involuntary muscles work together to force the food backwards. This is called vomiting or emesis.

The stomach is an elastic, muscular organ which holds the food while gastric enzymes and a strong acid turn food into a semiliquid state. From the stomach, the food passes into the small intestine. Enzymes in the intestinal juice are especially important in the digestive process. The liver produces bile which is necessary to absorb fat. Bile is produced in the liver but is stored in the gallbladder. Bile enters the small intestine and breaks up fats in the duodenum so they can be digested and absorbed. The duodenum is the

first 10 inches of the 19 to 20 feet small intestine. The jejunum is the second portion of the small intestine. It is about 9 feet long. The ileum is the third portion and is about 9 feet. The pancreas also releases a digestive pancreatic juice into the duodenum. Insulin, which controls sugar metabolism, is also released into the bloodstream from a specific area within the pancreas.

The digestive juices work together to break food down into a simpler form. The usable products of this breakdown are called nutrients. The nutrients are absorbed through the walls of the small intestine. The nutrients are then carried by the bloodstream to all parts of the body. Some portion of food remains in the small intestine because it cannot be broken down or absorbed. This remaining material moves into the large intestine in a semiliquid state. The large intestine, also called the colon, is about five feet long. In this area, much of the liquid from the food is absorbed into the body. This helps maintain the balance of fluids in the body. Persistalsis moves the remaining solid material into the lower part of the colon. When enough waste has collected, the voluntary muscles expel it through the anus. This is a normal bowel movement.

common disorders of the digestive system

constipation. A common problem with the bowels is constipation. This is a condition in which bowel movements are hard and difficult. Prevention might include exercise, an increase in fluids, and eating more bulky foods such as whole grain cereals, fruits, and vegetables. Prolonged or long-lasting constipation can cause feces (the technical name for the waste material of the body) to become lodged in the rectum **(impacted).** It may then be necessary for the person to receive an enema or a laxative.

Stools may have blood on the outside surface which may be the result of bleeding hemorrhoids or rectal cancer. If the stool looks dark, black, or tarry, internal bleeding in gastrointestinal system may be the cause. Brighter-colored blood in the stool may result from bleeding in the lower part of the intestinal tract. (Refer to the procedure for collecting stool specimens.)

diarrhea. Diarrhea is a condition in which feces are watery and frequent. Constipation and diarrhea may result from a number of causes. Proper diet, adequate exercise, and regular elimination of wastes help prevent both constipation and diarrhea.

heartburn. So-called "heartburn" results from a backflow of the digestive juices into the lower portion of the esophagus. These juices, because of their high acid content, cause irritation of the lining of the esophagus. Those affected experience a burning sensation.

the urinary system

The urinary system consists of the kidneys, ureters, bladder, and urethra, figure 6-17. The kidneys are the primary organs of this system. Their function is to filter waste material from the bloodstream. As the blood passes through the kidneys, it undergoes a purifying and recycling process; waste material and excess water are filtered from it. As the blood continues through the kidneys, much of the filtered water and some minerals are reabsorbed into the bloodstream. This reabsorption is necessary in order to maintain the body's liquid balance. The waste material and excess water (now called urine) pass from the kidneys into the bladder by way of ducts called ureters. The bladder is a muscular organ for storing urine. When the bladder has accumulated about a pint of urine, a nerve senses discomfort. Involuntary muscle contractions of the bladder then empty the urine into the urethra, from which it is expelled. These muscular contractions can

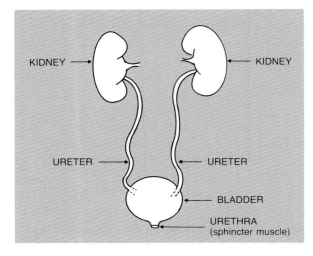

Figure 6-17 The urinary system

be controlled and do become voluntary to a large extent. The normal daily output of urine is between 1500 to 2000 milliliters (1½ to 2 quarts).

common disorders of the urinary system

incontinence.
Some individuals have no voluntary control of their bladder muscles. This causes them to be **incontinent;** they wet themselves. Incontinence occurs in babies prior to toilet training because they have not yet developed control over the muscles in the urethra. Similarly, a person who has had a stroke may not have normal bladder control. (Normal urine flow is 30 cc per hour.)

cystitis.
Cystitis occurs when the membrane lining of the urinary bladder becomes inflamed. It can be caused by bacterial infection or a kidney inflammation which has spread to the bladder. This condition usually results in painful urination. It is generally treated with antibiotics.

kidney stones.
Kidney stones are usually caused by an excess of calcium. The urine becomes crystallized and stones may block the ureters and cause painful urination.

reproductive system

The reproductive system consists of organs that are needed to produce a new life, figure 6-18. The male reproductive system manufactures sperm which fertilizes the ovum (egg) produced by the female reproductive system. Sperm is released into the female vagina during sexual intercourse. When the sperm comes together with the female egg, usually in the upper part of the uterine tube, the egg is said to be fertilized. The fertilized egg travels to the female uterus and begins to develop into a new individual. In this way the human race continues from generation to generation.

It normally takes 280 days from conception (when egg and sperm meet) until an

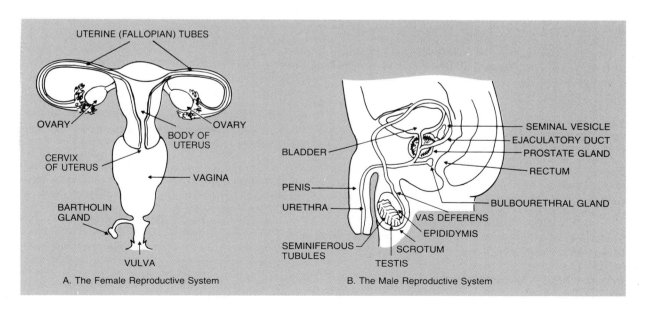

A. The Female Reproductive System

B. The Male Reproductive System

Figure 6-18   The female and male reproductive systems

infant is born. The menstrual cycle is interrupted for nine months of pregnancy. It may be six weeks after delivery before the cycle begins again. The menstrual cycle continues until menopause occurs later in life when eggs are no longer released.

common disorders of the reproductive system

The incidence of cancer affecting the reproductive system in both males and females is quite significant. Care of cancer patients is discussed more fully in a later unit. In addition, sterility, or infertility (inability to have children) often is the result of an abnormality of this body system. There are also several conditions which may be transmitted by sexual intercourse.

sexually transmitted diseases

Gonorrhea, syphilis, and other infections passed through sexual contact are called venereal diseases (V.D.). Over the past several years there has been an alarming increase in sexually transmitted diseases. In today's society, it is not unusual for people to be sexually active with several partners. This increases the chance for contact and incidence of venereal diseases. In some areas of the country, V.D. has reached epidemic proportions. The pathogens can be passed on to anyone who has sexual intercourse with an infected person. Direct contact with an infected person is the most common way in which gonorrhea is spread. Towels, bed sheets, or clothing contaminated with the discharge may transmit the infection, although this indirect method of transfer is rare.

gonorrhea. Gonorrhea can develop within 48 hours after contact. Usually the first sign of the infection in males is painful burning urine. The next stage is a yellowish green discharge from the penis. The female's symptoms include a burning sensation and painful urination; the vaginal area may become red and tender, with a discharge present. It is common for the female to have no symptoms at all. This absence of symptoms is dangerous since the woman will not know that she needs treatment. The symptoms may go away within a few days, but the pathogens may move into the reproductive system and do further damage. Untreated gonorrhea can cause permanent damage to the reproductive organs (pelvic inflammatory disease or PID) and even cause sterility. A person who suspects exposure to gonorrhea should have an examination at once. In order to detect the gonorrhea pathogen, a laboratory test is done on the discharge. A large dose of penicillin is usually an effective treatment for gonorrhea.

Babies born to mothers infected with gonorrhea may become blind as a result of contact with the bacteria causing gonorrhea in the vagina during birth. The eyedrops given to the newborn in the delivery room help to prevent blindness.

syphilis. Syphilis shows up very quickly in males. Open sores develop on the penis very early in the course of syphilis. If the pathogens are not killed early in the illness, they spread throughout the body. Secondary skin lesions (sores) may appear on the face. From contact with these open sores, the pathogens can be passed from person to person. Untreated syphilis can lead to severe brain damage, mental illness, heart disease, and death. In the female, syphilis is not as easy to detect, the pathogens continue to invade the body while the female is unaware of it. Women who have syphilis and become pregnant can pass syphilis to the fetus. Children born with active syphilis may be born with birth defects. Blindness is a frequent syphilitic complication at birth. In the United States and some other countries, a couple planning to marry are required to have a blood test before a license is issued. Negative blood tests ensure that neither partner has syphilis at the time they are married.

acquired immune deficiency syndrome (AIDS).

Acquired immune deficiency syndrome was first diagnosed in 1981 following an alarming outbreak of unexplained sickness among homosexual men in the United States. The disease breaks down the body's natural immune system, causing its victims to fall prey to almost any infection that comes along. A rare form of skin cancer (Kaposi's Sarcoma) is a complication of AIDS and will be discussed more fully in the unit on infectious diseases.

There is still a great deal that is not known about AIDS, and a health care worker must take special precautions. First, it is essential that you be informed that your client has AIDS. You have the right to refuse to care for such a client. If you choose to take on such a client then you must follow instructions from the physician and your supervisor completely.

- Wear disposable gloves when handling bloody secretions (such as urine, vomitus, sputum, or fecal material).
- Use a solution of one part household bleach to 10 parts water when wiping spilled body fluids or cleaning the bathroom.
- If you have open cuts be sure they do not come in contact with blood. WEAR GLOVES.
- WASH YOUR HANDS CAREFULLY before and after all client care procedures.

Just as it is important for a home health aide to protect his or her own health when caring for an AIDS client or a client with AIDS related complex (ARC), it is equally important to consider the AIDS client. If, for example, an aide develops a severe cold or other ailment, it would be foolhardy to expose the AIDS client to further risk. Remember, the immune system of the AIDS victim is not able to fight off infections.

herpes.

Herpes is another viral infection that can be transmitted during sexual contact. This virus has been known for at least 2000 years. It recurs periodically and, to date, cannot be cured. It is estimated that 20 million Americans now have genital herpes, with an annual increase of half a million new cases.

There are two types of herpes. Type I is the cause of cold sores on the lips. The more serious Type II causes genital lesions (sores). It has been found that ordinary cold sores (Type I) can be transferred to the genitals by finger or mouth contact and become a venereal disease. Oral sex may be one reason for the dramatic increase in the spread of herpes.

The first symptoms may be a tingling or itching sensation. Blisters may appear within two to fifteen days after infection. The first episode lasts on the average of three weeks. Subsequent attacks usually last around five days. The blisters may be accompanied by malaise.

While untreated syphilis and gonorrhea do far more damage, herpes is still an uncomfortable and annoying problem. It is generally suggested that sexual contact be avoided during the active stages of the disease.

the endocrine system

The endocrine system is made up of ductless glands which secrete substances within the body called hormones, figures 6-19 and 6-20. The glands in this system do not have **ducts** (little tubes) and are, therefore, unlike tear and sweat glands. Hormones are chemicals that are secreted directly into the blood or lymph. They are carried throughout the body to regulate and control specific body functions. They are very powerful substances and direct the functions of other systems. Each hormone has a

Pituitary Gland	Once called "master gland" of the body; secretes a number of hormones which regulate many bodily processes. The pituitary is completely controlled by the hypothalamus, a part of the brain.
Thyroid Gland	Helps to regulate the metabolic rate and growth process.
Parathyroid Glands	Regulate metabolism of calcium and phosphorous.
Thymus Gland	Regulates immunity to infectious diseases during infancy and early childhood; becomes smaller as body ages.
Adrenal Glands	Adjust body to crisis and stress; increases blood pressure; speeds reactions; metabolizes carbohydrates and proteins.
Islets of Langerhans	Produces insulin needed to burn sugar in body. (Too little insulin causes diabetes; too much insulin causes hyperglycemia.) Also produces glucagon to raise blood sugar.
Ovaries	Produce ovum (egg) for reproduction; secretes estrogen and progesterone which develop and maintain secondary sexual characteristics (breasts, pubic and underarm hair, etc.).
Testes	Produce sperm to fertilize ovum; secrete male hormones called testosterone.

Figure 6-19   Functions of the glands of the endocrine system

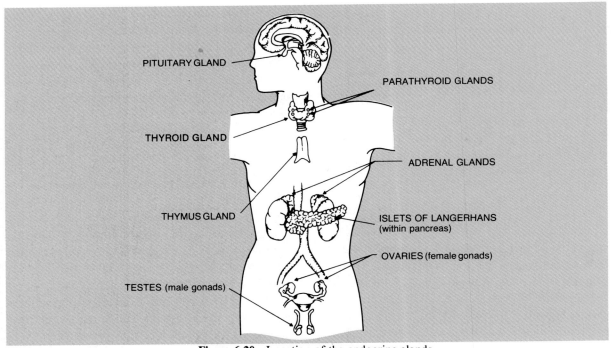

Figure 6-20   Location of the endocrine glands

special job to do. It only takes a small amount of hormone to trigger a body reaction. Most scientists agree that the brain sends messages to the endocrine glands. This message causes the gland to secrete the hormone needed by the body. For instance, in a time of physical danger the adrenal gland secretes a hormone called adrenalin. The adrenalin causes the heart rate to increase. This forces more blood through the body, which increases the nourishment to the muscles. Sugar is released into the body giving it quick energy. The adrenalin also speeds up the body's reflexes. All of these changes occur rapidly making the body able to react and save itself or others from harm.

The thyroid gland in the endocrine system regulates the metabolic rate of the body. This determines the speed that food is turned into energy.

common disorders of the endocrine system

hyperthyroidism and hypothyroidism.

The activity level of the thyroid has a direct influence on the body's metabolism. Some people are able to eat large quantities of food without gaining weight. They have an overactive thyroid gland and their food metabolizes (burns up) quickly. These people tend to be restless and irritable. When the thyroid gland is underactive, food is not used fast enough and is converted into fat. The person with an underactive thyroid gland becomes sluggish and slow moving and tired. One of the excuses used by many overweight people is that they "have a thyroid condition." However, most people who are overweight simply overeat.

goiter.

A goiter is a thyroid disorder which the aide may see when caring for clients. In this condition, the thyroid gland becomes enlarged to such an extent that it is visible as a swelling at the front of the neck. This enlargement is usually the result of iodine deficiency. Goiters rarely occur among people who live near the ocean, probably because there is a great deal of natural iodine in the coastal soil.

diabetes.

The endocrine gland of most interest to the home health aide is the pancreas. The endocrine part is known as the islets of Langerhans and is involved in the condition called diabetes.

The islets of Langerhans secrete insulin and glucagon. They control the use and distribution of sugar to the body. When insulin is not produced, the body metabolism is thrown off balance. A condition called diabetes may develop. Diabetes is a chronic disorder which can be controlled by medication, and/or proper diet and regular exercise. Diabetes is described more completely in a later unit.

the remarkable body

Imagine how hard it would be if, each second of the day, you had to consciously perform every body function. Most people take their bodies for granted as long as everything seems to be in good working order. Think of all the activities constantly taking place and all of the things that could go wrong. Maintaining a state of wellness seems miraculous.

The human body is remarkable because it can continue to work when some of its parts break down. Damaged brain cells cannot be "repaired," but there are so many brain cells that new ones can be trained to take over. Many of the body structures are in "pairs." A body has two arms, two legs, two kidneys, two eyes. In the well body all of the parts work together.

What happens when one of a pair becomes diseased? In the case of kidneys, one can be removed surgically and the other will take over the work. The person with only one kidney must be more careful with diet and generally take more health precautions than the average person. A person can return to a state of wellness with even one kidney. The human body and mind are able to adapt. The home health aide's job is important in helping a client adapt both physically, mentally, and emotionally, figure 6-21.

factors which influence body development

Bodies come in all shapes and sizes. There are records of men who have been as tall as 9 feet and as short as 26½ inches. These statistics are interesting because they show the tremendous contrasts possible within the human body. Just as there are contrasts in size, there are other individual differences. Heredity is the passing of traits from parents to their children. Heredity can determine height, weight, general appearance, skin color, talents and abilities, basic physical wellness, and many other things. All children get half of their heredity from each parent. However, some traits are more dominant than others. This explains why some children are more like one parent than another.

Another factor which helps determine body size, shape and wellness is environment. Environment is the sum total of the circumstances, conditions and surroundings affecting the development of an organism. Some environmental factors which may affect growth are nutrition, financial conditions, climate, number of children in the family, and the parents' ages and occupations. The child who is born healthy with good hereditary characteristics is likely to start life as a well person. If the child grows up in a healthy environment where it is well fed, clothed, sheltered, respected and loved, the child will continue to be well physically and mentally. An identical twin with the same heredity would not be as likely to develop into a well person if the twin was raised in an unhealthy environment. Many argue about which is more important, heredity or environment. One side believes that good heredity can overcome poor environment. The other side claims that good environment can rescue a child with poor heredity. It is clear, however, that both contribute to a person's development. Ways to control heredity are limited; however, environment can, to some extent, be controlled. The role of the home health aide is involved in improving environmental conditions for the client.

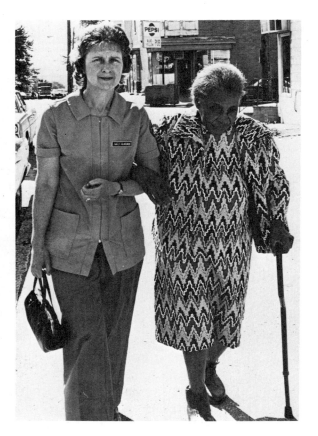

Figure 6-21 Walking increases the activity of all body systems.

- As one begins to understand the way the body works when it is well, the effects of illness are easier to grasp.
- Mental outlook, healthy body cells, proper nutrition, rest, exercise and good relationships with others are all part of wellness.
- The body systems work together and depend on one another to make the body function, figure 6-21.
- The body functions are affected by both heredity and environment. Changes in the environment which may lead to illness affect all body systems in some way.

review

1. Name the nine body systems.
2. Name one function of each body system.
3. List one disorder for each of the nine body systems.
4. What is the largest organ of the body?
5. What might be suspected if a red, warm-looking spot appears on a bony prominence?
6. What is the difference between hereditary and environmental factors?

Understanding Human Development and Age-Related Health Problems

Unit 7
Infancy to Adolescence

key terms

cesarean section	low-birth-weight	identical twin
conception	sibling rivalry	fraternal twin
gestation period	adolescence	lethargy
immunity	puberty	
premature		

learning objectives

After studying this unit, you should be able to:
- Name five basic needs of the newborn infant.
- Identify three immunizations necessary for infants.
- List six abnormal conditions of the infant.
- Give the normal weight gain for an infant during the first year of life.
- Recognize definitions for five of the key terms listed.
- Name two health problems which may affect adolescents.
- Identify changes which occur at puberty.

An aide who is assigned to care for a newborn infant and the mother is usually going into a happy environment. If it is a first child, both parents will hover over the baby and watch its every move. Of course, the newness wears off, and suddenly they are faced with a demanding, helpless human being for whom they are entirely responsible. Even so, this is still one of the most pleasant assignments you can be given.

Conception is the fertilization of the female egg by male sperm. This union forms the beginning of a new individual. When two eggs are fertilized by two sperm, twins develop. These are called **fraternal twins.** Fraternal twins can be a boy and a girl, two boys, or two girls. If only one egg is fertilized by one sperm and then divides in half, **identical twins** develop. Identical twins are always of the same sex and look very much like each other. Triplets, quadruplets, and quintuplets also may develop, but are less common. The doctor is usually able to tell if more than one fetus is growing before birth. The time from conception to birth is called the **gestation period.**

Amniocentesis is a procedure in which a long needle is inserted into the amniotic fluid so that a sample can be removed for testing. This procedure is done in cases where the pregnant mother may have been exposed to German measles (rubella), for instance, during the first two months of the pregnancy and then came down with the disease. This could cause malformation of the fetus. Tests of the amniotic fluid after the first three months might show if the fetus had been harmed. Amniocentesis is also often performed on those who have a family history of a congenital defect or first-time mothers of 35 years or older. The results might show if a child would be born with Down's Syndrome. At that point, the pregnancy could be terminated.

labor and delivery

Infants are most often delivered by a doctor in the hospital. However, in some areas, this situation is changing. The use of midwives to perform deliveries is increasing. Also, in certain regions, homelike clinics may be used instead of hospitals. Normally, a woman goes into labor and delivers the baby with little assistance. The baby moves from the uterus into the vagina and passes out of the body. This normal process is eased, however, by use of medications, health facilities, and trained personnel.

In some cases it may be necessary to deliver the baby by **cesarean section.** This is a surgical technique in which an abdominal incision is made and the infant is lifted out. After a cesarean section, the mother needs extra time to recover. The incision site must be kept clean to prevent infection. The aide may be instructed to assist the mother to clean the wound and apply clean dressings.

normal infant growth and development

As an infant grows, both physical and mental abilities develop. In the first month, infants are quite helpless. They totally depend on others to meet their basic needs, figure 7-1. Infants need to be kept warm and dry and they need to be fed and allowed to sleep. Giving love to the infant also fulfills a basic need, figure 7-2. Infants need to be held, cuddled, and crooned to as much as possible.

By two months, babies can raise their heads and cry when they want to be picked up. They notice lights and sounds and begin to babble. They get used to certain patterns, especially the time to eat and time to sleep. Usually by the fourth month an infant sleeps 8 to 12 hours at night and naps during the day. Regular schedules of meals, activity and sleep are needed.

normal weight gain

Normally, infants weigh between 5 to 8 pounds (2.3 to 3.6 kilograms) at birth. During the first five days, a weight loss of several ounces is expected. Until birth, all the baby's needs are supplied within the uterus through the umbilical cord. Birth is a shock to the baby's system and it takes a few days for the infant's body to adjust. When the body starts to function, a weight gain of 6 to 8 ounces (0.17 to 0.23 kilograms) a week is normal. Birth weight is usually tripled by one year. In the second year, the weight increases at a rate of ½ pound (0.23 kilograms) per month.

Nutritionists believe that a child's weight should be controlled. The formation of too many fat cells in childhood can lead to obesity in adulthood. It is important for children to eat a well-balanced diet. All of the body's systems need the right foods so that they will develop in a strong and healthy way.

immunizations

Babies are born with natural **immunities.** This means that they have some built-in resistance to pathogens for one to three months. However, once born, a child's body is exposed to many new pathogens. To protect infants from common childhood diseases they are given vaccines. At two, four, and six months, an infant should be given vaccines against diphtheria, pertussis (whooping cough), and tetanus. These three vaccines are combined, and given in one injection called a DPT shot. An oral vaccine for poliomyelitis is also given

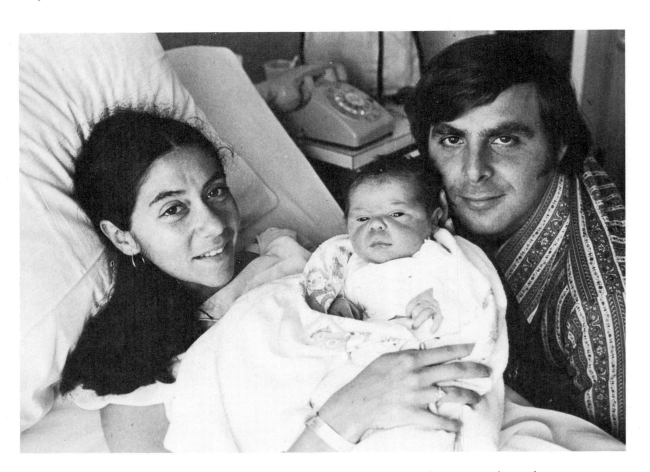

Figure 7-1 The newborn is totally helpless and depends on others to meet its needs.

at two, four, and six months. Vaccines for measles, mumps, and rubella are given after a child is one year old. A test for tuberculosis is given at one year in addition to the vaccines. Boosters of DPT and polio vaccines are given two more times before the child enters school. Many states do not permit children to begin school until they are properly immunized. Parents should keep records of their children's immunizations. They should also record the childhood diseases contracted by their children and the age of the child when they occurred.

common health problems in infancy

One common problem with newborns is premature birth. An infant born before full

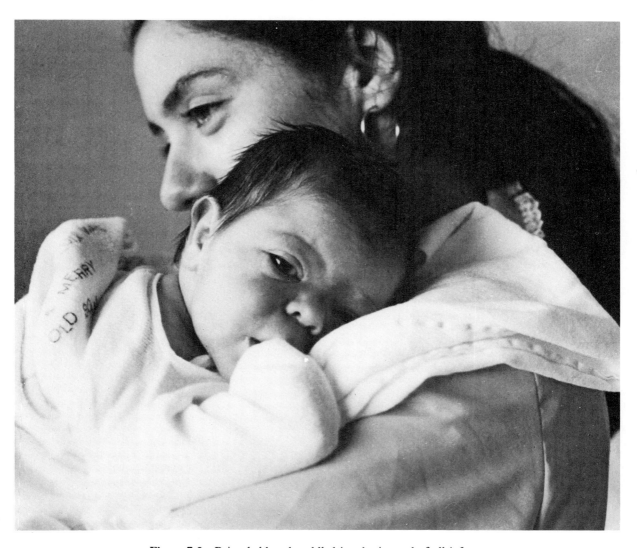

Figure 7-2 Being held and cuddled is a basic need of all infants.

Condition	Description	Treatment
PKU (phenylketonuria)	Body is unable to break down a certain amino acid. Mental retardation, convulsions, and eczema are common.	Specific diet begun early in infancy prevents symptoms.
Cerebral palsy	Defect, injury, or disease of the brain tissue which causes lack of muscle coordination and possible paralysis; person has shaking and muscle spasms with poor balance.	No cure but treatment varies and may include muscle relaxants, orthopedic surgery, use of casts or braces, exercises.
Congenital heart disease	Malformation of vessels, valves, or chambers in the heart; results in faulty circulation and usually cyanosis.	Surgery is often successful in restoring normal functioning.
Down's syndrome (Mongolism)	Chromosome abnormality causing retardation and typical physical malformation.	No treatment but many persons can be taught to live with some independence.
Hydrocephalus	Defect in the absorption of cerebrospinal fluid; fluid builds up and increases the size of the head. Increased weight of the head limits infant's mobility and may result in decubitus ulcer formation. Malnutrition is common.	Common treatment is with surgery. Shunts are commonly used to divert fluid away from brain and into the abdomen.
Sickle cell anemia	Abnormal sickle-shaped red blood cells break down easily and cannot transport oxygen efficiently; fever, blackouts, and pain. (Black population)	Blood transfusions. No cure; administration of oxygen and fluids may prolong life.
Cooley's anemia	Poorly formed red blood cells immature and easily ruptured. Person has stunted growth, with enlarged spleen and jaundice.	No cure; blood transfusions are necessary to support life.
Leukemia	Overproduction of immature white blood cells; anemia, internal bleeding. Person has increased risk of infection, fever, pain in the joints and swelling of the lymph nodes, spleen, and liver.	No cure; transfusions, X-ray treatments, antibiotics and other drugs may prolong life.
Tay-Sachs	Degeneration of the central nervous system; infant does not develop mentally; disease affects those of Jewish ancestry.	No cure; infant usually does not live beyond one year.
Cystic fibrosis	Inherited malfunction of the pancreas, intestinal, and sweat glands, and the respiratory system. Child fails to gain weight and has chronic cough and respiratory problems.	No cure; special diet and respiratory care prolongs life.
Congenital hip dislocation	Fetal hip does not form properly; causes crippling.	Orthopedic surgery highly successful; body and leg cast help bones to heal in proper alignment.
Clubfoot	Fetal distortion; extension, and inward rotation of foot.	Foot is realigned with plaster boots which are applied soon after birth. Surgery may also be required.
Cleft lip/cleft palate	Fetal growth incomplete. Infant may have problems feeding. Cleft palate may alter tooth formation and cause speech problems.	Surgical repair, special feeding nipples and special therapy.

Figure 7-3 Abnormal conditions which exist in infancy may require medical attention and sometimes long-term adjustments for the infant and family.

term (before 37 weeks of gestation) is considered **premature.** Some also judge prematurity by low birth weight. A newborn weighing less than five pounds may be premature. However, some babies are full term yet weigh less than five pounds. A newborn in this condition is called a **low-birth-weight** baby.

Some infants are born with diseases, injuries, or malformations. These abnormalities may be inherited through the parents' genes. Conditions also may result from diseases or drugs present in the mother's body during pregnancy. The most common abnormal infant conditions are described in figure 7-3. Children with one of these conditions need special medical and emotional care. The aide may need to help the mother and family members adjust to meeting the child's special needs.

responsibilities of the home health aide

Often a mother must leave one or more children at home while she is at the hospital. The aide may be assigned to attend to the children then or after the mother has returned home with the newborn. The children are likely to want to be near the mother and may want to play with the baby. Sometimes older children are too rough with the baby even though they do not intend to be. The children also may be jealous of the new member of the family. This jealousy is called **sibling rivalry.** At these times, the home health aide should give the children extra attention. The aide can make the children feel important by giving them chores to do for the baby or mother. They should be praised for being helpful. Children may need help adjusting to the role of being a big brother or sister. The aide should be sure that the older children wash their hands before touching the baby. If they have colds they should be kept away from the baby until they are no longer contagious.

Besides the older children, the aide cares for the mother and the newborn. These duties include:

- bathing the infant
- diapering
- feeding the infant
- preparing the formula
- doing added laundry such as diapers and crib sheets
- caring for the mother
- assisting the mother if she is breastfeeding
- accident prevention

handling visitors

Many visitors will likely come to see a newborn child. One of the aide's duties is to make sure that the mother does not get over tired. A new mother should rest for a period in the morning and afternoon. Most mothers are happy to show off their newborn child. However, it is a good idea to plan ahead with the mother as to how to handle visitors. Visitors should not stay too long and should not come in great numbers. The home health aide must encourage the mother to set the standards as to who can and cannot hold the baby. Visitors who have colds or similar infections should be discouraged from going near the baby. The mother and home health aide should wear a disposable mask if they are coughing or have a cold. Babies are born with some natural immunity to pathogens. However, it is unwise to expose them to disease when it can be avoided.

toddlers and preschoolers

Ages one and two are known as the toddler stage. The toddler approaches life with a great deal of interest, figure 7-4. A favorite activity is exploring the immediate environment. As the infant grows into a toddler, muscle coordination increases, and physical skills expand

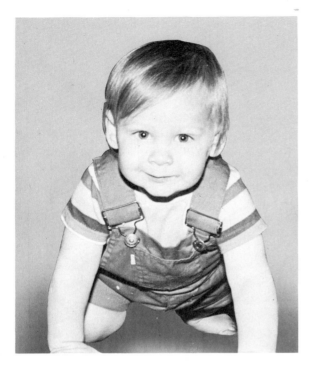

Figure 7-4 The toddler faces most activity with great interest.

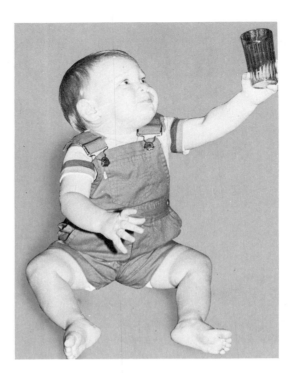

Figure 7-5 The toddler shows increased muscle coordination by successfully holding a glass.

and improve greatly, figure 7-5. Toddlers learn to walk and to feed themselves. Social skills and language become more meaningful.

Ages three through five are considered the preschool age group. The preschool years are a time of slower physical growth but a time of increased motor skill development and an increase in language and social skills. By age three, the child plays alongside other children of the same age. Toilet training is usually mastered by the time the child is five and ready to start school. The preschooler is learning to be less dependent, figure 7-6.

school-age children

A child beginning school often needs time to adjust to the new situation. Some children find it difficult to leave the familiarity of home. However, most children enjoy being with other children. A school-aged child should be able to follow simple instructions. It is important that children be given small jobs so that they feel a sense of responsibility. Praise for achievements is better than punishments for mistakes.

adolescence

Adolescence is the age period between 13 and 18 years of age. **Puberty** marks the beginning of the time when the body is capable of reproduction. Adolescence and puberty may be difficult periods of self-exploration. Physical changes in the body occur rapidly and emotional needs are demanding.

An adolescent wants to feel independent, but needs to know that the family can be depended upon. This is a time when parental guidance and love are extremely important.

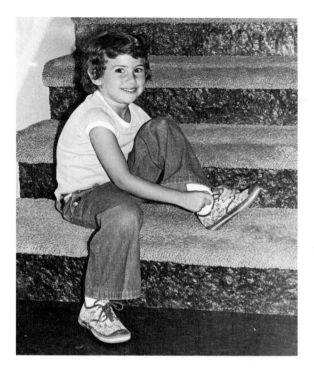

Figure 7-6 Learning to tie shoelaces is an important move toward independence for preschoolers.

During adolescence, a child is strongly influenced by the peer group (those of the same age), figure 7-7. Parents should be aware of who their children are with. Showing a loving concern for their well-being is important.

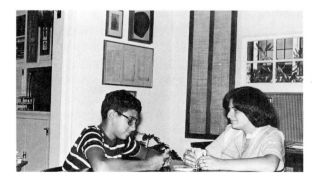

Figure 7-7 Peer group interaction is important to an adolescent.

physical changes in puberty

Puberty begins sometime between the ages of 10 and 15 when the endocrine system releases hormones in both males and females. At this time, the secondary sexual characteristics begin to mature. In boys, the beard, underarm and pubic hair starts to grow and the voice deepens. There is usually a marked growth rate of both height and weight. At puberty, the male is able to produce sperm and have an orgasm to deposit the sperm in the female.

In young females, the breasts develop and pubic and underarm hair grows. A 28- to 35-day menstrual cycle also begins at puberty. About every 28 days the mature female reproductive system releases one or more eggs (ova). During sexual intercourse the ovum may come in contact with the sperm. If the sperm fertilizes the ovum, a fetus begins to grow.

common health problems in adolescence

Adolescents are at an age of experimentation. They often express their independence by trying new things. For some adolescents, this experimentation leads to abuse of drugs or alcohol. Many adolescents also become curious about their sexuality.

Sex-related health problems are especially common with adolescents. An active sex life may pose emotional problems. Diseases which are passed through sexual contact also may bring about additional problems. The female, in particular, must consider the possibility of becoming pregnant. Sex-related health problems often result from the adolescent having inadequate information. It is often difficult for young people to set reasonable limits on sexual behavior.

teenage pregnancy. In addition to an increase in sexually-transmitted diseases among adolescents, an increase in teenage pregnancies has also occurred. It is currently estimated that two of every five girls now 14 years old will become pregnant before they are 20 and that one of those five will bear a child. In 1971, unmarried teens had 124,000 abortions; today, that number has surpassed 444,000. It is now estimated that 42 percent of teenagers are sexually active. Most of these teenagers have sex without contraceptives, and when they do go to family planning services, it is often too late.

Few teenagers are ready to handle the responsibilities that accompany pregnancy and parenthood. The decision to raise a child, place the child for adoption, or have an abortion is usually a difficult decision for a teenage girl.

Teenage girls are still growing themselves, both emotionally and physically. Even a healthy, well-adjusted teenager will feel the stress that pregnancy puts on her body. A teenage father may feel emotional stress. The financial and practical aspects of parenthood are usually too much for a teenager to handle.

Pregnancy can be prevented through use of planned birth control methods as well as abstinence from sexual intercourse. Teenagers who desire to be sexually active should be made aware of the methods available. The most common methods are the oral contraceptive pill, the diaphragm, the condom, and foam spermaticides. The rhythm method is also practiced by some.

Religious practice may determine the type of birth control used. In any case, it is wise to consult a medical doctor when choosing a method. The only advice a home health aide should offer is that a doctor be consulted. Giving any other information would be in poor taste. In addition, the parents of a teenager may regard the action as interference.

substance abuse. Drug use among adolescents has been on the increase over the past twenty years. It is recognized that "pot" smoking, "pill popping," and the use of hard drugs has increased the crime rate and caused serious health problems, both physically and mentally. Many families have been destroyed because of the aftermath of drug abuse by its members. Drug awareness programs are run in schools to alert young people to the dangers involved. Legislation has been passed in an effort to stop drug abuse. Television and radio programs continue to tell of the harmful effects of drug abuse.

Parents should see that their children are well informed about the dangers and effects of drug abuse. A loving home environment where the child feels accepted and is able to talk about concerns and feelings helps to deter drug abuse. If a parent sees physical or emotional signs—extreme mood swings, **lethargy,** overactivity, nervousness, red eyes, sniffling, needle marks, or other unaccountable signals—professional help should be sought.

In America today there is another "drug" being used more and more by young people. Alcohol abuse has become a major problem. Children as young as six and seven years of age are abusing alcohol. In fact, according to one recent report, among youth the average drinking age nationwide is eleven and one half years. Parents often are not as concerned about drinking as they are about other drugs. They seem to feel that alcohol is less harmful than drug abuse. Unfortunately, the truth is that youthful drinking is a serious and dangerous problem. Drinking can lead to cirrhosis of the liver, which is irreversible. It can also lead to permanent brain damage. Moreover, drinking is a major cause of death on the highway due to driving while intoxicated (DWI). The fact that it is illegal to drink below the age of 18, or 21 in some states, has not slowed down the consumption of alcohol by minors. Alcohol is an accepted part of our adult society but all too often its negative influence reaches the younger generation. Organizations such as Al-Anon and Alateen are helping to educate drinkers and re-program them to stop drinking for at least "one day at a time."

summary

- Life begins with the uniting of a sperm and an ovum.

- An infant is born and continues to develop through adolescence.
- A home health aide's job in caring for children is to help the family meet the difficult or everyday problems. By understanding the needs of each age group, the aide can prepare for possible problems.

review

1. What are the five basic needs of a newborn?
2. List three immunizations recommended for infants.
3. Name two health problems that affect adolescents.
4. What physical changes occur at puberty?
5. What is a cleft palate?
6. Why is it important for the aide to allow the mother to assume as much care of the newborn baby as possible? What would you look for and document relating to the mother's "bonding" with her infant?
7. What kind of observations would you be likely to make in caring for a newborn infant? An older baby? A toddler?

Unit 8

Early and Middle Adulthood

learning objectives

After studying this unit, you should be able to:
- List the causes of health problems in the early adult years.
- Describe the adjustments that often must be dealt with in the middle adult years.
- State why preventative health measures are important.
- List the physical effects of aging.
- Describe the changes that occur during the early and middle adult years in terms of family relationships.

early adulthood

Adolescence is followed by early adulthood. This is the time of life when formal education is usually completed. Most young adults enter the labor force and begin to assume the responsibilities of daily life.

During early adulthood, most individuals are concerned with bettering themselves. They may change jobs often. Many look forward to better jobs, higher wages, and greater opportunities. As young people make these changes, they must constantly make personal adjustments.

Also, during early adulthood, close personal relationships take on greater significance.

Some young adults choose to marry; some also choose to start a family. If both partners are working, they need to arrange their personal lives around their jobs. This effort helps produce harmonious relations with each other. They must learn to share duties and work together as a team.

Today, many young couples choose to delay the start of a family. When they do decide to have children, the mother may find it difficult to leave the work environment. As a result, the child is often left in the care of others. As the family grows, each stage of infancy and childhood brings its own challenges and problems.

health problems in early adulthood

During early adulthood, the body normally works efficiently. It remains at a high level of health for about thirty or forty years. The body heals quickly through childhood, adolescence, and early and middle adulthood.

Health problems in early adulthood often accompany parenthood. For example, an infant may be born with a birth defect. The physical problems of the child can create severe psychological stress and financial burdens for the parents. For a woman, the pregnancy itself can endanger her health. Normal pregnancy, pregnancy with complications, and reproductive system disorders can occur in the adult female. Such problems should be cared for by a physician.

As a **preventative health measure,** all persons should have an annual physical examination. Illness can be detected and treated in the early stages. The early detection of diseases such as cancer, heart disease, diabetes, and emotional stress often leads to the condition being treated before it becomes more serious. Also, women should have breast examinations and a periodic vaginal examination that includes a **Pap smear** once a year. The American Cancer Society recommends that women undergo routine radiological breast examinations (mammograms) after age 35, beginning with one every several years and increasing the frequency to a yearly examination after age 50. These examinations are especially important during and after the childbearing years. Other health problems can result from conditions related to auto accidents and job-related injuries.

Alcoholism is a problem among adults, as well as among adolescents. Social drinking can, in some cases, lead to alcoholism. For many years, alcoholism among men has been studied. Special programs have been designed to assist persons with this illness. Organizations such as Alcoholics Anonymous have been very helpful. There are auxiliary groups such as Al-Anon for the spouses of alcoholics. Alateen groups are for children of alcoholics. Within the past 15 years, society has become aware of a high increase in alcoholism among women. Because women stayed in the home, they could hide their illness. The problem among women is not new, but it is now out in the open. As a result of this greater awareness there is a better chance that cures can be initiated.

middle adulthood

Society places great demands on a person in the middle adult years. It is during this period that people are expected to be highly successful and productive as well as financially secure. If a woman has chosen to remain at home with her children, this may be the time when she decides to re-enter the work force.

During the middle adult years, people often assess their accomplishments. Some may question how worthwhile their work or other achievements have been and seek a change. This change may take the form of a different life-style—a separation from their marriage partner, or a change in career or place of residence.

Physically, those in their middle adult years will notice some changes. Their hair may turn grey or recede and their eyesight may diminish. Weight gains may occur as a result of a general slowing of metabolism. Hormonal changes that occur during **menopause** may result in mood swings, changes in sleeping patterns, increased anxiety, and other physical symptoms.

adjustments during the middle adult years

There are several major adjustments which the person in the middle adult years may have to make. These adjustments are in response to a change in some area of their lives.

family relationships. The middle years is generally the time when grown children leave the home. Parents who have been very involved in their children's lives may feel at a loss when this occurs. As the children mature and gain independence, their own roles and responsibilities may become first priorities, and their ties with their family may become more remote. This can be a time when parents and children form close, adult relationships with each other. This can also be a time of freedom and creativity for the parents as they find they have more time to spend with each other and more time to develop their own mutual interests.

Individuals in middle adulthood may have to assume responsibility for caring for an elderly parent. If the elderly parent is brought into the home, **intergenerational conflicts** (conflicts between younger and older generations) may result. For instance, young children may not understand why their mother or father spends so much time with "grandma" and not with them, and they may come to resent the older person. Also, the stress of caring for an ailing parent is often great, especially if one has not developed a strong emotional support system, or if it is not possible to periodically take a break from responsibility. If the decision is made to place an elderly parent in a nursing home or other extended care facility, one must deal with the guilt that that decision may cause.

retirement. When a person retires from an active career, a major adjustment must be made. Often, an individual's identity and sense of **self-esteem** is closely linked with his or her job. Retirement from gainful employment may erode one's self-esteem. It may also remove a person from close relationships formed in the workplace. Loss of income may also present a problem if adequate financial plans have not been made previously. Those who retire may

find it difficult to adjust to a fixed, decreased income, and may even find it necessary to seek financial support from their families or from welfare. Conversely, if an individual or couple have planned for retirement, it may be a pleasant, rewarding time during which they can pursue personal interests and activities.

change in social status. The American culture is a youth-oriented culture. As a result, older people are often not valued, and their opinions and ideas are often considered outmoded and unacceptable. They may come to feel outcast from the mainstream of living, and may withdraw from people altogether, or from all but people their own age.

death of a spouse. The middle adult years may be a time when an individual is increasingly aware of the advance of age and the threat of death. Certainly, the death of a spouse is a shattering experience which may lead to increased dependence on others, isolation, and loneliness, figure 8-1. Plans that were made mutually by both partners may be abandoned. If

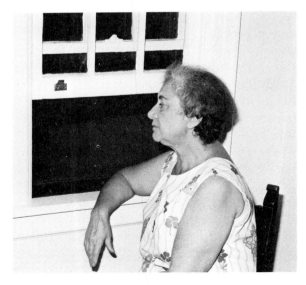

Figure 8-1 The death of a spouse may result in feelings of loneliness and despair.

the grieving process is not worked through, the surviving partner may become severely depressed and lose interest in all activities and relationships.

illness and disability. As a person reaches middle adulthood, the ability to remain independent may decline due to illness or disability. It is commonly a time when **debilitating** illnesses, such as stroke, heart failure, high blood pressure, arthritis, and cancer arise. Financial resources may be drained by expensive treatments and hospitalization. Even if major illness is not a factor, the effects of aging may be felt in terms of muscle weakness, decreased mobility, and sensory deficits.

summary

- Changes that may occur in early and middle adulthood require a major adjustment.
- The home health aide should always try to be sensitive to those who are affected by these changes.
- A supportive, caring attitude may help the individual to successfully adapt to shifting life patterns.

review

1. Name three causes of health problems in the early adult years.
2. List three adjustments that may need to be made during the middle adult years.
3. What period of life does society expect the most from an individual?
4. Why are preventative health measures important?
5. Name three physical effects of aging.

Unit 9
Late Adulthood

key terms

senescence	reality orientation	masturbate
Alzheimer's disease	chronological	

learning objectives

After studying this unit, you should be able to:

- Name some of the physical and emotional effects of the aging process.
- Identify the reasons for establishing regular schedules for elderly clients.
- Identify the effects of Alzheimer's disease.
- List three reality orientation techniques.
- Describe the problems of persons confined to bed.

It cannot be definitely stated at what time in life people become old, for age is more a matter of physical and mental aging than it is of **chronological** processes. Tremendous variations exist. Some people are physically and mentally old at age thirty-five; others are still young at the age of sixty-five.

The terms **aging** and **aged** must also be clarified. Aging is a process which begins with conception and ends with death. The term aged means old or mature. Because of today's increased life expectancy, our perceptions of the age at which an individual is old may not be entirely accurate. Today, if a person lives to be sixty-five and is in reasonably good health, that individual can expect to live 14 to 20 more years. Moreover, women often outlive men by several years. The most recent statistics show that there are over 26 million Americans over the age of 65. By the year 2000, that number is expected to rise to 35 million. These figures have special meaning for anyone entering the field of home health care. Many of these older citizens will probably have need of the services of a home health aide.

In the past, most of the statistics concerning the aged were based on the chronically ill and elderly persons in hospitals, nursing homes, and other institutions. The largest proportion of the aged population, though, are healthy, alert, able, working and contributing members of society, figure 9-1. They have made adequate adjustments to the physical, mental, and emotional changes associated with the aging process. For some of them, home care extends the time in which they can enjoy living at home, figure 9-2.

What is it like to become old? One per-

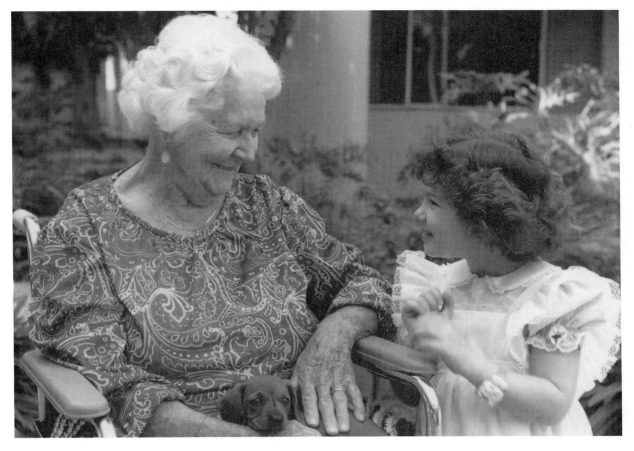

Figure 9-1 This client enjoys the company of her granddaughter. There is no generation gap here!

son described it in this way: "Smear dirt on your glasses, stuff cotton in your ears, put on heavy shoes that are too big, and wear gloves; then try to spend the day in a normal way." Older people admit that they find it harder to do many of the things they like to do and become impatient with themselves and others just because they find it difficult to accept the loss of their independence. Imagine how an older individual who is in ill health must resent these added problems. A home health aide must become "tuned in" to the special needs of such a person.

effects of aging on the body systems

As the body grows older, the machinery begins to run down. The body loses its ability to bounce back after illness. Healing takes longer after surgery, illness, or injury. The body becomes less able to fight off infections.

Each body system shows some signs of age, figure 9-3. The nervous system reacts slower to stimuli. Hearing and sight may fail. Slowed circulation to the brain may cause damage. The nerves of the feet and fingers

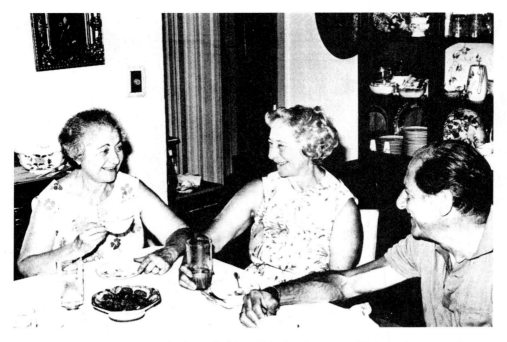

Figure 9-2 Home care extends the period in which the pleasures of living at home continue to be enjoyed.

may be less sensitive. As a result, the body may not sense that the bath water is scalding hot, or that the toes are cold and frostbitten. Aging can affect recent memory. There may be a buildup of fat in the circulatory system causing the blood vessels to clog up. Slowed circulation weakens the functioning of many other systems. Aging causes the tiny air sacs in the lungs to stretch. This reduces the oxygen exchange and causes the person to feel breathless.

Another system affected by age is the integumentary system, figure 9-4. The skin becomes dry and flaky because the oil glands secrete less oil. The body hair becomes thin and starts to fall out. In addition, the urinary system filters wastes less effectively. Falls occur more often and are more serious in the elderly. This is because the bones are more brittle and the muscles less elastic. Many factors of aging cause the healing time to increase. The diges-

tive system is less active. Some foods cannot be digested at all. As a person eats less, there is less available energy, figure 9-5. The other body systems suffer from poor nutrition.

The female reproductive system no longer produces eggs after menopause. Among older males, the sperm count is decreased. This means that there is less chance that the sperm will fertilize a female's egg. Sexual activity may slow down as people grow older. However, the sex drive is still a normal part of their lives. It is not unusual for older people to **masturbate** (stimulate themselves sexually) when they no longer have a sex partner.

A home health aide must recognize that older clients do still have sexual desires. This may cause minor problems, particularly if the client is of the opposite sex. If the client should make a pass or try to take advantage of the home health aide, he or she should firmly say "no." The aide should not shout at clients or

Observable

Hair: Thins and whitens

Vision: Declines; three out of five persons 75+ are affected to some degree, and more often in females than males.

Kidneys:
Eventually lose up to 50 percent of their capacity to filter body wastes. This major system shows the greatest decline with age.

Heart:
1st—Between ages 20-90 the amount of blood pumped by the heart decreases 50 percent.
2nd—Muscle fibers contract more slowly.
3rd—Heart and blood vessels are more vulnerable to disease.

Bones: At 40+, the body no longer absorbs calcium efficiently, which contributes to fractures in more than 25 percent of all elderly women.

Joints: 1st—Begin to stiffen, particularly the hips and knees.
2nd—Compressed spinal discs shorten the body and cause a bent posture. Height loss of 1-3 inches is common.

Nervous System: 1st—Hardening of blood vessels create circulatory problems in the brain.
2nd—Aging reduces the speed with which the nervous system can process information or send signals for action.

Circulatory System: Failure in this system is the most common cause of death. Death from cardiovascular disease at age 75 is 150 times higher than at 35.

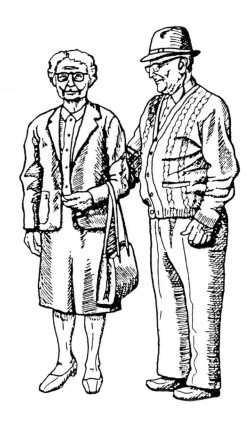

Nonobservable

Hearing:
1st—Ability to hear high pitches is more difficult.
2nd—Normal sound levels are more difficult to understand.

Skin:
1st—Fine lines around eyes and mouth.
2nd—Lines deepen into wrinkles.
3rd—Skin loses elasticity and smoothness.
4th—Spots of dark pigment.

Lungs:
1st—Between ages 30-75, the amount of air inhaled and exhaled drop by 45 percent.
2nd—Between ages 30-75, the amount of oxygen passing into the blood decreases about 50 percent.

Hormones:
1st—Decline in hormonal flow from the adrenal gland, located atop the kidney, lowers the ability of the elderly to respond to stress.
2nd—For women, menstruation ceases.

Immune System: This system becomes less efficient and therefore lowers the body's resistance to disease.

Muscles:
1st—There is a loss of muscle strength, which reduces coordination.
2nd—Lack of muscle tone causes a sagging of muscles.

Figure 9-3 Changes in the body over time (Reprinted by permission from *Aging in America* by Sandra Zins, © 1987 by Delmar Publishers, Inc.)

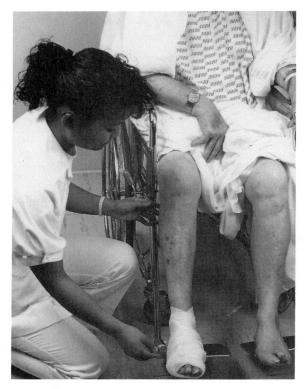

Figure 9-4 Note the signs of aging of the skin in this client. The skin is blemished and discolored; the knees are puffy due to edema resulting from arthritis; toes are deformed; toenails are thick and grow unevenly.

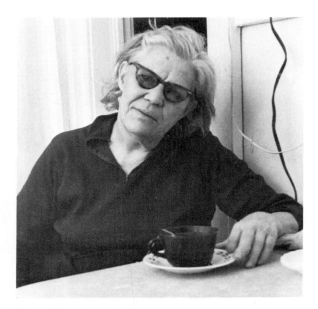

Figure 9-5 As people grow older, they often eat less and have less energy.

angrily scold them. Telling them "no" and walking away is the best action to take. Because the sex drive does continue in later life, it is important for older people to have social contact with members of the opposite sex. Just being with the peer group provides an outlet for sexual needs.

chronic illness, physical health problems, and aging

Although the problems associated with chronic illness and those associated with aging and the aged are not identical, the two areas overlap extensively. Aging in itself is not neces- sarily accompanied by chronic illness; most of the disabilities and limitations experienced by elderly persons are a result of chronic, pro- gressive disease and not a result of aging alone. Figure 9-6 identifies some of the health prob- lems common among the aged. Many condi- tions result from a natural aging process; others arise from chronic health problems developed earlier in life.

care of the bedridden client

A client who is confined to bed needs special care no matter what the reason for the bedrest may be. Inactivity, especially in the eld- erly, leads to conditions such as constipation pneumonia, and decubitus ulcers. Constant pressure on certain skin areas can easily lead to the formation of bedsores. Lying in the same position for a long time or poor posture can cause the muscles to become weak and deformed. The deformed condition (a muscle contracture) becomes permanent if not cor-

CONDITION	SYMPTOMS AND TREATMENT	HOME CARE REQUIRED
GLAUCOMA	**Symptoms:** Accompanied by severe pain causing partial loss of vision or total blindness. May be chronic or acute and may be a complication of diabetes. It is a buildup of pressure of fluid in the eyeball which causes damage to the optic nerve. **Treatment:** The condition cannot be cured but it can be controlled with prescribed medication taken daily.	The home health aide should assist the client in the activities of daily living. Help client adjust to the diminished vision as much as possible. Make sure that the medication is taken as prescribed. If client is diabetic, make certain that the diet is carefully followed.
CATARACTS	**Symptoms:** A person suffers a gradual loss of vision as the lens of the eye becomes thick and hard. The lens appears milky or opaque. This prevents light rays from reaching the retina. **Treatment:** Laser—outpatient clinics Surgery may restore partial or total vision. Surgery cannot be performed until the cataract is "ripe." Contact lenses may be implanted into the eye itself.	The client may be fitted with hard or soft contact lenses. The home health aide may assist in the care of the lenses or assist the client with the eyeglasses prescribed. If client has only partial vision, the aide assists in the activities of daily living as recommended by the doctor or supervisor.
DEAFNESS	**Symptoms:** A person may gradually suffer mild to total loss of hearing. Deafness may be the result of an ear injury, a congential defect, or simply be a process of aging. **Treatment:** A hearing aide may be prescribed. In some cases surgery may restore partial or total hearing.	The home health aide should follow medical instructions. It is important to speak clearly, slowly and distinctly when communicating with a deaf person. The aide may assist the client with care of the hearing aide. Make sure that the batteries are working and that the volume control is operating.
PARKINSON'S DISEASE	**Symptoms:** A person develops tremors and may walk in a shuffling manner. There is a loss of muscle control and a slowly spreading tremor with muscular weakness and rigidity. This can be one-sided only, or may affect both sides at once. The face may become expressionless, the body may bend forward and the arms may be flexed. There is no decrease in awareness or intelligence. Speech may be affected because of vocal cord involvement; the person may mumble or speak indistinctly. **Treatment:** Medication may be prescribed to control the condition. In some cases surgery is performed to reduce tremors.	The client *may* require a special diet. The aide should make every effort to prevent accidental falls. The client should be encouraged to be as active as possible. This activity includes eating, bathing, and walking. The aide must show patience because frequently the client is extremely frustrated and depressed. Clients often become hysterical and cry easily. Remember, however, *they are not mentally ill.* Their minds are just as sharp as they were prior to the disease. Medication should *not* be taken with meals because the medication will not take effect.

Figure 9-6 Medical conditions common among older adults

CONDITION	SYMPTOMS AND TREATMENT	HOME CARE REQUIRED
FRACTURES	**Symptoms:** A fracture is a break in a bone. After an accidental fall, a person may complain of pain. Swelling may occur around the injured part. Fractures among the aging are the result of loss of muscle tone and brittle bones. The most frequent sites for breaks are the shoulder, arm, collarbone, and hip. **Treatment:** Treatment is determined by the location and severity of the break. Some breaks are put in a light plastic cast, others are set surgically using metal pins; in some cases a joint may be replaced.	The doctor may order a high-calcium diet. The aide can provide this and make the environment safe so that other falls can be prevented. The aide follows any other instructions given by the doctor. The aide should observe the color and temperature of the affected extremity. Look for signs of blood on the cast. The client may complain of pain inside the cast. These signs should be reported at once. Use care in transfer techniques.
ARTHRITIS	**Symptoms:** There are many types of arthritis. The person complains of pain and muscle spasms or cramps. Arthritis is an inflammation of the joints; in some cases there is a change in the structure. The fingers become bent and gnarled. There is often heat and swelling of the joints. **Treatment:** Bedrest in acute stages. There is no cure, but it may be controlled by medication. Heat treatment may be prescribed. Splints may be applied to prevent permanent deformities.	The home health aide should follow the doctor's instructions. Client should be kept as comfortable as possible. Passive range of motion exercises may be required. For the client on bedrest, the prevention of decubiti is most important. Suitable recreation may be provided to keep the client more content. Arthritic clients should have a well-balanced, nutritious diet.
CEREBRAL VASCULAR ACCIDENT (Arteriosclerosis and arteriosclerotic brain changes)	**Symptoms:** A person may suffer a one-sided weakness, drool, and become unable to speak clearly. Because of a buildup of deposits in the arteries, hemorrhage, an embolism or thrombus, or an aneurysm, the brain is deprived of blood. This may lead to a stroke leaving the person with one-sided paralysis, aphasia, etc. Blood pressure becomes very high. Arteriosclerotic brain changes may lead to senile dementia. The person may develop personality changes and behave in a peculiar or inappropriate manner. Such persons may not be aware of time or place. **Treatment:** CVA (stroke) patients are started on physical therapy at once. Diet and skin care are vital. Medication may be of some help.	The home health aide must show patience and kindness while following doctor's instructions. It is important to assist the client in self-help. Clients with arterial problems are usually placed on a low-sodium diet. Skin care is extremely important for the paralyzed client. Special mouth care is also vital. For clients suffering emotional disturbances or confusion, the aide is expected to watch them carefully so they will not harm themselves. These clients are often impatient. Follow instructions for medicating such clients.
COLDS, VIRUSES, PNEUMONIA	**Symptoms:** A person suffers upper respiratory discomfort, often accompanied by high temperature, chest pains, and labored respirations. Pneumonia may be a complication of colds or flu. It may be viral or bacterial. **Treatment:** Medication may be prescribed. Oxygen is sometimes needed. A vaporizer may be set up in the person's room. Bedrest and diet modifications.	An aide may be asked to take cardinal signs regularly and report changes to the doctor. Fluid intake is usually increased; a high-caloric diet may be recommended. The client should be kept comfortable. Aseptic techniques should be used in handling linens, tissues and body wastes.

Figure 9-6 *(Continued)*

CONDITION	SYMPTOMS AND TREATMENT	HOME CARE REQUIRED
HEART DISEASE (coronary occlusion, heart block fibrillation, emboli, congestive heart failure)	**Symptoms:** A person develops shortness of breath, may have angina (severe pain), complain of coldness of extremities. Such persons tire easily, may feel they have severe indigestion, develop kidney symptoms and feel pain when breathing. **Treatment:** Medications as prescribed, bedrest, oxygen, rehabilitation within limits ordered by doctor, psychological support.	When caring for a client with a heart condition, the aide should observe the client for changes in color, pain, or sudden changes in cardinal signs. Medical instructions should be carefully followed. Clients are usually on a restricted low-sodium, soft diet. It is important to help the client maintain a positive outlook.
CHRONIC OBSTRUCTIVE PULMONARY DISEASE (COPD)	**Symptoms:** A person suffers shortness of breath and tires easily after physical activity. Some advanced cases bring about a physical change in that the person becomes barrel chested. Breathing is labored (dyspnea), and the person may become dizzy and cyanotic. In this condition the lung tissue is damaged and the exchange of gases within the lungs is affected. Once emphysema has developed, it is irreversible. Efforts must be made to slow its progress. **Treatment:** Oxygen (O_2) therapy, no smoking, avoid exposure to respiratory infections. Flu shots are recommended. I.P.P.B. (Intermittent Positive Pressure Breathing) using a breathing machine which combines oxygen with medication. Special nasal sprays to open or dilate bronchi and increase oxygen supply to body.	The COPD client must limit physical activities. The home health aide should observe the client for signs of distress and follow medical instructions as given. Keep visitors from smoking so that the air is not contaminated. The fluid intake may be increased to liquify sputum and help client to cough up the sputum. Portable O_2 tanks allow the client more mobility.
OSTEOPOROSIS	**Symptoms:** Decreased density (thickness) of the bones caused by an imbalance of bone formation and reabsorption. As the bones become thinner, there is a loss of strength and the bones become porous and brittle. This may lead to collapse of the vertebrae and bone deformity. As a woman reaches menopause, hormonal changes occur. The decrease in the hormone, estrogen, makes postmenopausal women more prone to this condition. Low back pain and backaches may be the first symptoms. In later stages, a "dowager's hump" may appear. (This is a rounded hump between the shoulder blades often seen in older women.) **Treatment:** Calcium additives, Vitamin D, Vitamin E and sodium fluoride, combined with regular exercise and physical activity.	The aide must help the client to avoid accidental falls. Extreme caution and attention to the client's safety is crucial. . Balanced diet with increased calcium intake. The doctor may order calcium daily, plus hormone drug administration daily. Check the order of medication for your client. Orders may vary with the client or doctor. You may assist with these self-administered medications.

Figure 9-6 *(Continued)*

rected early. The following care techniques help prevent complications of long periods of bedrest:

- Change the client's body position at least every two hours.
- Massage the skin around the bony prominences to prevent decubitus ulcers.
- Keep the client's skin clean and dry.
- Place a bed cradle over the client's feet to take the weight of the bedcovers off the feet.
- Use a footboard and pillows to align the body.
- Assist the client to do range of motion exercises.
- Record the frequency of the client's bowel movements to check for constipation. The doctor may order an enema if the client is constipated. Diet changes may include an increase in high fiber foods and increased fluid intake, as well as increased mobility.
- Provide the client with a radio, television or some form of entertainment. Diversion reduces boredom and takes the client's mind off the pain and discomfort.
- If limited use of a wheelchair, walker or cane is permitted, encourage the client to use it.

emotional and psychological effects of aging

Aging is a general winding down of the life forces. The process of growing old is called **senescence.** For many people this is a welcome time of life. They have led productive, busy lives and their work is done. They look forward to relaxing and enjoying their final years. Some older people are very spry. They still have energy and can do many things. They have good health habits and their bodies are strong. They eat nutritious foods. They can find many outlets for passing the time, figure 9-7.

Other elderly people cannot enjoy their later years. Loneliness overcomes many of the

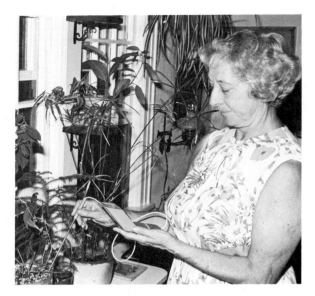

Figure 9-7 Senescence may provide more time for hobbies and interests.

elderly. Some who sincerely desire to work may be physically unable. Lacking a sense of purpose is a common problem. Many senior citizens live on a fixed income. They may not be able to pay rent, buy warm clothing or nutritious foods. They may have no living relatives to help them. When they become ill there is no one to care for them. Most of the home health aide's clients are elderly. Understanding a client's home situation helps in evaluating related health problems. Common emotional and behavioral problems that sometimes occur with aging are listed in figure 9-8.

general effects

Aging should be expected as a normal part of the life process. However, depression and sadness often accompany aging. The depression felt by many older people comes from the discouragement of having nothing to do that gives them a feeling of success and achievement. Older persons must be encouraged to

- Memory changes
- Differences in personality due to arteriosclerotic changes (hardening of the arteries).
- Unusual or bizarre behavioral patterns
- Withdrawal from usual life patterns
- Sense of anxiety, stress, frustration
- Recurring grief over loss of family and friends; loneliness
- Fear about the future (i.e., economic dependency, illness, loss of time concept)
- Inability to accept change
- Lack of motivation
- Tendency to recount life experiences

Figure 9-8 Emotional and behavioral problems commonly associated with the aging process

find new outlets. If they can no longer drive, then when riding in the car they should be reminded to look around and see the changing of the seasons, watch people walking, enjoy the children playing along the way. If older persons spend all of their time regretting what they cannot do, there will be no time to expand their horizons and they will surely become depressed.

A person who was once active in the garden but can no longer perform the heavy work involved should be encouraged to have a windowsill garden. A person who enjoyed reading but whose eyesight is failing can get tapes and records of "listening books" from the library and keep up on new literature through the sound medium.

Setting up a daily schedule is very important in old age. A regular pattern of rising, dressing, eating, doing chores, working on hobbies, and visiting with friends and family should be arranged. This kind of planning allows for variety and keeps the person from sinking into a depression where sleep becomes a way of escaping from boredom. When an older person sleeps away the day, it is hard to get a restful night's sleep. This causes anxiety and sets up a cycle of fear, anger, and resentment. The elderly must find a rhythm of daily activity that lets them feel alive, useful, and content based on their physical capacities.

Some elderly persons become mentally confused. This confusion may be the result of pneumonia, cardiac failure, too much medication, abuse or misuse of alcohol, strokes, dehydration, anemia, malignancy, or some other physical process or disease. Even a minor change in the individual's environment may bring about a state of confusion. The home health aide should make every attempt to provide a secure, supportive environment for confused clients.

more about growing old

Geriatrics, according to the dictionary, is that branch of medicine that deals with the structural changes, physiology, diseases, and hygiene of old age. That covers a wide area. What does the term *geriatric* mean to the home health aide? When does an individual qualify as a geriatric patient—at age 50, 60, 70, or older? What are the structural changes that can and do occur? What are the vital processes, or physiology, of aging? Which are the diseases most often associated with the geriatric patient? What is meant by the hygiene of old age?

These are not easy questions and there are no answers that apply to every older individual. As has been noted before, it is not possible to generalize. Each and every person goes through the aging process in his or her own way. Environmental and hereditary factors play a large part in what happens to any one person.

Let us start with the home health aide's role, responsibilities, and reactions to the aging, ill client.

The majority of clients for whom you will provide care will be geriatric patients. The combinations of physical ailments, personality types, and environmental conditions are impossible to predict. This places a great deal of responsibility on the home health aide. Remember, one of the major traits a home health aide must develop is to remain flexible. (It might be mentioned here that physical and emotional flexibility is not one of the traits you can expect of your clients. You must keep in mind that as individuals grow older, they lose the ability to "go with the flow" or to adjust to new and changing conditions. They also lose physical flexibility, their bones are brittle, muscles may be weak, and diseases such as arthritis and osteoporosis limit movement. Thus, they can't bend, move, or function as well as younger persons.)

Devise a care plan for the client described in the case study on page 105. The client lives in a two-story house; the bedrooms and bath are upstairs. The doctor advises no more than one trip upstairs per day. There is a toilet on the main floor. The client must be assisted in bathing. Laundry must be done. Beds need to be changed and meals prepared. A medications chart has been set up by the visiting nurse. (The aide is to work four hours per day, five days a week.)

Write a narrative for a typical day's activities in this home. Some of the areas you might want to include are: how the couple relate to each other and to you; successes or failures in getting them to eat properly; whether the medications were taken properly; how the wife responded to personal care; the energy level of the wife; the mental status of the husband; what you said or did to build their self-confidence; any progress in getting them to agree to removing some of the accumulated "stuff." (You would always want to be sure the client understood and agreed to having any of the accumulated items thrown away. Remember "one man's trash is another man's treasure." Often what may look like junk to an outsider is an object with great sentimental value to the owner.)

One of the hardest adjustments that an elderly person must make is that his body just isn't functioning as well as it did only a few months earlier. It takes longer to get up from a chair; it is harder to take care of hair grooming; and it becomes a chore to plan meals and prepare and clean up after them. As body functions become less efficient, an individual becomes fearful. "What if I should fall?" "Did I take my medicine?" "Did I turn off the iron?" Fear is a negative emotion, and it feeds on itself. Suddenly, the aging individual can become afraid of anything and everything. They become uncertain about writing checks to pay bills and worry whether they did actually pay the bills. They wonder if they have enough money to last the rest of their lives. Then, when an illness strikes, they become even more fearful. One elderly patient said she felt like the song "Ole Man River"—"Tired of livin' and feared of dyin'." One of the jobs of a home health aide is to help the client regain self-confidence and remind them of how much progress they have made.

Very often elderly individuals become depressed. They remember how active they were just a short time ago and compare their active days to the restricted lives they now lead. This is particularly true when illness or a physical condition is also present. Depression feeds on itself and as they become more depressed, they feel worse physically. Their appetites become poorer, they give in to the fear of dying. These feelings of hopelessness lead to helplessness.

It has been proven that laughter can be good medicine in cases such as this. Norman Cousins, who was diagnosed as having a ter-

Here is an example of an actual situation faced by a home health aide. CLIENT: Female, 83 years of age, mildly diabetic with high blood pressure, angina, and arthritis, develops an ulcer due to medication to ease the arthritic pain, is anemic, is diagnosed as having hardening of the arteries, and her spine is disintegrating, causing great pain.

Until recently, this individual has been functioning at a reasonable level, caring for her 84-year-old husband and herself in their own home. Suddenly she becomes aware that her husband is short of breath, his sleep pattern has changed, his walk is slow and appears to be painful. He says he just doesn't feel well. This change in her husband causes her to become fearful. What will she do if he dies? In her own words, she can't sleep at night because she is afraid that her husband will die at night. He isn't sleeping; she isn't sleeping.

They are dependent upon each other. She feels inadequate and is fearful that she is losing her mind. It becomes a chore to decide what to eat so she stops planning and cooking regular meals. As a result, neither of them are eating nutritionally proper food. They both become weak. He sits in a chair all day watching television and nodding off to sleep. She finds herself becoming dizzy and falling down. She is restless and unable to find a comfortable spot for herself. It is hard for her to get dressed in the morning. Over a four month period, she has been out of the house only to go to the doctor or the grocery store, perhaps only two times a month in all. They start bickering with each other, each blaming the other for anything and everything. Both are getting weaker each day. As one sees the other not functioning, fear grows. Are they dying? If so, what will happen to the other one?

What else is going on in that situation? The housework is not being done. Dust and clutter are everywhere. Neither has the energy to vacuum. The kitchen is a mess. Dishes are not washed because she is too tired and possibly because she can't see too well. Although there is a clothes washer and dryer in the basement, she is unable to go up and down the stairs to do the laundry. He wears his clothes until they are stiff with dirt. Finally, he takes the dirty clothing to the basement and does the washing. The clothing is stained with bits of food that have dropped. The stains don't come out because he either can't see the stains or he hasn't the strength to take the extra effort required to remove them.

Neither of them is willing to throw out anything. So the house is piled high with "things"—old, stained, and torn clothing, bedding, and pillows; unopened gifts; and furniture that should have been discarded. They have every television set ever brought into the house, as well as coats, shoes, and clothing from the past twenty years. They do not have the strength to get such junk out of the house.

She is taking five kinds of medicine, including nitroglycerine, ulcer pills costing $1.45 each, two separate medications for blood pressure, and pain pills (cortisone and muscle relaxants) to ease the arthritic and spinal discomfort. She can't remember which pills she has taken and when she is due for another.

Neither of them eat very much. She says she has no appetite and everything tastes like sawdust. She is controlling the diabetes by watching her intake of sugar. So far she has kept her blood sugar within the normal range and her urine tests are negative. However, her hemoglobin count is down, the cholesterol count is up, and her blood pressure is too high. She also is chronically constipated and has hemorrhoids.

She has just returned from the hospital where the ulcer was diagnosed when the homemaker/home health aide is assigned to the case.

The homemaker/home health aide's primary responsibility is the 83-year-old woman. Where does she start? What are the limits of her responsibilities?

Ideally, the supervising doctor, nurse, or nutrition therapist will determine what foods should be consumed. This is particularly true in a case in which there are so many special requirements. There are many factors to be considered. Since the client is a diabetic, she will need a diet that is balanced and low in sugar. Since she has an ulcer, the diet must be bland and must not include acidic foods. In addition, she must be encouraged to eat many small, frequent meals instead of several large ones. Because she has high blood pressure she needs a sodium-free diet. Although her cholesterol level indicates that her diet should not include red meat, liver, cream, whole milk and butter, her low hemoglobin indicates that she eat red meat and liver, as well as apricots and other foods high in iron. Although her ulcer indicates that she should eat bland foods, her chronic constipation requires a diet high in bulk and fiber. Finally, her poor appetite needs to be counteracted with small, good-tasting, attractively served meals.

As you can see, filling all of these needs will not be easy. The client has lost her appetite and "all foods taste like sawdust." A skilled dietician or nutritional therapist should be consulted to set up appropriate menus for this client.

It should also be noted that certain of the prescriptions are to be taken at different times: either before, after, or at the same time meals are given. Check with the supervising nurse for the correct time each drug should be taken.

(Using the diets listed in the unit on nutrition, plan a suitable menu for two days under the above-listed circumstances.)

This client lives on a fixed income which averages approximately $15,000 a year. Basic medical expenses are covered by Blue Cross/Blue Shield and government major medical (Medicare). Let us look at the way this money is spent:

Total Income		$15,000.00
(Social Security and Investments)		
Property Taxes	$2,000.00	
Food ($60.00 per week)	3,120.00	
Insurance (car and house)	1,350.00	
Monthly car payments (gas/oil)	2,000.00	
Medical insurance (Blue Cross/Blue Shield/ Major Medical $200.00 Deductible)	2,400.00	
Clothing/shoes	600.00	
Oil Heat	1,300.00	
Electricity	300.00	
Water	140.00	
Telephone	280.00	
Newspaper/magazine subscriptions	275.00	
Total budgeted expenses		$13,765.00

$200.00 prescriptions not covered by major medical, emergencies—new tires for car, replacements of furniture or other unbudgeted items $1,235.00

Home health care is *not* covered by the insurance plan so that means that if the total costs through the health care agency amount to $120.00 per week, this client will be left with no emergency money cushion after only ten weeks of home health care. Just imagine if the client had to have three shifts of home health aides seven days a week. That alone can run as much as $1,500 in just one week.

minal illness, had a very positive attitude about himself and about life in general. He refused to become depressed and give in to his illness. He deliberately set out to find things that would make him laugh because he discovered when he laughed he felt better.

Recent experiments in nursing homes have reinforced the idea of laughter being good medicine. Patients were shown movies and videotapes of Charlie Chaplin films, Buster Keaton, the Keystone Kops, Laurel and Hardy and the Marx Brothers—all of whom, it should be noted, produce the "slapstick" variety of comedy.

Recent research has shown that depressed people respond positively to sunlight. Experiments have proven that clinically depressed individuals who spend several hours a day in a specially lighted room have shown remarkable improvement and have expressed how much better they feel. If such treatment works for those who are psychologically impaired, just imagine how helpful "sunlight" treatment might be for a homebound client.

Write a brief description of an imaginary encounter with the client described in the case study on page 109 in which she accuses you, the aide, of stealing her watch. (You find the watch later in the kitchen cabinet).

Write a second brief description of a situation where the same client told you what a miserably rude and uncaring person the previous aide had been. What else would you do besides document this?

The New York Bell Telephone Company provides some special services for handicapped individuals. For example, for this client, the agency requested specially magnified dials for the phone so that, even with limited vision, the client can dial her phone. In addition she has been given "operator assistance" at no extra charge. If she needs to make a call and does not know the number, all she has to do is dial "0" and the operator will look up the number and complete the call.

There is also available a "medic alert" which is a button the patient wears at all times. In case she should fall while alone, she can press the button and an emergency number will be dialed automatically. The phone will continue ringing the emergency number until someone answers and receives the message that there is an emergency at the client's address.

Another service available through the telephone company is a remote phone which the client can place in a bag on her walker. No matter where she is, she will have a phone within reach. For the individual who is alone in a home or apartment for any period of time during the day, these services are quite important.

Another service available in some areas is "medi-cab." For a very small sum (perhaps only a dollar each way), a client will be picked up and taken, for example, to medical appointments or to senior citizen functions. When the appointment is over, the medi-cab will return the client to her home. The home health aide or companion rides without charge. Many communities have special services for the disabled or elderly people.

Alzheimer's disease

An illness that has received a lot of publicity in the past few years is **Alzheimer's disease.** There is no known cause for this debilitating illness which is characterized by loss of memory and diminished mental capacity. The disease may eventually lead to a vegetablelike state in which the person has no control of mental or physical functions. Changes occur in nerve cells in the outer layer of the brain, producing almost unnoticeable symptoms at first. As the disease progresses, simple forgetfulness increases to greater memory loss. There are changes in thought patterns and personality. Those affected can no longer care for themselves or communicate their needs to others, see figure 9-9 on page 112. First diagnosed in 1906, Alzheimer's disease is now recognized as the most common cause of severe intellectual impairment in older adults.

According to experts on Alzheimer's, the terms presenile and senile dementia are used to describe any kind of severe mental impairment in older individuals. Approximately one-half of such persons are victims of Alzheimer's

disease. Another one-fourth have diseased blood vessels, and the rest suffer from conditions such as brain tumors, thyroid dysfunction, and pernicious anemia. In all cases, it is necessary for complete medical supervision to be provided.

Dementia, or loss of mental powers, is often irreversible. Once a client becomes confused, depressed, fearful, and suffers severe loss of memory, it may be that that individual is one of the 10 percent of those over age 65 or the 30 percent over age 80 who must be categorized as suffering from dementia. Of those, it is estimated that 60 percent to 70 percent can be diagnosed as having Alzheimer's disease. Between 15 percent and 25 percent of dementia cases are the result of a series of small cerebrovascular accidents that eventually bring about brain dysfunction.

Since Alzheimer's disease is the most common form of irreversible dementia, let's take a closer look at what it does to a client and family members. There is no known effective treatment when the disease reaches its advanced stages. Sedatives are prescribed to lessen agitation and perhaps allow the patient to sleep. Remember always that patients deserve to be treated with dignity and every effort should be made to keep the patient functioning at the highest level possible.

On the average, once Alzheimer's disease has been diagnosed, it may be twelve years until total degeneration occurs. It starts with simple memory lapses similar to that experienced by most individuals, figure 9-10 on page 113. All of us have put an item down and forgotten where we put it. At one time or another, everyone has started into another room to perform a task and suddenly found themselves unable to remember why they went there. We have all parked in a large parking lot and forgotten where the car was. Everyone has had such episodes, and they are momen-

This client is a 76-year-old female living alone in a co-op apartment. She has an inoperable brain tumor and suffered a CVA. After hospitalization and three months of rehabilitation at a nursing home, she is released to her home. The only relatives live out of state or out of the country. The medical recommendation is that twenty-four hour home health aide coverage be initiated. This requires the rotation of three aides daily, seven days per week; visits from public health or visiting nurses; regular visits from the agency supervisor and/or the agency nurse; a physical therapist three times a week; a speech therapist three times a week; and an occupational therapist three times a week.

The environment is a one-bedroom apartment in a pleasant suburban area. Prior to the CVA, the client's husband died. Following his death, the client first showed signs of mental disorientation when she collected every container, carton, wrapper, can, or bag that was brought into the house. She could not bring herself to throw out anything. As a result, the apartment was stacked high with boxes, cartons, piles of newspapers, magazines, and mail, leaving only an aisle in which to move from room to room.

Before the client was brought home, her attorney had arranged to have the apartment cleared out so that there would be room for a wheelchair, chair commode, and walker, as well as room for an aide to walk beside the client as she became more mobile.

During the first two months, three aides a day were provided by the agency. For the first few weeks, the client was so happy to be at home that she made no complaints about anything. The agency supervisor spoke daily with each aide. She discovered that the client was gossiping about each of the aides to the other two—making critical remarks and comparing them unfavorably. The client was also showing favoritism by offering extra money to one aide. (The aide immediately reported this to her supervisor, who called the client and explained that such behavior on her part was improper.)

At about this time, the client became very critical of the aides and called the supervisor to complain on a daily basis. The supervisor spoke with the aides individually and heard their side and recognized that it would be best to change their assignments. At first, when a new aide was assigned, the client would be very enthusiastic and tell the supervisor how wonderful the aide was. However, after two or three weeks, she would claim that money was missing or that the aide came in late or was lazy or just wasn't a nice person. The night time aide reported to the supervisor that the client told the aide to go to sleep as she wouldn't need her. Then she became aware that the client was trying to go to the bathroom by herself. Finally it was decided that the night time aide really wasn't needed and the client agreed to try coping alone for one, then two, then three, and finally a full week without an aide at night. At this point the client was progressing very well and again it was determined by the doctor and the agency supervisor that the aides' hours be cut back.

It has now been one year since the client was released from the nursing home. She no longer needs the wheelchair or commode and can use the walker very well. She prepares her own breakfast and dresses and undresses herself. Arrangements have been made for a neighbor to prepare her evening meal and do the grocery shopping. An aide comes in between nine A.M. and one P.M. Monday through Friday to go to the laundry room and do the laundry, change the bed, and assist with activities of daily living. This aide also prepares lunch, goes with the client to her appointments with the doctor and dentist, and takes the client out of doors when the weather permits.

The client has reported to the supervisor that she truly enjoys this aide because she really listens when the client talks. The aide explained to the supervisor that she asks the client questions about where she and her husband used to go on vacation, what movies or plays she saw— she gets the client involved in reminiscing about pleasant, past experiences. At the same time she will take out a dresser drawer and have the client "help" her rearrange, throw away, and clean the drawer. This aide has unlocked the secret of pleasing the client, who loves to talk. She has proved to be a creative and thoroughly professional aide.

What would happen if this client noticed that her eyesight was failing? After a visit to the opthalmologist, she learns that not only are cataracts developing, but, following the stroke, there was damage to the blood vessels of the eyes which is now getting worse. The doctor tells her that there is no corrective surgery and her eyesight will gradually fade completely.

1. She will require full-time aides.
2. She should start taking lessons in Braille so that she can read for pleasure.
3. While she is still able to get around easily, she could enroll in programs for the blind offered through the Lighthouse so that she would be better prepared to function and become as independent as possible when her eyesight is gone.

This client's annual income from investments and social security comes to just over $50,000 per year. During her first year of illness her medical expenses alone were over $100,000. Fortunately much of that was covered by insurance.

Health Care Not Covered By Insurance during past year	$35,955.00
Maintenance Fees (Co-op Apartment)	7,200.00
Electricity	580.00
Telephone	425.00
Food	2,800.00
Pharmacy (prescriptions and medications)	818.00
Insurance (health and property)	2,700.00
Charities (church, etc.)	2,000.00
Clothing	400.00
Dental care (not covered by insurance)	2,600.00
Transportation (cabs to doctor appointments)	345.00
Attorney's fees	2,000.00
(No taxes were due this year because of excessive medical expenses.)	
Television repair contract	230.00
	$58,478.00

This meant that she had to use nearly $8,000. of her capital to pay the bills for the past year. As a result, her income next year will be lower.

During the period when three, and later two, aides were assigned to work with this client, the need for accurate observing, reporting and documenting was of more than normal importance. This patient was a manipulative person, and each aide needed to be sure that the record of her own activities was complete so that if the patient complained about tasks not being done, the record would stand to refute that accusation. It was also important that activities and tasks were clearly recorded so that each aide could quickly learn what the aides on the preceding shifts had done, and what the patient's reactions had been. In this way, tasks would not be duplicated or omitted, and tips on successful interventions and methods could be passed on from aide to aide.

---

tarily frightening. These memory lapses occur more and more often to those with Alzheimer's disease (AD). As the disease progresses, they forget to pay bills, don't realize they have invited guests for dinner, arrive somewhere and don't know where they are or what they are doing there.

At this stage, AD patients become anxious, tense, nervous, and very uncomfortable. They can still perform all the basic activities of daily living, but should be supervised by family members in more complex social and daily situations. Financial supervision should be given and structured or supervised travel should be arranged. At this point it will probably be necessary to sew address labels in the patient's clothing, or provide identification bracelets in the event that the individual wanders off or becomes disoriented.

In the next stage, the patient can no longer function independently. The family must take over financial affairs, shopping, and even choosing proper clothing. The patient may forget to bathe and become careless about personal appearance. It may be that some clients are extremely fearful of being in water. Driving a car at this stage can be very danger-ous. If a client continues to want to drive, it is up to the caregiver to prevent the client from driving. Crying episodes, hyperactivity, and sleep disturbances may arise at this time and around-the-clock care becomes necessary.

As the disease progresses, the patient loses the ability to dress, feed himself or herself, bathe, and go to the toilet. This may first be noticed when the client puts on daytime clothing over pajamas or is unable to tie his shoes. The brain and body no longer function as a unit.

The caregiver can become extremely frustrated with the Alzheimer's disease client. The caregiver should try to imagine the frustration of the client, figure 9-11. During the course of the illness the client sometimes seems fully aware, recognizes family and friends and makes "sense." These "windows of reality" become smaller and smaller as the condition progresses. It finally reaches a point where the client becomes nonfunctioning and requires around-the-clock custodial care.

There is no point in trying to force the client to "make sense" or to become angry because the client is forgetful, personally sloppy, or appears to be "stubborn." What the

STAGE	SYMPTOMS	CARE PLAN
I.	Forgetfulness	Be supportive, provide reminders, make lists. Client is still competent in the activities of daily living. Client can work, drive, and socialize.
II.	Increase in memory lapses: forgets appointments, fails to pay bills. An increase in anxiety and tension—fear of new situations.	Sew labels in clothes; provide ID bracelet or prepare ID card to be kept in the wallet or purse. Supervise and structure travel. Avoid crowds, remove the client from stressful situations.
III.	Inability to function independently. Progressive loss of motor skills. Increasingly uncomfortable in complex situations where much activity is taking place. No longer able to hold job. Has tantrums, and very little emotional control—may run away.	Help client with money matters: shopping, choosing clothes, etc. Client may have difficulty using eating utensils, so finger foods should be given. Accept clients as they are, not how they ''should be.'' Clients must be treated with dignity.
IV.	Personal carelessness. Refuses to bathe. May refuse to eat, is restless, and may have sleep disturbances. May try to get dressed in the middle of night to go to work. Unable to button clothing, tie shoes, and dress appropriately.	Do not allow the client to drive. Provide slip-on shoes and simple clothing. Assist with eating and dressing. Protect client from self-harm.
V.	Crying episodes common. Hyperactivity increases. Days and nights completely confused. Decreased attention span, unable to follow instructions. Probably will become incontinent of both bowels and bladder. Unable to feed self and shows no interest in food.	Keep client as comfortable and calm as possible. Client requires full-time custodial care. Speak slowly and clearly, giving only one suggestion at a time. (''It's time to take a bath,'' ''Take off your shirt,'' ''Take off your shoes,'' etc.) Handle one item at a time to avoid making the client feel threatened. If a caretaker demands instant responses, the client will become terribly distressed and stubborn. The aide must *always* remember the client is not in control of his emotions, therefore, the aide must retain *self-control*. Keep client clean and dry. Feed client small amounts as often as possible or provide liquids and liquified or puréed foods.
VI.	Incontinence of bladder and bowel. Inability to speak or feed self. Increased agitation, complete helplessness	Installment in a health care facility with 24-hour supervision. Medical assistance from doctors. Intravenous feeding and sedation are required. Client may lose consciousness and sink into a coma.

Figure 9-9 Stages and symptoms of Alzheimer's disease

- Memory loss
- Difficulty in finding the right word to use in conversation
- Difficulty in speaking or understanding what is said
- Poor judgment and loss of logical reasoning ability
- Loss of mathematical ability
- Change in visual perceptions
- Inability to recognize faces or objects

Figure 9-10 Early signs of Alzheimer's Disease

home health aide and the family must understand is that the victim of Alzheimer's disease has no control over what is happening. They cannot force the client to admit to confusion. They must accept the person just as he or she is. The client must have the freedom to be old and confused. Don't make a tug-of-war over meals and sleeping time. All an aide can do is make sure the client is clean, fed, warm, and safe.

Alzheimer's clients must be weighed on a regular basis and any significant changes in weight—more than five pounds either way in six weeks—must be reported to the supervisor. If a decrease in weight occurs, changes in meal patterns may be required, such as smaller, more frequent meals, or the use of finger food so that the patient can self-feed.

- Problem solving ability
- Patience
- Caring attitude
- Empathy
- Ability to relate to clients and to family members

Figure 9-11 To care for the Alzheimer's Disease client, the homemaker/home health aide must possess these essential characteristics

Avoid sweets and other empty calories. As the disease progresses, regular eating patterns may be refused by the client. They become confused with the knife, fork, or spoon and will have to be fed by the aide. If the client refuses to eat, it may be necessary to turn to finger foods, liquid nutritional supplements or puréed foods. When oral feeding becomes impossible, the patient will probably require placement in a nursing home.

Alzheimer clients may become incontinent. Regular toileting schedules can be set up when incontinence first occurs; this gives the patient more dignity. Be sure the bathroom is clearly marked and the client knows where to go. Don't try to limit fluids because dehydration might occur. When incontinence cannot be controlled by medical treatment or regular toileting, there are products that can be recommended by the pharmacist. Protective panties or briefs can protect the furniture and avoid embarrassment to the client. Diapers and underpads can be used at night or for the bedbound client. There may come a time when an in-dwelling catheter will be required. (See catheter care in unit 29.)

There are support groups in many communities. Family members can meet to share common problems and learn more about how to cope with their parent or relative as well as face up to their own feelings and fears.

In some areas there are special "day care" centers where Alzheimer's disease clients can be taken for a few hours a day. These centers are well supervised and patients will often entertain each other by talking, playing cards, playing the piano, or singing. Since the progress of the disease is uneven, clients may have "good" days or weeks when they function reasonably well at such centers. On the other hand, if the group activities have a bad effect on the client and make him or her more agitated or fearful, the activity should be stopped immediately.

THE ALZHEIMER'S DISEASE

CLIENT	HHHA ACTIONS/RESPONSIBILITIES
Has difficulty communicating . . .	• Approach the client with a friendly facial expression • Be calm • Stand in front of the client • Try to maintain eye contact; touch the client to attract attention or regain it • Speak in a low, calm, reassuring tone of voice (if the client has a hearing problem, follow the instructions in the care plan) • Speak slowly and give the client time to answer • If necessary, repeat the statement or question—do not change the wording • Keep the language simple and express only one idea at a time • Lead the client in answering if he can't find the right words—point to objects to provide cues • Do not become impatient
Has difficulty walking . .	• Provide a safe environment —Remove scatter rugs —Do not wax floors —Pick up and put away objects the client may not see and thus trip over such as small footstools, doorstops, plants, pet toys, and dishes —The client is to use only chairs with arms for support • Show the client what you want him/her to do and provide support • Do not hurry the client • If the client is unsteady and is using an aid (cane, walker) do not let the client out of your sight • Be sure the client's shoes fit properly • Always use proper body mechanics when helping the client • Keep the client walking as long as possible (as the disease progresses)
Experiences changes in eating patterns . . .	• Meals must be served at the same time each day • Meals should look appetizing and be served at the proper temperature • Give the client one course and one utensil at a time; do not give the client a choice of foods • If the client must be fed, do so slowly and cut the food into small pieces • Nutritious snacks should be kept on hand • Always encourage fluids • As the client loses the ability to chew, soft foods are introduced; a blender can be used to liquify foods

Figure 9-12 Guidelines for working with the Alzheimer's disease client (up to terminal stage)* (courtesy of Foundation of Hospice and Homecare)

CLIENT	HHHA ACTIONS/RESPONSIBILITIES
	• As the client loses the ability to use utensils, finger foods can be used
	• Maintain the diet plan included in the overall care plan
	• Weigh the client regularly (at least once weekly) and record the weight
Tends to wander . . .	• Be sure the client wears an ID bracelet or necklace
	• Sew labels to each piece of clothing—labels should have the name of the client, address, and telephone number
	• Keep doors locked; make sure the bell or chimes are in working order
	• Place large print signs on doors—"DO NOT GO OUT," "TURN AROUND"
	• If the client insists on going out, do not argue—go with him (lock the door and take keys)
	• After a few minutes, suggest returning to the house to rest
	• Try to distract the client from leaving—try another activity you know the client enjoys (Alzheimer's Disease clients often respond to music)
	• Keep a recent photograph of the client at hand in the event the client does wander off and is not in the immediate neighborhood
	• If the client does leave unnoticed and you can't find him—call family members, police, and your agency
Experiences incontinence . . .	• Remember that the client cannot control this behavior
	• Do not scold or punish the client
	• Treat the client with respect
	• Set up a regular schedule for toileting and follow it
	• Encourage fluids as usual to prevent dehydration
	• Mark the bathroom clearly with a large print sign and a picture
	• Keep the client clean and dry; use simple washable clothing
	• Recognize the client's verbal and nonverbal language
	• Check the skin regularly for signs of irritation
Exhibits restlessness and agitation in late afternoon (sundown syndrome) . . .	• Decrease the level of activity in late afternoon to reduce potential stress
	• Play soft, soothing music
	• Do not try to reason the client out of this behavior—the client has no control over his/her actions
	• Do not institute sudden changes into the routine which will confuse and upset the client
	• Appointments and trips should be scheduled for morning and early afternoon
	• Do not restrain or argue with the client

Figure 9-12 (*Continued*)

CLIENT	HHHA ACTIONS/RESPONSIBILITIES
	• Try to distract the client with quiet, simple activities • Make sure the client has adequate exercise during the day
Experiences sleeping disturbances . . .	• The client may exhibit less need for sleep • Try to keep the client active during the day so he/she will feel the need for sleep • The client should drink caffeine-free beverages • Establish a bedtime routine and follow it • Make sure the client is toileted before going to bed • Make sure there are no loud noises; soft music may help • The client may feel more secure with a night-light • Keep a night-light on in the bathroom and keep the door open
Needs help with bathing and oral hygiene . . .	• Permit the client to do as much as he/she can—suggest steps if necessary • Ensure the client's safety when bathing—use hand holds, nonslip mats, tub seats, etc. • Organize all the necessary equipment before you bring the client to the bathroom • Stay calm and pleasant; try to make this a pleasurable experience for the client • Do not leave the client alone when bathing • Schedule bathing when the client is least agitated • Do not force the client into bathing; wait until the client is calm and try again • Give the client a sponge bath if all attempts to tub bathe or shower fail • Cleanliness must be maintained—consult with your supervisor if the client continues to exhibit resistance to bathing • If the client cannot provide oral care, even with coaxing, brush his/her teeth yourself or clean the dentures
Experiences delusions, hallucinations and inappropriate (catastrophic) reactions to normal events . . .	• What the client sees or hears is real to him • Do not argue or reason with the client • Maintain a calm, ordered environment • Reassure the client that you are there to protect him • If the client becomes violent, stay out of his/her way • If the client becomes agitated, try to distract him/her with an activity you know he/she likes; a small snack of a favorite food may distract him/her sufficiently to restore calm • If the client attacks you verbally, do not take it personally • The client may accuse you of stealing; again, do not take it personally
Exhibits improper sexual behavior . . .	• Remember, the client is confused and disoriented • Do not overreact—remain calm

Figure 9-12 *(Continued)*

CLIENT	HHHA ACTIONS/RESPONSIBILITIES
	• Do not scold or argue with the client • Do not try to reason with the client • If the client undresses, provide a robe or redress him/her • If the client is in public when inappropriate behavior takes place, distract the client and remove him/her from the scene • Plan ahead ways you can distract the client • Provide appropriate touching to show that you care for and value the client

Figure 9-12 *(Continued)*

* Adapted from ''How to Care for the Alzheimer's Disease Patient: A Comprehensive Training Manual for Homemaker-Home Health Aides'' copyright 1986 by the Foundation for Hospice and Homecare.

The home health aide helps the family members by providing respite care, figure 9-12, pages 114–117. That is, while the home health aide provides care, the family may take advantage of these few hours to take care of errands or just experience the freedom from care-giving responsibilities.

For further information about Alzheimer's disease contact

Alzheimer's Disease and Related Disorders Association
70 East Lake Street
Chicago, Illinois 60601

To view ''Do You Remember Love,'' a CBS made-for-TV-movie, contact

CBS Television
51 West 52nd Street
New York, New York
(212) 975-4321

reality orientation

Activities for clients with mental impairments should be maintained at as normal a level as possible. It may be helpful to provide simple memory aids to assist the client in day-to-day living: a prominent calendar, lists of daily tasks, written reminders about routine safety measures, and other "memory joggers." This process is known as **reality orientation.**

A legend attributed to the American Indians states that, in order to understand how another person feels, you should walk a mile in that person's "moccasins." Too often, people do not stop to think about how other people feel, and often expect others to react as they would. As people grow older, their normal response time slows down. This does not make them less worthwhile as an individual. They know they do not respond as quickly, think as fast, or move as fast as they once did. This is frightening to the elderly and they also resent it.

The elderly often seem to dwell in the past. They are sometimes confused and may think a grandchild is their son or daughter. They may forget what day it is or what task they were doing. Forgetting what they are doing can be dangerous. Suppose an older person puts the teakettle filled with water on the stove to heat and then goes to another room and forgets about it. The teakettle could boil dry and explode, or the gas stove pilot light could be extinguished causing gas fumes to fill the home.

the home health aide's role in reality orientation

Following are a few suggestions the home health aide can use to help a confused client become better oriented to the immediate surroundings:

1. Repeat the confused client's name often throughout the day. Remind the client of your name, the date and day, the client's location, what the next meal will be, etc. If you know your client is confused you might say: "Good morning, Mrs. Johnson. Remember me? I'm Elsie, your aide. Are you ready for your breakfast? It's 8:30 in the morning, May 13, 1989 and we have many things to do today."

2. Visitors, friends, neighbors, and even young children should be asked to use basic reality orientation techniques. All correction of the client must be done in a respectful way. You might say: "Mrs. Johnson, your neighbor, Mrs. Martin is here. Isn't it nice to see her?" If Mrs. Johnson should call someone by the wrong name, gently remind her of the correct name, e.g., "This isn't your son, Don; this is your grandson, Tommy. You remember Tommy, don't you?"

3. Get into the habit of announcing events. "It is time for your bath, Mrs. Johnson. This is the way to the bathroom. Let me push your chair to the bathroom, Mrs. Johnson."

4. Correct your client immediately when disoriented remarks are made. "You just had your breakfast, Mrs. Johnson. We won't have supper until 5:30."

5. Keep changes to a minimum. Do not move furniture around. Help the confused person keep belongings in a regular location. Reinforce this as often as necessary.

6. Spend 10 or 15 minutes each day talking with the disoriented client. Talk about a favorite family member, or the trip to the doctor. Get input as to what the client would like to eat at the next meal or what plans the client has for the upcoming holiday.

7. Allow the client to reminisce and talk about the past, but try to keep the facts straight, if possible.

8. Assist the client in self-care, even if it takes more time than if you did it yourself. This builds a sense of personal pride and allows the client to feel successful.

9. Do not patronize or talk down to the client. Be respectful, firm, matter-of-fact, and kind, figure 9-13.

10. Provide a change of scene occasionally, but describe the location. "We're going to the doctor's office. There's your church on that corner. Do you remember the minister's name? Oh, there is Reverend Thomas."

Caring for the elderly can be very demanding and sometimes it is easy to lose patience, figure 9-14. There have been reports that lonely, aged persons have been mistreated by their families and by those caring for them. This kind of abuse from a home health aide is unethical and grounds for dismissal.

Many people make the mistake of putting all elderly people into the category of "se-

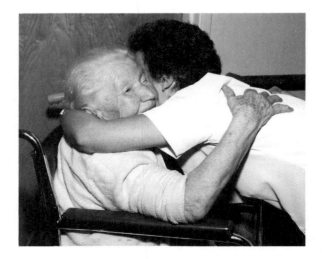

Figure 9-13 Clients need affection.

This poem was found in the bedside table at a geriatric ward in a hospital in Ireland. It appeared in the Christmas issue of *Beacon House News*, the magazine of the Northern Ireland Association for Mental Health.

What do you see nurses, what do you see?
are you thinking when you are looking at me
a crabbit old woman, not very wise,
Uncertain of habit, with far-away eyes,
Who dribbles her food and makes no reply
When you say in a loud voice, "I do wish you would try".
Who seems not to notice the things that you do,
And forever is losing a stocking or shoe,
Who unresisting or not, lets you do as you will,
With bathing and feeding, the long day to fill.
Is that what you are thinking, is that what you see?
Then open your eyes, nurse, you are not looking at me.

I will tell you who I am as I sit here so still,
As I use at your bidding, as I eat at your will,
I am a small child of ten with a father and mother,
Brothers and sisters, who love one another.
A young girl of sixteen with wings on her feet,
Dreaming that soon now a lover she will meet,
A bride soon at twenty, my heart gives a leap,
Remembering the vows that I promised to keep.
At twenty-five now I have young of my own,
Who need me to build a secure, happy home.
A woman of thirty, my young now grow fast,
Bound to each other with ties that should last,
At forty my young sons now grown and will be gone,
But my man stays beside me to see I do not mourn,
At fifty once more babies play round my knee,
Again we know children, my loved one and me.
Dark days are upon me, my husband is dead,
I look at the future, I shudder with dread.
For my young are all busy rearing young of their own,
And I think of the years and the love that I have known.
I am an old woman now and nature is cruel,
"This her jest to make old age look like a fool."
The body it crumbles, grace and vigor depart,
There is now a stone where I once had a heart;
But inside this carcass a young girl still dwells,
And now and again my battered heart swells,
I remember the joys, I remember the pain,
And I am loving and living life over again.
I think of the years all too few, gone too fast,
And I accept the stark fact that nothing can last.
So open your eyes, nurses, open and see,
Not a crabbit old woman, look closer—see ME.

—Anonymous

Figure 9-14 A Crabbit Old Woman

nile." It is rude and unnecessary to make a remark such as, "I'm taking care of this senile old lady." Remember, just as you expect to be treated with respect, so do those who are aging.

Someone once said, "We can foresee the needs and the problems of aging, but we cannot forefeel them." Therefore, we need imagination, much patience, kindness, and understanding in order to give the elderly the service and care which really meets their needs.

summary

- Each stage of life offers its own rewards and has its own special problems.
- As the body ages, it is slower to return to wellness after injury or illness.
- Depression, loss of self-esteem, loneliness, anxiety, and boredom can become more common as elderly persons face the process of aging and illness.
- The deaths of relatives and friends, as well as other crises, add to the problems of old age.
- The home health aide must draw on many areas of learning in order to provide the care needed for each client.
- The home health aide must keep in mind that some of the problems generally referred to as senile dementia can be treated and cured. Others, like Alzheimer's disease, can only be treated to minimize symptoms, without hope of restoring lost brain function.
- Helping the client keep in touch with day-to-day reality and keeping to a daily schedule are very important duties of the aide.

review

1. What is osteoporosis?
2. Name two emotional problems that the elderly may have to deal with.
3. What are the characteristics of Alzheimer's disease?
4. Name three memory aids used to help orient elderly clients.
5. List four common ailments of older clients.

Promoting Health and Understanding Illness

Unit 10
Mental Health

key terms		
psychology	defense mechanism	denial
adjustment	rationalization	compensation
internal stimulus	projection	phobia
external stimulus	displacement	fantasizing
emotion	conversion reaction	anxiety
temperament	withdrawal	

learning objectives

After studying this unit, you should be able to:
— Identify an example of a defense mechanism.
— Identify several common emotions.
— Identify how a physical response can result from an emotional reaction.
— Identify the meanings of psychology, temperament and adjustment.
— Differentiate between external and internal stimuli.

Psychology is the science of human behavior. It is the study of the way the mind works and how emotions and feelings affect human behavior. Just as no two bodies are exactly alike, no two minds react in the same way. **Adjustment** is the change a person makes in behavior in order to deal with a situation. A well-adjusted person is able to handle the daily problems of living, taking bad times in stride and coping with crises. The well-adjusted person has a good self-image and can be flexible when meeting new or difficult obstacles. It takes less time for a well-adjusted person to recover from a difficult situation. People can adjust easily to some situations and not to others. A person does not have to be strong all the time.

The well-adjusted person is able to make life work in a way that is both personally and socially acceptable.

To understand basic psychology it is necessary to review the nervous system. The brain acts as the body's communication center. All messages (called stimuli) from the five senses are carried to the brain where they are received and acted upon. There are both internal and external stimuli. Example: The stomach is empty so the nerve endings in the stomach send a message to the brain. The brain translates the impulses, and the individual thinks "I'm hungry" and looks for food. This is an **internal stimulus.** On the other hand, upon entering a room where food is being cooked, a person might smell a pleasant aroma or see an attractive piece of fruit. The sight and smell of the food can stimulate the nerve endings and the person might think "I'm hungry" and eat the food even though it was not mealtime. This is an **external stimulus.**

Internal stimuli cause automatic or unconscious reactions within the body. External stimuli come from outside the body and bring about a conscious reaction. Psychology relates to both internal and external stimuli. In some conditions, chemical imbalances within the body or brain and nerve cell damage can cause changes in behavior. In other cases, environmental conditions may have a direct effect upon emotional health.

understanding emotions

Emotions are common to all humans and are neither good nor bad. An **emotion** is a strong generalized feeling. The way a person shows emotion may be healthy or unhealthy. There is a wide range of acceptable levels of emotional behavior. Well-adjusted people most often use emotions in a healthy way to serve their purposes; they can control emotions so

as not to harm themselves or others. Fear, anger, and grief are necessary to all people. Those who claim that they "never lose their temper" or have "never been afraid" or "do not feel grief" are fooling themselves. Whether emotional behavior is healthy depends on where and how the person expresses these emotions. Anger and happiness can be healthy reactions in some situations while not in others.

Emotions may cause physical reactions. Anger and fear sometimes cause the heart to beat faster, respirations to increase, and chemical changes to take place within the body. The mouth may become dry, the person may become pale and start to shake. Such physical changes are common and usually of short duration. Emotions can trigger the release of hormones and produce unusual results. For example, a 34-year-old man was traveling in an airplane which crashed. The plane burst into flames and hundreds of people were trapped inside. This man, who was injured himself, pulled ten victims from the plane before he collapsed. In spite of his upset mental and physical state, his body was able to function at an unusually high level.

Individuals develop a pattern of emotional response. This may partly be a hereditary characteristic. Some babies, for instance, seem calmer and happier than others. It is generally felt that most behavior is learned and, therefore, a result of environment. The social environment of a family determines whether a baby's early experiences are pleasant or unpleasant. As years pass, the child's successes and failures in daily life influence the child's emotional patterns. The child who is healthy and who is given tender, loving attention from birth has a good chance of growing up to be well adjusted.

The type of emotion (pleasant or unpleasant) that a person feels most of the time often determines temperament. A **temperament** is the usual mood of an individual. An optimis-

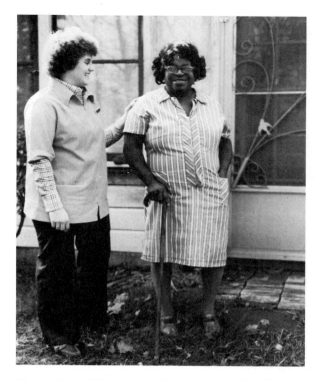

Figure 10-1 The homemaker-home health aide who presents a cheerful outlook can transfer this pleasant mood to the client.

tic person probably feels more pleasant emotions and, therefore, has a brighter outlook than a pessimist. The aide who has a cheerful outlook can transfer this pleasant mood to the client, figure 10-1. Words, tone of voice, actions and facial expression show how a person looks at life. This often exposes the person's inner feelings. Pessimists may be just as well adjusted as optimists but their viewpoints differ.

People have mood changes or emotional cycles. It is normal to feel high or low from time to time. In some people, this mood swing is more noticeable than in others. The well-adjusted person is able to function in both highs and lows. A less stable person has extremes of highs and lows. Emotional cycles can be affected by the time of day or season of the year or the weather. For example, some people are happiest and function best early in the day. Others, who are sometimes called night people, are more alert in the evening hours. Many people also allow the seasons to affect their feelings. Some dislike the winter and feel depressed; others dislike the summer months.

Well-adjusted people learn to make their emotions work for them. One can deal with unhealthy emotions in a positive way. When a home health aide gets angry with a client, the aide cannot have a tantrum. Strong outbursts of emotion are not acceptable while on duty. Sometimes anger must be expressed but it should be done in a way which is constructive. A home health aide must not only deal with her own emotional needs, but must also be aware of the emotional needs and reactions of the client. This requires a great deal of self-control and self-discipline. The

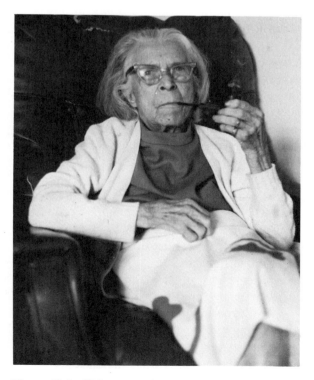

Figure 10-2 This woman is showing her independence by smoking a pipe.

home health aide must be sensitive to the emotions of the client. Clients are often frightened and worried about their health. The home health aide must be kind and understanding and think of the client's needs first. Illness can cause temporary changes in the client's personality. This often requires the client to make adjustments. It takes time to accept the physical changes which may be caused by a disease. The home health aide must be willing to allow clients to express their emotions, figure 10-2. The well-adjusted aide will be able to endure the client's emotional storms without becoming a part of them.

defense mechanisms

Defense mechanisms are specific techniques used to protect oneself from unpleasantness, shame, anxiety or loss of self-esteem. Some are common and are unknowingly used when a person feels uncomfortable.

Rationalization is the use of excuses to substitute for the real reasons behind an action. An example of this would be a girl trying out for a lead in the school play and not being accepted. She might say, "I had a headache and just couldn't do my best at the tryouts."

Projection is blaming someone else to cover up personal failure. The child who fails a math test might say, "The teacher hates me. That's why I failed."

Displacement is taking anger or frustration out on someone else. A woman might be very angry at her husband but too afraid to let it show. Instead, she exhibits her anger with one of her children by overreacting to a minor incident or by scolding the child.

Fantasizing or daydreaming is a way of avoiding reality. A woman who is 30 pounds overweight and on a weight-reducing diet might fantasize that she won a beauty contest. If the fantasy helped her stay on the diet, it could have positive effects. However, fantasies often just delay action needed to make a change.

Escape into illness or **conversion reaction** is a device used to avoid doing something unpleasant by becoming physically ill. People most commonly develop a headache or a stomachache. However, a more serious reaction can also occur. In this case, the person has been so severely upset that blindness, deafness, or paralysis may occur. For example, a person witnessing a murder of a close relative might shut out the incident and actually become blind.

Withdrawal or isolation is removing oneself physically from an uncomfortable or frightening situation. Children who hear and see their parents fight might go to their room and close the door.

Denial is the defense mechanism used to avoid facing the truth. Glen Cunningham, the first man in history to run the mile in four minutes, was severely burned and was told by doctors that he would never walk again. He refused to believe the doctors—he denied being severely injured. In this case, denial was a positive reaction and the man overcame hardships to reach success. However, if a child lost a parent in an accident and denied the truth, it could cause deep psychological problems.

Compensation is making up for a weakness by becoming very good in some other area. The physically weak person may become a good student to compensate for not being good in sports.

Most people are anxious and concerned from time to time. **Anxiety** is an unpleasant emotional or psychological state of constant fear or apprehension. Anxiety can be severe and cause a person to stop functioning. There are people who are afraid to board an airplane. They have such a **phobia** (fear) that they refuse to go near a plane. Others may be uncomfortable about flying but decide to fly in spite of their fear.

People make many adjustments within the course of one day. There are always new problems which arise and choices which must be made. Well-adjusted people accept the fact that they will make errors of judgment. Making mistakes is part of life. Adjustments come about easier when people accept that they are not perfect. They learn to do the best they can with what they have.

the effects of emotions on health

Wellness means different things to different people; people feel better on some days than on others. Temporary discomforts are not necessarily a health hazard or danger. Life can be compared to a roller coaster ride—it has its ups and downs. After a very hard day at work, an argument with a close friend, or the death of a loved one, people may feel unwell. A tension headache caused by an emotional crisis can make a person feel ill for a short time. When the upset is resolved, the person forgets the pain and feels well again, figure 10-3. Persons who are acutely or chronically ill also have good and bad days. To a great extent these changes are related to their emotional outlook. When routines have gone smoothly or when a special friend has called or visited, a person may feel very well in spite of physical problems. On a day when the home health aide comes late and is in a bad mood, the client may complain of feeling much worse than the physical condition warrants.

No two people react the same to external stimuli. The stressful situation causing one person to feel unwell may have no effect on another person in a like situation. People react to personal crisis in their own way. It has been proven that an emotionally depressed person is more likely to catch a cold or develop a physical disorder. Wellness may be described as freedom from discomfort—both physical

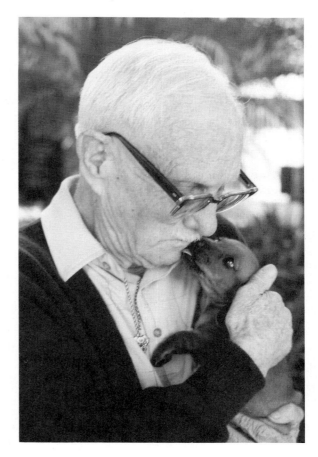

Figure 10-3. The elderly and the lonely often find that the attentions of a loving pet can promote a sense of well-being.

and mental. Emotional health may strongly influence a person's state of wellness.

Mental illness and developmental disabilities have been handled in many different ways over the years. Mental illness, sometimes called "insanity," refers to those who are unable to cope with life because of severe emotional problems. Developmentally disabled refers to those who are born with brain damage or deficiencies that make it impossible for them to grow intellectually. But, it must be noted that with proper care, loving attention, and special education, developmentally disabled individuals can learn and be able to function at varying levels of self-sufficiency.

At one time, those who were mentally ill were regarded as being possessed of the devil and were greatly feared. In Medieval England, the mentally ill were thrown into a prison-like hospital. They were literally discarded, ignored, and forced to survive under impossible conditions. They were treated with less care than animals on a farm. The screaming, crying, and yelling of these poor creatures caused the London mental institution's nickname, Bedlam, to mean a place of noisy confusion.

Developmentally disabled children were sometimes hidden away in the family attic or basement because the family was ashamed of them. Gradually, however, society came to realize that the mentally ill and developmentally disabled are human beings with the same needs and desires as the general population. Special institutions were opened where families could take their severely retarded or emotionally disturbed relatives.

Unfortunately, many of these mental hospitals gave only custodial care. In other words, they kept the inmates fed and kept a roof over their heads. They did not provide guidance, psychological support, training programs, or rehabilitation so that these people could possibly re-enter the mainstream of society. In many instances, it was discovered that inmates of these institutions were mistreated, beaten, sexually abused, forced to lie in their own feces, and required to take medications to "keep them quiet."

Within the past twenty years, many of these institutions have been closed. Some "half-way houses" were started so that the mentally ill could live with others who were being returned to the "real world." In these houses they lived under the supervision of psychiatrists, psychologists, and house supervisors.

Some of these "half-way houses" have proven successful. However, the majority of the mentally ill were simply released in the hope that family members would provide shelter and take care of them. Many have ended up on the street.

Group homes have also been set up for the developmentally disabled so that they can live in a family-like situation and work together to provide for their common needs. However, there are not enough half-way houses or group homes.

There are a great many emotionally ill and developmentally disabled individuals living with their families. When caring for such persons, an aide must be well briefed by the nurse or supervisor and must follow instructions very carefully. If any problems should arise, the aide should contact the supervisor immediately.

Several in-service courses should be taken before an aide works with the mentally ill or with a developmentally disabled individuals.

summary

- The field of psychology can be quite complex. However, the aide does not need to study the many mental disorders in order to care for clients.
- The aide should develop an awareness of the ways in which emotions affect behavior.
- Psychology is concerned with making reasonable adjustments. The human body and mind are both able to adapt to new situations.
- A home health aide's job is important in helping a client adapt both physically and mentally by giving proper care.
- While each individual is different, there are reasonable limits of acceptable behavior for all.

- Each person experiences the same emotions—fear, anger, joy, sorrow, contentment, pleasure. However, people may show their emotions in different ways. As long as emotional responses are within reasonable limits they are acceptable. In other words, a person's emotional responses should not cause personal harm or harm to others. Mood swings are normal to all persons.
- The aide should keep personal emotions in balance when caring for a client. At the same time the aide must recognize the emotional needs of the client.

review

1. Define adjustment.
2. What is the difference between an internal stimulus and an external stimulus?
3. What is meant by conversion reaction?
4. Name five defense mechanisms. Give an example of each.

Unit 11
Nutritional Guidelines

learning objectives

After studying this unit, you should be able to:
- List the Basic Four food groups and give two examples of each group.
- State the number of servings recommended daily in each of the Basic Four food groups.
- Identify the special diets used for at least five medical conditions.
- Name six things to keep in mind when planning and preparing meals.
- Name eight special diets which may be prescribed for your client, and describe the types of foods that are usually permitted for each.

Nutrition is the sum of those processes which use food for growth, development and maintenance of the body. The body needs food for energy, cell growth, and to feel comfortable and satisfied. The single most important use of food is to provide proper nutrition to the body.

Since the field of nutrition is so very complex, it is recommended that home health aides take in-service courses to learn more about this vital health area. One of the most rapidly growing fields in health care is in nutrition. Hospitals have nutritionists on staff as do other health care facilities such as nursing homes. It is becoming a common practice for hospitals and nursing homes to provide a nutritionally sound plan to patients as part of their discharge instructions. The nutritionist takes into account the age, weight, sex, and medical condition of the patient when setting up a food plan. It is the responsibility of the home health aide to follow this plan.

Some nutritionists recommend that the average diet consist of the following:

25%–30% fat
15% protein
15% simple sugars (such as fruits)
40% complex carbohydrates (pasta, rice, potatoes, and grains)

They further suggest that the amount of fiber, found in whole grains, leafy vegetables, fruits, beans, and peas, be increased in the daily diet. It is thought that fiber flushes out food wastes and may help to prevent cancer of the colon.

In addition, these nutritionists feel that the average individual should have a regular exercise program. A half-hour walk three times a week would be beneficial to keep the body trim. Nutritional therapists know that individual diets must take into account a person's ethnic background and food likes and dislikes. Also to be considered is any physical condition which prevents a client from eating certain foods and requires certain foods as part of the care plan.

the four food groups

There are four basic food groups which must be included in the daily diet, figure 11-1. These food groups are the fruits and vegetables group, the dairy products group, the breads and cereals group, and the meat and meat substitutes group. Each individual needs the nutrients that can only come from a proper balance of the **Basic Four.**

the fruits and vegetables food group

Four servings are recommended daily from the fruits and vegetables group. One or more servings should be of green, leafy vegetables or yellow vegetables. At least one serving of citrus fruit should be eaten daily. Citrus fruits are high in vitamin C. Fruits and vegetables provide roughage to stimulate the digestive system and are high in vitamins and minerals. (Figure 11-2 on page 132 shows good sources of various vitamins.)

the dairy products food group

The dairy products food group consists of milk and milk products. For adults, two servings daily are necessary. Children should have at least three servings. Servings may include butter, cheese, yogurt, skim milk, buttermilk or ice cream. The calcium from milk products is needed to develop strong bones. Other nutrients provided are protein and vitamin D.

the breads and cereals food group

Four daily servings are recommended from the breads and cereals food group. Enriched grain products give iron, protein, carbohydrates and other nutrients used by the body, figure 11-3 on page 134. Foods from this group provide bulk. Bulk makes the stomach feel full and is needed for proper elimination.

the meat and meat substitutes food group

Two daily servings consisting of three ounces each are recommended from the meat and meat substitutes group. Meats or meat substitutes are high protein foods. Lean meats are better for the body. Excess fat should be trimmed away before the meat is cooked. Some fat is needed by the body, but too much can cause a buildup in the veins and arteries. This buildup forces the heart to work much harder to pump blood throughout the body. Eggs are meat substitutes high in iron and protein. The fat substances in eggs cause health problems for certain people. Some authorities advise people to eat only two eggs a week. However, opinions differ on the recommended intake of eggs. Dried beans, legumes and nuts are also substitutes which can add variety to the menu. An excellent source of protein to include one or more times a week is fish.

1. VEGETABLES AND FRUITS

One should select 4 or more servings and include dark green or yellow vegetables and citrus fruit or tomatoes. Usually one-half cup of cooked vegetables, fruits, fruit juices, or small pieces of fresh fruit constitute one serving.

DARK GREEN AND DEEP YELLOW VEGETABLES

Use vegetables raw, cooked, frozen, or canned. This group provides vitamins A, B-complex, C, and E; the minerals calcium, phosphorus, iron, and magnesium and some carbohydrates.

One or more servings daily

asparagus, green	endive, green	peas, green	squash, butternut
broccoli	escarole	peppers, green	sweet potatoes
carrots	kale	and red	turnip greens
chard	mustard greens	pumpkin	wild greens
collards	parsley	spinach	other greens, including salad greens

CITRUS FRUIT AND TOMATOES

This group consists of foods high in vitamin C. It also provides some vitamin A, sugar and cellulose.

One or more servings daily   The best sources are *

cantaloupe	*grapefruit juice	limes	pineapple, raw
watermelon	kumquats	*oranges	*tangerines
*grapefruit	lemons	strawberries, raw	tomatoes and juice

POTATOES AND OTHER VEGETABLES AND FRUITS

Use foods in this group raw, cooked, frozen, canned, or dried. When eaten in fairly large amounts, foods from this group provide carbohydrates, vitamins A, B-complex, C, and K, and some calcium and magnesium.

Two or more servings daily

apples	cabbage, white	eggplant	peaches	radishes
apricots	cauliflower	figs	pears	raisins
artichokes	celery	grapes	persimmons	rhubarb
avocados	cherries	leeks	pineapple, canned	salsify (oyster plant)
bananas	corn, sweet	lettuce	pineapple juice	sauerkraut
beans	cranberries	mushrooms	canned	squash, summer
beets	cucumbers	okra	plums	turnips
berries	currants	onions	potatoes	
brussel sprouts	dates	parsnips	prunes	

2. DAIRY FOODS

Children and pregnant women 3–4 glasses milk; teenagers and lactating mothers 4 or more glasses; adults 2 or more glasses. Cheese and other milk-made foods can be substituted for part of the milk requirement. This group provides proteins, fats, carbohydrate (the latter in the form of lactose), calcium, phosphorus, vitamin A, riboflavin, and vitamin D (in fortified milk). The following dairy foods contain calcium equal to that in one cup of milk.

1 1/3 ounces cheddar-type cheese		
1 pound cream cheese	Milk is available in the following forms:	
1 1/2 cups creamed cottage cheese	whole evaporated	buttermilk
1 cup yogurt	skim condensed	dried

Figure 11-1 The four food groups

3. BREADS AND CEREALS

One should select 4 or more servings. Enriched or whole grain foods with added milk improve nutritional values. This group provides carbohydrates, thiamine, riboflavin, niacin, vitamin B_6, iron, phosphorus, and magnesium.

Four or more servings daily

One serving depends on the particular product. For example, each of the following constitutes one serving: 1 slice of bread, 1 roll, 1 biscuit, about 2/3 cup of cooked cereal, and 1 cup of dry cereal.

breads:	rolls or biscuits made	oatmeal bread	converted rice
whole wheat	with whole wheat or	grits, enriched	other cereals, if
dark rye	enriched flour	cereals:	whole grain or
enriched	flour, enriched	whole wheat	restored
cornmeal, whole	whole wheat, other	rolled oats	noodles, spaghetti,
grain or enriched	whole grain	brown rice	macaroni

4. MEAT GROUP

Select 4 ounces daily. Alternate dried beans, peas or nuts. (Incomplete protein) This group provides protein, iron, copper, phosphorus, vitamins A, B-complex, D and K.

One serving daily (lean meat, poultry, fish)

Usually about 2–3 ounces cooked weight, constitutes one serving. Remove fat and poultry skin.

beef	pork, except	brains, tongue,	fish, shellfish
lamb	bacon and	sweetbreads	lunch meats
mutton	fatback	poultry, such as	such as
veal	variety meats, such as	chicken, duck,	bologna
game	heart, liver, kidney	goose, turkey	liverwurst

Two or more servings weekly (dried beans and peas, nuts, and peanut butter)

dried beans	lentils	peanuts	soya flour and grits
dried peas	nuts	peanut butter	soybeans

Two or more servings weekly (eggs)

Figure 11-1 (*Continued*)

developing good eating habits

Is it possible to look at a person and tell whether that person's body is well nourished? A well-nourished person usually has shiny hair, clear skin, good posture and firm flesh. The person also appears alert and energetic. In order to be well nourished, people must select the correct foods. Lower forms of animals seem to have a natural body wisdom. They eat only those foods which are good for them and they do not overeat. People, however, have so many foods to choose from that they often make mistakes.

Often people living alone do not get the proper nourishment. They may not have the desire to eat, or they may not have the knowledge or energy to prepare nutritious meals, figure 11-4 on page 135.

empty calorie foods

Favorite foods are often oversalted, oversweetened, or high in fat content. Examples of such favorite foods are potato chips, candy, soda, and french fries. Teenagers especially have a tendency to eat these foods. In

VITAMINS	BEST SOURCES	FUNCTIONS
Fat-Soluble Vitamins		
Vitamin A	Vegetables (dark green and deep yellow) Fish liver oils Liver Egg yolk Fruits (yellow)	Essential for: Growth Health of eyes Structure and functioning of the cells of the skin and mucous membranes
Vitamin D	Sunshine Fish liver oil Milk (irradiated) Egg yolk Liver	Essential for: Growth Regulating calcium and phophorus metabolism Building and maintaining normal bones and teeth
Vitamin E	Wheat germ and wheat germ oils Vegetable oils Margarine Legumes Nuts Dark green, leafy vegetables	Not conclusively defined in humans; may affect the red blood cells Recommended for middle-age women as it helps in the metabolism of calcium
Vitamin K	Spinach Kale Cabbage Cauliflower Pork liver	Essential for: Normal clotting of blood
Water-Soluble Vitamins		
Vitamin C (Ascorbic Acid)	Citrus fruits, pineapple Melons and berries Tomatoes Broccoli Green peppers	Essential for: Maintaining strength of blood vessels Health of the teeth and gums Aids in wound healing
Thiamine (B_1)	Wheat germ Lean pork Yeast Legumes Whole grain and enriched cereal products Liver: other organ meats	Essential for: Carbohydrate metabolism Healthy appetite Functioning of nerves

Figure 11-2 Many foods contain more than one vitamin.

VITAMINS	BEST SOURCES	FUNCTIONS
Riboflavin (B$_2$)	Milk, cheese Enriched bread and cereals Yeast Green, leafy vegetables Eggs Liver, kidney, heart	Essential for: Health of skin, eyes and mouth Carbohydrate, fat, and protein metabolism
Niacin (Nicotinic Acid)	Meats (especially organ meats) Poultry and fish Yeast Enriched breads and cereals Peanuts	Essential for: Prevention of pellagra Carbohydrate, fat, and protein metabolism
Vitamin B$_6$ (Pyridoxine)	Wheat germ Liver and kidney Meats Whole grain cereals Soybeans and peanuts	Essential for: Metabolism of proteins
Pantothenic Acid	Heart, liver, kidney Eggs Peanuts Whole grain cereals	Aids various steps in metabolism
Biotin	Organ meats Yeast Mushrooms Peanuts	Aids various steps in metabolism
Vitamin B$_{12}$ (Cobalamin)	Liver, kidney Muscle meats Milk, cheese Eggs	Essential for: Metabolism Healthy red blood cells Treatment of pernicious anemia
Folacin (Folic Acid)	Dark green, leafy vegetables Liver, kidney Yeast	Essential for: The blood-forming system Metabolism

Figure 11-2   (*Continued*)

WORD	DEFINITION	EXAMPLES
CARBOHYDRATES	Sugars or starches which are made up of carbon, hydrogen and oxygen and deliver quick energy to the body.	Found in grains, potatoes, corn, fruits, and sweets
PROTEINS	Compounds composed of amino acids needed for growth and tissue repair.	Found in meats, fish, milk, eggs, nuts, dried beans
FATS	Oily substances made up of glycerin and fatty acids which provide stored energy to the body, and protect vital organs.	Present in meats, butter, milk, peanuts
MINERALS	Inorganic elements essential in tissue building and in regulation of body fluids.	Iron, calcium, sodium, and zinc
VITAMINS	Organic substances which are vital to certain metabolic functions and are needed to prevent deficiency disease. Vitamins are needed only in small amounts but must be obtained from food sources since they are not produced in the body.	Vitamins A, C, B_{12}
WATER	A tasteless, odorless liquid compound of hydrogen and oxygen necessary in the digestive process and to regulate body processes.	
CALORIE	A measure of heat produced by the body when utilizing a specific portion of food.	
METABOLISM	Sum total of processes needed for the breakdown of food and absorption of nutrients.	

Figure 11-3 Knowing terms used in nutrition helps us to understand how the body uses food.

every day language, these foods are called junk foods but the proper descriptive name for them is **empty calorie** foods or hollow calorie foods. Empty calorie foods are high in carbohydrates and fats; they are very low in proteins, minerals, and vitamins—all of which are necessary for good nutrition. Overindulgence in these empty calorie foods leads to poor nutrition.

overeating

Another dietary problem is overeating. Normally, the body can only burn or use a certain number of calories every day. Those calories that are not used are turned into fat tissue. In the United States it has been estimated that as much as 60 percent of the population is ten or more pounds overweight. Excess weight forces the heart to work harder and is a major cause of heart disease.

degenerative diseases

Many degenerative diseases can be traced directly to the kinds and amounts of food eaten. **Degenerative diseases** are those which cause tissues or organs to weaken and become diseased. Included in this category are

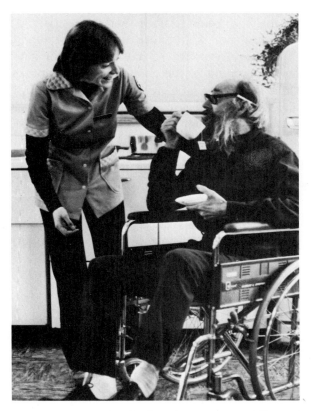

Figure 11-4 People who live alone may especially need encouragement to eat and drink.

diabetes and arteriosclerosis. The most common of all degenerative diseases is tooth decay. Strong, healthy teeth are very important for the proper digestion of food. Eating too much sugar is a main cause of tooth decay.

malnutrition

Malnutrition is poor nourishment which most often occurs when the body does not get a full, balanced diet. Early signs of malnutrition include muscle weakness and a constant feeling of tiredness or fatigue. Later symptoms include a distended or swollen abdomen, a dull film over the eyes, hair that is dry and brittle, and bones that become deformed. A state of malnutrition may occur after a person has gone on a severe weight-reducing diet. This condition is most often found among teenage girls who diet without first consulting a doctor. After a time the lack of nutrients causes serious body fluid imbalances. It can reach a point that the dieter is unable to eat at all, and the body rejects all foods. It may be necessary to hospitalize the person and provide liquid nourishment through intravenous tubes. A long time may be needed before the body systems are again in balance.

the importance of water

One item that many people overlook in their daily diet is water. It is generally recommended that each individual drink between six to ten glasses of water daily. This is necessary for proper digestion; it also helps to maintain proper elimination. Wastes are eliminated from the body by the kidneys. This flushing process is helped by the amount of water taken into the body. Water keeps feces from becoming hardened and decreases the chances of constipation. Water also prevents dehydration.

general guidelines for meal planning

There are some general rules to follow when planning nutritious meals for clients. (Specific strategies for planning and preparing meals and storing foods are discussed in a later unit.) In addition to the general rules listed, the aide should see that an emergency food supply is on hand, figure 11-5. The homemaker/home health aide should take into consideration the ethnic and regional preferences of the client when planning a menu, figure 11-6. A recommended meal planning guide is shown in figure 11-7 on page 139.

The Meat and Meat Substitutes Food Group	Canned meats, poultry, fish, beans, stews, chowders, or other mixed dishes; soups with meat; peanut butter
The Fruits and Vegetables Food Group	Canned vegetables Canned vegetable juices Instant potatoes Instant soups Canned fruits Canned fruit juices Dried fruits
The Dairy Products Food Group	Evaporated milk Dry milk Instant Cocoa Instant or canned puddings
The Breads and Cereals Food Group	Crackers Instant hot cereals Dry cereals (low sugar) Pasta

- Keep a one to two day supply of easily stored quickly prepared food on hand.
- Be sure there are foods from each food group on hand.
- Rotate supplies of food.
- Restock food supply regularly.

Figure 11-5 An emergency food supply for times when the weather is bad or there isn't time to cook. By following this storage plan, the aide will be prepared for the unexpected and be able to meet nutritional needs as well.

eating patterns

Generally, people expect to have three meals a day—breakfast, lunch (dinner), dinner (supper). The midday and evening meals are a cultural choice. For example, farmers who work hard during planting and harvesting often expect and need a hot, full meal at noon. They expend so much effort in the morning that they need to replace energy at noon so they can go back to work. Office workers usually do not need nor want more than a light lunch. They usually prefer to have their main meal in the evening in the comfort of their homes. This gives them a chance to be with their families as they all enjoy a hot meal.

Some older people find that eating the main meal in the evening makes them uncomfortable. They find that they feel better having their main meal at midday and then eating a light meal in the evening. This relieves the feeling of heaviness and discomfort when they go to bed. **Meals-On-Wheels** (a service that brings hot meals to shut-ins and the elderly) usually provide the food at midday for this reason.

Some people prefer to have five or six smaller meals which can be divided into a light breakfast, an early light lunch, a midafternoon snack, a small dinner and a late night snack. Cancer patients are often encouraged to follow this practice. The aide should also remember that persons who are ill may lose their appetites as a result of their condition, figure 11-8.

food allergies

Some foods cause an allergic reaction in certain people. There are individuals whose bodies cannot digest milk or milk products. Others may be unable to eat eggs, strawberries, or foods made with wheat, (Celiac disease). Substitute foods must be found to provide the nutrients normally provided by these foods. Allergies may be a result of an emotional reaction. It may not be possible to determine the emotional cause of the allergy, but substitute foods will have to be used by these persons.

food preparation and appeal

Foods may be prepared in a number of ways. They may be eaten raw. Some can be broiled, baked, fried, boiled, or steamed. Overcooking causes the loss of minerals, vita-

ETHNIC GROUP	BREAD AND CEREAL	EGGS, MEAT FISH, POULTRY	DAIRY PRODUCTS	FRUITS AND VEGETABLES	SEASONINGS, ETC.
Chinese	Rice, Wheat, Millet, Corn, Noodles	Little meat and no beef, Fish, including raw fish, Eggs of hen, duck and pigeon	Water buffalo milk occasionally, Soybean milk, Cheese	Soybeans, soybean sprouts, bamboo sprouts, soy curd cooked in lime water, radish leaves, legumes, vegetables, fruits	Sesame seeds, ginger, almonds, soy sauce
American Black	Hot breads, Cookies, Pastries, cakes, Cereals, White rice corn breads	Chicken, Salt pork, ham, bacon, sausage, Salted salmon, salt herring, fish	Milk and milk products Little cheese	Kale, mustard, turnip greens Cabbage, Hominy grits Dandilion greens	Molasses
Jewish	Noodles Crusty white seeded Rolls Rye bread Pumpernickel bread chalah	Koshered meat (from forequarters and organs from beef, lamb, veal), Milk not eaten at same meal (not a rule for all Jewish people) Fish	Milk and milk products Cheese	Vegetables (sometimes cooked with meat) Fruits	Salt, garlic, dill, parsley
Italian	Crusty white bread Cornmeal and rice (Northern Italy) Pasta (Southern Italy)	Beef veal Chicken Eggs Fish	Milk in coffee Cheese (many different kinds)	Broccoli, zucchini, other squash, eggplant, artichokes, string beans, tomatoes, peppers, asparagus, fresh fruit	Olive oil, vinegar, salt, pepper, garlic

Figure 11-6 Traditional ethnic, regional, and racial food patterns according to the basic four food groups (to be considered in nutritional teaching)

ETHNIC GROUP	BREAD AND CEREAL	EGGS, MEAT FISH, POULTRY	DAIRY PRODUCTS	FRUITS AND VEGETABLES	SEASONINGS, ETC.
Puerto Rican	Rice, beans, noodles, spaghetti, oatmeal, cornmeal	Dry salted codfish, meat, salt pork, sausage, chicken, beef	Coffee with hot milk	Starchy root vegetables, green bananas, plantain, legumes, tomatoes, green pepper, onion, pineapple, papaya, citrus fruits	Lard, herbs, oil, vinegar
Near Eastern	Bulgur (wheat)	Lamb, Mutton, Chicken, fish, eggs	Fermented milk Sour cream, Yogurt, Cheese	Nuts, grape leaves	Sheep's butter, olive oil
Greek	Plain wheat bread	Lamb, Fresh fruit, Pork, poultry, eggs Organ meats	Yogurt, Cheeses, Butter	Onions, tomatoes, legumes	Olive oil, parsley, lemon, vinegar
Mexican	Lime-treated corn	Little meat (ground beef or pork), Poultry, Fish	Cheese, Evaporated milk as beverage for infants	Pinto beans, tomatoes, potatoes, onions, lettuce	Chili pepper, salt, garlic, herbs

Figure 11-6 (*Continued*)

mins and other nutrients. Some meats, particularly pork and chicken, must be thoroughly cooked.

When planning and preparing food the home health aide must always remember that a menu should provide proper nutrition. This is the most important rule. Foods selected must fall within the limits of those foods allowed by the client's medical condition.

When planning and preparing meals, a home health aide should keep the following in mind:

- variety
- appearance
- flavor and aroma
- satiety (hunger satisfaction)
- individual preferences
- food costs
- four food groups

variety. Variety is necessary to avoid dulling the appetite. People become bored with the same menu day after day. This can cause a loss of interest in food. It is important for sick people to receive appealing meals. The same nutrients can usually be obtained from a variety of foods. Variety in the menu helps improve the client's interest in eating.

appearance. Appearance is the way food looks when it is served. Nicely arranged food

Breakfast
1 serving vitamin C-rich fruit or vegetable
1–2 servings Breads and Cereals Group
1 serving Dairy Products Group
Coffee or tea (optional)

Lunch or Supper
½–1 serving Meat and Meat Substitutes Group
1 serving Fruits and Vegetables Group
1 serving Breads and Cereals Group
1 serving Dairy Products Group
Coffee or tea (optional)

Dinner
1 serving Meat and Meat Substitutes Group
2 servings Fruits and Vegetables Group (try to
    have dark green leafy or orange vegetables and
    fruit 3–4 times a week)
1–2 servings Breads and Cereals Group
Coffee or tea (optional)

Dessert and Snack Suggestions

Yogurt	Vegetables
Ice cream	Bread or crackers
Pudding	Meat
Cheese	Nuts
Fruit	

Figure 11-7   Recommended meal planning guide

adds to the pleasure and enjoyment of eating. When foods are overcooked they become mushy and unappetizing to look at. At the same time overcooking destroys many of the nutrients. Overcooked meats become tough and lose flavor. Foods that appeal to the eye perk up the appetite. Properly cooked vegetables, for example, retain their natural color. The color enhances the appearance of the vegetables on the plate. The attractiveness of the meal can be illustrated by two examples. Imagine a plate of food consisting of a chicken breast, mashed potatoes, white bread and cauliflower. This meal would be nutritious but it would

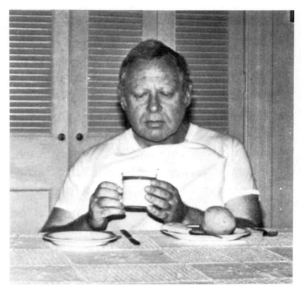

Figure 11-8   Illness often causes a loss of appetite.

look dull and colorless. If the potatoes and cauliflower were replaced by a garden salad and string beans, the meal would look much brighter and more appealing.

flavor and aroma.   Flavor and aroma set the digestive juices into action. Seasonings most often used are salt, pepper and garlic. However, there are many herbs, such as thyme, rosemary, parsley and sage which can be added to bring out the aroma and sharpen the flavor. Often these herbs and spices can be used when a client is on a salt-free diet. Fresh lemon juice can be squeezed over meat and vegetables also. Since both sight and smell affect the appetite, proper use of seasonings can be of value in planning a menu.

satiety.   Satisfying the pangs of hunger is another reason people eat. There are some foods which make the stomach feel full but not uncomfortable. This feeling is called **satiety.** If daily menus are well planned, the satiety value will be provided. Bulk foods such as bread, macaroni, beans and spaghetti are good fillers.

individual preferences. A very important factor in meal planning is providing foods that the person likes to eat. There is no logic to explain why some people like certain foods and dislike others. There are individuals who want steak served rare, while others will only eat it well done. Some people dislike spinach, cabbage, beets or mushrooms. The home health aide must try to prepare those foods which the client likes, cooked as the client likes them.

food costs. In most homes, it is necessary to work within a budget. Therefore, it is important to check newspaper ads for daily specials and seasonal bargains. Fresh fruits and vegetables are lower in price during the summer and fall. At other times it is more economical to purchase frozen, canned or dried items, such as powdered milk. If money is a consideration, then planning and purchasing must be worked around the prices. Careful planning makes it possible to meet nutritional needs while keeping costs at a minimum.

diet therapy

There are medical conditions which require special diets. The home health aide must carefully follow directions in preparing special diets. The aide should try to vary the menus and make the food look attractive. Flavor and aroma of the food should be maintained. Meals should satisfy hunger while taking into consideration the client's food preferences. However, it may not always be possible to meet all of these conditions. There may be times when the client begs the home health aide for "just a little taste" of a forbidden food. At such times, the aide should gently and kindly refuse the client's request. An answer to such a plea might be, "I know you would rather have something else, but it would not be wise to go off your special diet. See if the doctor will add new foods." An attractively arranged tray may stimulate the appetite of a client whose diet is limited.

special diets

Special diets may be ordered by the doctor to meet a client's specific health needs. A description of some special diets follows. Figure 11-9 lists recommended foods and foods to avoid for these special diets.

low-fat (fat-controlled) diet. A low-fat diet is required for those with gallbladder conditions, heart disease and hypertension.

diabetic diet. A **diabetic diet** calls for using measured amounts of the Basic Four food groups. All foods must be carefully measured. Sugar or foods high in sugar such as sugar-cured ham and many sweetened, dry cereals must be limited or avoided. A prescribed diet list is supplied by the doctor.

calorie-controlled diet. A **calorie-controlled diet** may be ordered for an obese person or a malnourished person. The calorie count is very low for the obese person and high for the person who is underweight. The individual client's needs and characteristics (age, sex, height, type of work done, and weight) determine the size of the portion served and the total intake of calories. Whatever the size of the servings or the prescribed caloric intake, proper selections must be made from the Basic Four food groups. It should be remembered that very active children burn more calories per day than an aging person who is confined to bed.

bland diet. A person with a peptic ulcer is kept on a **bland diet.** The foods allowed are served without strong spices, and usually contain milk and milk products.

low-residue diet. A **low-residue diet** is one in which tough fiber foods are kept at a

DIET	GENERAL USE	FOODS ALLOWED	FOODS TO AVOID
Low-calorie	Overweight	skim milk, fresh fruits, lean meat or fish, vegetables, 1–2 servings cereal per day	fried foods, rich gravies and sauces, jams, jellies, rich desserts
High-calorie	Underweight	peanut butter, egg nog, jellies, ice cream, desserts, frequent snacks, milk shakes	none
Bland	stomach or intestinal problems; ulcers	milk, cream, buttermilk, cottage cheese, cream cheese, mild cheddar cheese, butter, eggs (not fried), beef, lamb, veal, chicken, fish, liver (only tender meats, roasted, boiled or broiled), refined cereals, macaroni, white rolls, crackers (unsalted), cream soups, white potatoes, peas, tender carrots, most fruit juices, canned fruits, peaches, pears, puddings, custards	highly seasoned, fried foods, raw vegetables and fruit, whole grains and cereals
Diabetic	diabetes	canned fruits without sugar, fresh fruits, regular meat, vegetables, bread, sugarless gelatin, custards	foods containing sugar, alcoholic beverages, gravy, sauces, chocolate, carbonated beverages
Low-sodium	fluid retention; heart problems	foods cooked without salt, regular meat, vegetables, fruits, salt substitute if doctor prescribes	smoked, cured, canned meats, cold cuts, cheese, potato chips, pickles, bouillon, prepared mustard, catsup, commercial salad dressings, soy sauce
Low-fat	gallbladder; liver disease; heart disease; hypertension	veal, poultry, fish, skim milk, buttermilk, yogurt, low-fat cottage cheese, fat-free soup broth, fresh fruits and vegetables, cereals, gelatin, angel cake, ices, carbonated beverages, coffee, tea, jams, jellies	fatty meats, bacon, butter, whole milk, cheese, kidney, liver, heart, fried foods, rich desserts, sauces
Clear-liquid	postoperative	tea or black coffee with sugar, apple juice, plain gelatin (no fruit), fat-free broth	solid foods
Full-liquid	convalescents; chewing problems	all foods in clear-liquid diet, strained juices, milk, cream, buttermilk, eggnog, strained cream soups, strained cereal (gruel), cocoa, carbonated beverages, ices, ice cream, gelatin, custard puddings, sherbets, milk shakes, bouillon	solid foods
Soft	convalescents; gastrointestinal conditions; chewing problems	milk, cream, butter, mild cheeses (cottage, cream cheeses), eggs, (not fried), soup, broth, strained cream soups, tender cooked vegetables, fruit juices, cooked fruits, bananas, grapefruit and oranges peeled with all section skins removed, enriched white bread, refined cereals, cooked cereals, spaghetti, noodles, macaroni, pasta, tea, coffee, carbonated beverages, sherbets, ices, sponge cake, tender chicken, fish, ground beef or lamb, only small amounts of salt and spices	fibrous meat, coarse cereals, fried foods, raw fruits and vegetables, rich pastries

Figure 11-9 Special diets

DIET	GENERAL USE	FOODS ALLOWED	FOODS TO AVOID
Low-residue	postoperative; colitis	milk, buttermilk (2 cups daily), butter, mild cheeses, tender chicken, fish, ground beef, ground lamb, soup broths, fruit juices, refined breads and cereals, macaroni, noodles, custards, sherbet, vanilla ice cream, tapioca pudding, sponge cake, plain cookies, mild flavored vegetables	fried foods, fresh fruits and vegetables, fibrous meats, nuts
High-bulk	constipation	whole grain breads and cereals, raw and cooked vegetables, fruit juices, water, milk, protein-rich foods, bran or bran flakes	
High-potassium	potassium loss due to medication; kidney disease	fresh fruits and vegetables, especially bananas and raisins	canned tomato juice, raw clams, sardines, frozen lima beans, frozen peas, canned spinach, canned carrots

Note: This chart is a general guide to special diets. Always follow the doctor's prescribed diet plan.

Figure 11-9 *(Continued)*

minimum. It is low in vitamins and is used only as long as needed to clear up a condition in the intestinal tract. Clients with colitis or diverticulitis may be on low residue diets. There is very little waste product in this diet. Examples of food allowed in the low-residue diet are strained and cooked vegetables, custards, mild cheeses and tender meats. As soon as possible, normal bulk foods are added.

high-potassium diet. Persons with high blood pressure are treated with a drug called a **diuretic.** A diuretic helps to lower blood pressure by washing salt from the body. However, it also causes potassium to be flushed from the body. The loss of potassium may cause muscle cramps and muscular weakness. Some older persons not taking diuretics, persons with kidney disease, or persons taking the drug digitalis may also need added potassium in their diets. Very often this can be provided by eating foods high in potassium.

Most fruits are high in potassium; bananas and raisins are especially high in potassium. Fresh vegetables, raw or cooked, are also good sources of natural potassium and are included in a high potassium diet.

liquid diets. A person recovering from an illness, injury or a surgical wound may require a light, easily digested diet. Especially after surgery, the body needs to be treated very carefully. Postsurgical patients are usually put on a **clear liquid diet.** Liquids which are light and easy to digest such as broth, tea, and apple juice are given. As the patient becomes better, a **full-liquid diet** is prescribed. Milk, pudding and strained cream soups are added to the clear liquid diet.

soft diet. After the patient is able to tolerate a full liquid diet, the **soft diet** is prescribed. Soft boiled eggs, toast and other easily digested foods are added. As the body heals, the patient can gradually return to eating a regular diet. Clients with chewing problems or gastrointestinal conditions may also be on a soft diet.

high-bulk diet. Another special diet is the **high-bulk diet.** Elderly clients or clients on bedrest are often prescribed high-bulk diets. Bulk is helpful for providing good bowel elimination.

1. Use foods from the Four Food Groups, however, use no salt in preparation.

2. All foods contain natural sodium. Some have a higher salt content than others and should not be served at all or else should be served only in small quantities.

3. Examples of foods that **ARE** permitted:
   - Regular meats
   - Fresh vegetables and fruits (except celery, beets, beet greens, kale, spinach, sauerkraut)
   - Low-sodium bread and rolls
   - Oatmeal, puffed rice, puffed wheat, shredded wheat
   - Fresh fruit juices
   - Fresh fish
   - Macaroni, spaghetti
   - Honey, jellies,
   - Unsalted nuts

   (A list of acceptable foods is usually provided by the doctor.)

4. Examples of foods that should be **AVOIDED**:
   - Salt at table or in cooking.
   - Crackers and other baked products with salt toppings.
   - American and all other processed cheeses, cheese foods, cheese spreads. Highly salted cheeses such as camembert, parmesan, roquefort. (Natural cheeses such as brie, cheddar, mozzarella, muenster, port du salut, swiss, cottage cheese, cream cheese, ricotta may be used in moderation.)
   - Bacon, bacon fat, salt pork.
   - Salty or smoked fish such as anchovies, caviar, salted and dried cod, herring, sardines.
   - Salty or smoked meats such as bacon, ham, pastrami, corned beef, smoked tongue, lunch meats (cold cuts), frankfurters, sausages. Meats koshered by salting. Frozen and canned dinners, stews, hash, etc.
   - Salted popcorn, salted nuts, potato chips and pretzels with salt coatings. Party spreads and dips and other salted snacks and appetizers.
   - Canned, dried or frozen soups; cube, powdered or liquid bouillon.
   - Sauerkraut and pickled vegetables.
   - Seasonings and relishes such as barbecue sauce, bouillon made with salt, catsup, celery salt, chili sauce, cooking wine, garlic salt, meat and vegetable extracts, meat sauces, meat tenderizers, monosodium glutamate, prepared mustard, olives, onion salt, pickles, pickle and tomato relishes, soy sauce, Worcestershire sauce.

Figure 11-10 Guidelines for a low-sodium diet. (Adapted from *Your Mild Sodium-Restricted Diet,* American Heart Association, 1973.)

low-sodium (sodium-restricted) diet. **Low-sodium diets** are prepared without salt. **They may be prescribed when the client has a heart condition, kidney disease, or suffers from hypertension. Some clients on a low-sodium diet are able to use salt substitutes. Guidelines for a low-sodium diet are given in figure 11-10.**

- Food is a major part of recreation and is sometimes the main feature of a social occasion. However, the true purpose of food is to provide the fuel needed by the body in order to keep the body machinery working.

- A practicing home health aide must be aware of the client's need for suitable nutrition.
- The aide must be able to prepare and serve those foods which are best for each client.
- Aides should also understand the importance of maintaining the right kind of nutrition needed by their own bodies. The kind of foods eaten determine how well the body systems function.
- A home health aide can provide better care for clients by making sure that the necessary nutrients are being provided.
- The aide must also know the special diets that may be required by some clients.

review

1. Foods from the Basic Four food groups must be included in the daily diet.
   a. List the Basic Four food groups.
   b. Indicate the number of daily servings recommended from each food group.
   c. Give two examples of foods included in each food group.
2. Name four considerations for making the client's meals appealing.
3. Name six special diets that may be ordered to meet a client's specific health needs.
4. A client with a gallbladder problem may be placed on what type of special diet?
5. Foods cooked without salt are to be included in what type of special diet?

Unit 12
Principles of Safety and Body Mechanics

key terms

hazard	immobilize	extinguish
body mechanics	cyanosis	evacuate

learning objectives

After studying this unit, you should be able to:
- Identify five causes of accidents around the home.
- Name two conditions in aging which may contribute to the incidence of accidents.
- State the basic rules to follow in the event of a home fire.
- Define and demonstrate good body mechanics.

According to the National Safety Council, at least 4 million persons are injured each year in home accidents. This means that about one person in 50 suffers some kind of injury as a result of an accident that takes place in the person's home. As many as 8000 people die each year because of falls.

common hazards

In addition to actual physical hazards, there are human factors which are directly related to many home accidents. Statistics show that certain kinds of accidents happen most often in some age groups. Most of the accidents identified in figure 12-1 could be avoided. Young children must be carefully watched at all times. Parents should be aware of the actions of teenagers. Adults should use good judgment and not attempt to do too many things at one time. Carelessness and accidents go hand-in-hand. Since home health aides are caring for clients in the home, they should be aware of potential **hazards** in this environment.

An aide should be aware of the effects of medication on the client. Sometimes muscle relaxants or tranquilizers can cause the client to become unsteady so that they may fall if they get up from a chair or bed without assistance. If an aide observes that a client becomes disoriented and loses balance easily after taking medication, she/he should inform the supervisor immediately. Sometimes clients are over-medicated because of too many med-

Age	Accidents
Infants up to 1 year are physically active and willing to touch or taste most anything.	Falls from a bed or table Burns from stoves or heaters Swallowing small objects Small objects stuffed in ears Smothering in bedding/pillows Cuts from sharp pointed toys Choking on candies or food, toys or coins
Preschool children are curious and extremely active. They explore most everything by looking, tasting, and touching. They have few fears and no judgment.	Scalding from pulling pot handles on stove. Electrocution from playing with electrical cords and outlets Burns from stove or radiators or playing with matches Poisoning from pesticides or cleaning supplies, lead based paint chips, medicines Falls from chairs, tables, countertops, open windows or falls into deep holes in ground Drowning in unattended pools Smothering in discarded refrigerators, freezers, and plastic bags Cuts from kitchen knives
Preteen children are adventurous and not aware of dangers. They become involved in play and do not watch for hazards.	Injuries from bicycle and auto accidents. Hit by car when darting into street or between parked cars Poisoning Drowning
Teenagers like to experiment and are influenced by their peers (others in their age group). They like to show off and are careless.	Injuries from auto, motorbike, or bicycle accidents because of carelessness, drunkenness, or drug abuse Wounds from accidents with guns Burns from careless smoking habits Injuries from carelessness with tools and machinery Drug overdose
Adults have fewer accidents since learning is based on experiences. Self-control and judgment are better developed, but overconfidence, negligence, and carelessness may cause accidents.	Burns from careless use of outside fire, and inside fireplace; from overloading electrical circuits; from smoking in bed Electrical shock from attempting to repair home appliances Using table or chair for climbing instead of sturdy ladder Automobile accidents from carelessness or drunkenness Poisoning or drug abuse from failure to read labels
Old age causes many changes within the body; bones are brittle, eyesight and hearing may fail. Minor accidents may cause great bodily harm.	Falls Burns Cuts and bruises Poisoning because labels can't be seen due to poor eyesight

Figure 12-1   Age-group related accidents

ications or too high a dosage of a single medicine. If no one tells the doctor, the client may be in danger.

The aide must also watch out for a client who may try to take additional medication. Clients that are confused will not remember if they have taken a particular medication. For this reason, it is best to keep medications out of such clients' rooms and bring them the proper medicine at the prescribed time. Overmedication can be just as bad as undermedication.

falls

As the human body ages, the bones become brittle and break easily. Broken hips are a common disability of the elderly.

Many clients cared for may need canes, walkers or wheelchairs. There are a number of accidents that may happen to persons using these aids. Before allowing the client to use a cane, walker, crutches, or other device, make certain that each rubber tip is firmly in place and has not worn through.

Some hazards may be avoided by providing a safer environment. Stairways and landings should be kept uncluttered. Children's toys, such as skateboards, balls, blocks, and roller skates, must be put away after use. Waxed and polished floors and stairways can be very dangerous. Scatter rugs in hallways should have a skid-proof backing or be removed if older people are in the home. Spills on kitchen and bathroom floors should be wiped up at once so that falls may be avoided.

Do not permit the client to walk about with untied shoelaces, figure 12-2. Tripping over the laces can result in serious injury in the elderly. If the client cannot reach the laces to tie them, even with the use of aids designed for this purpose, the homemaker/home health

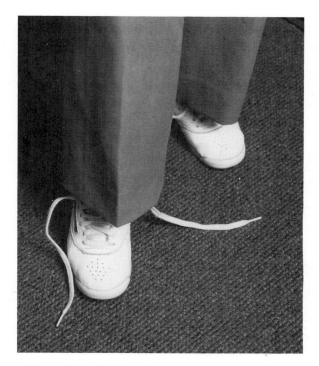

Figure 12-2 Tie those laces and prevent an accident

aide should tie the laces so they do not present a hazard.

The bathroom is one of the most dangerous rooms in the house as far as accidents are concerned. Bath mats should have a rubber backing so they won't skid. Bathtubs should be equipped with nonskid rubber strips to decrease the danger of slipping when getting in and out of the bath. For older persons, special hand rails should be installed to assist them as they use the tub or shower, figure 12-3. A bath chair should be provided for some elderly clients. Faucets for hot water should be clearly marked so that accidental scalding will not occur. Special elevated toilet seats and handrails make it easier for clients to use the toilet safely, figure 12-4a and 12-4b.

When transferring a client from bed to wheelchair, the home health aide must remember to lock the wheels, figure 12-5. The client

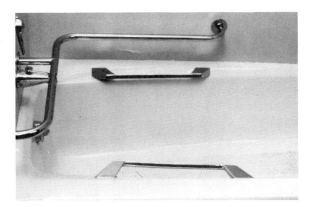

Figure 12-3 Safety features for the tub may include several types of bars and nonskid strips to allow the client to get into and out of the tub safely.

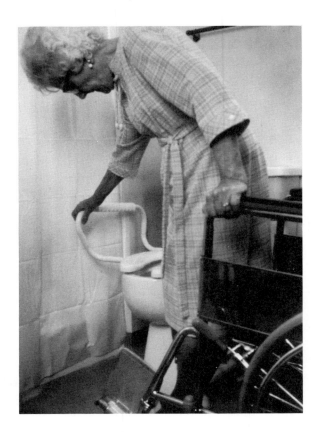

Figure 12-4b Client transferring from a wheelchair to the toilet finds the handrails helpful in providing stability.

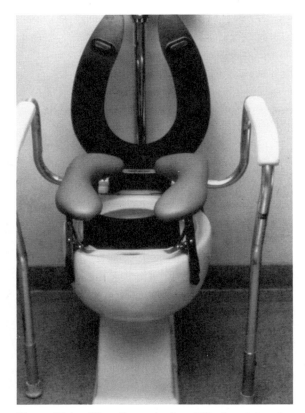

Figure 12-4a The client who has difficulty sitting down finds it easier to use the toilet because of the elevated seat and handrails.

is less likely to fall if the chair remains still. Carelessness on the part of a home health aide can cause accidents, either to the client or to the home health aide.

If a client does suffer a fall and if a cast is used to *immobilize* the broken bones, the home health aide should check the skin around the cast frequently for signs of irritation such as redness or swelling. Skin areas below the cast must be observed for signs of *cyanosis,* unusual coldness, or any unusual odor which may indicate a serious problem. These signs and any complaints of numbness should be reported to the supervisor.

Elderly or debilitated clients may need assistance in sitting safely in chairs or wheel-

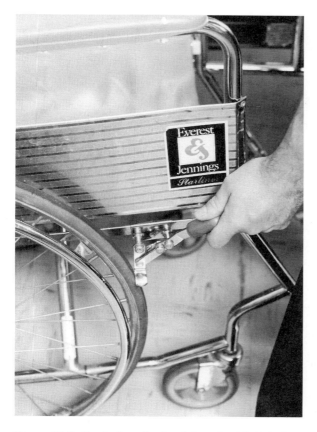

Figure 12-5 Lock the wheels of the wheelchair before transferring the client to the chair

chairs or to keep from falling out of bed. Numerous safety products are available for these situations, figures 12-6 to 12-8. The home health aide must be aware, however, that the physician must order the use of the safety product. The care plan for the client will indicate if the use of safety products has been approved by the physician. Under no circumstances is the home health aide to initiate the use of such items.

fire

Few words are more frightening to hear than "fire, fire!" The smell of smoke or the flash of flames from the kitchen stove can cause

panic. Some people are stunned and unable to function. Others rush around wildly trying to save their belongings. Figure 12-9 on page 153 gives safety precautions which can help prevent fires in the home. The homemaker/home health aide should advise the client and/or the client's family whenever a fire safety problem is noticed. If necessary, report your concerns to your supervisor so the family can be notified.

As a home health aide, there are basic rules to follow in case a client's home, or something in it, catches on fire, figure 12-10 on page 156. Remaining calm is the first and most important rule. Lives can be saved if an emergency plan has been made beforehand. A home health aide, upon entering a client's home, should make note of the nearest exit from each room. The telephone number of the fire department should be placed close to the telephone, figure 12-11 on page 157.

The aide must consider the client's condition and decide the best way to move the client in case of a fire. At the time of the fire, other decisions must also be made:

1. Decide if the client or family members are in immediate danger. If so, *evacuate* them at once.
2. If the client cannot be safely moved, place a damp towel over the client's mouth and nose to lessen the danger of smoke inhalation. If there is heavy smoke, try to move the client's bed to a less smoky area, or move the client to the floor where the smoke is less concentrated. Remember, smoke rises, and if it is inhaled for a long period, it can cause death.
3. Determine if the fire is major. If it is minor, put it out at once, following the directions given in figure 12-10.
4. Decide if there is time to call the fire department before evacuating the client. If there is no time, move the client and call the fire department from a phone outside the house.

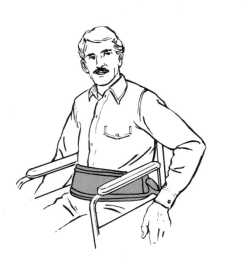

SOFT BELT
For bed or wheelchair

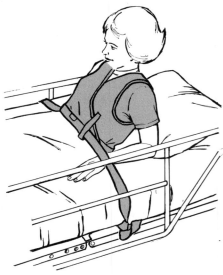

BUDGET VEST
For bed or wheelchair

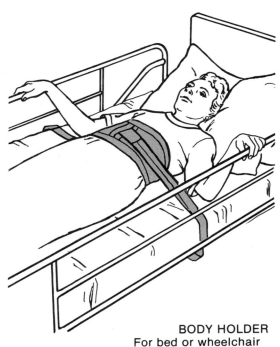

BODY HOLDER
For bed or wheelchair

HOUDINI
For bed or wheelchair

Figure 12-6 Patient safety products (courtesy of J. T. Posey Company, Arcadia, CA)

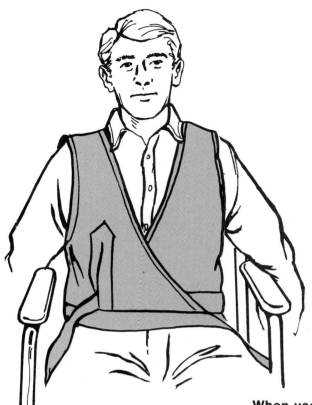

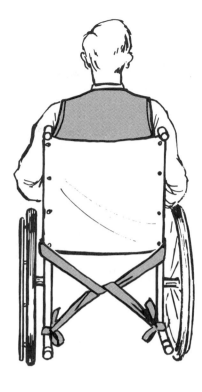

1 Always put the vest on so the straps criss-cross in front.

Be sure that the vest is the proper size for the patient. The vertical seams under the arm holes should be under the patient's arms. All Posey vests are color-coded by size:

SIZE	COLOR	WEIGHT
Small	Pink/Red	To 130 lbs.
Medium	Green	120-170 lbs.
Large	Yellow	160-210 lbs.
X-Large	Blue	200 lbs. and up

Belts are not color-coded but are sized the same.

2 When used for a patient in a wheelchair, position the patient's hips at the rear of the seat, and pass vest straps through the slots at the sides of the seat. From behind the wheelchair, draw the straps toward the back, bringing them around the rear legs, crossing over each other, and then secure them to the kick spurs.

IMPORTANT: Be sure that the vest is not too tight. You should be able to place four fingers (with your hand flat) between the patient's abdomen and the bottom of the vest.

When used for a patient in bed, position the patient so that his or her hips are at the center of the bed— where they would be if the bed were elevated. Bring the straps directly over the sides of the bed, wrap once or twice around the bed spring frame, then secure the end of the straps about 6-8″ toward the foot of the bed and 6-8″ in from the sides of the bed.*

IMPORTANT: Do not angle the straps toward the head or foot of the bed. If the patient slides up or down in bed the straps will loosen.

* See figure 12-8 for correct method of tying straps to the bed springs.

Figure 12-7 Correct application of patient safety products (courtesy of J. T. Posey Company, Arcadia, CA)

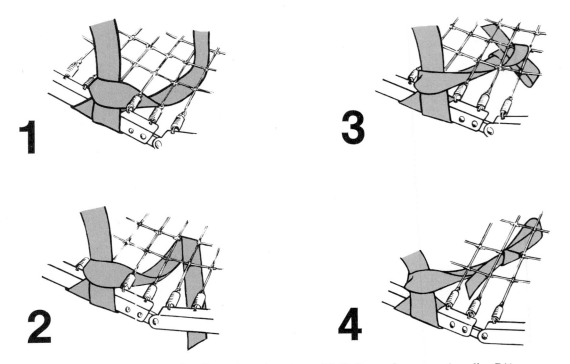

Figure 12-8   How to tie a Posey knot (courtesy of J. T. Posey Company, Arcadia, CA)

Waiting for the fire department to arrive is difficult for the aide and family members. Under no circumstances should the home health aide return to the burning building. Family members and neighbors should also be stopped from returning to the building. No personal possession is valuable enough to risk a human life.

fire extinguishers.   Small fires may be extinguished by using a fire extinguisher. There are four main types of fire extinguishers, each of which is used for a specific type of fire.

1. **Class A extinguishers** contain water that is under pressure. They are used to douse fires involving paper, wood, or cloth.

2. **Class B extinguishers** contain carbon dioxide. They are used to put out fires caused by igniting gasoline, oil, paints or other liquids, and cooking fats. These types of fires would spread if water were used to extinguish them. The carbon dioxide smothers the fire, leaving a snowy residue. These extinguishers should be used with caution, since the residue they leave may irritate the skin and eyes. Fumes may also be dangerous to inhale.

3. **Class C extinguishers** contain dry chemicals and are used on electrical fires.

4. **Class ABC** or **combination extinguishers** contain a graphitelike chemical. They can be used on any type of fire. The residue that results from their use can cause irritation of the skin and eyes.

Here's how to be
BURN WISE!

The majority of burns *can* be prevented. Being *burn wise* is the best way to avoid serious burns. Burn prevention is the most effective way to be *burn wise* but knowing what to do if you are burned is also important. The National Fire Protection Association suggests three ways to protect your client:

1. correct any household hazards you find
2. practice client escape planning
3. teach your client fire-safe behavior

Here are some information and activities to make you *burn wise*.

Safety Tips to Tell Your Client

The Kitchen
- Never leave small appliances with the cords hanging over the edge or within sight of a child.
- Never leave heat-producing appliances (such as a toaster oven) plugged in. If the starter button is accidentally hit, it could start a fire. This is especially dangerous if it is covered with a decorative cover.
- Pot handles should always be turned inward so that they cannot be pulled down by a child or knocked off by an adult.
- Never use the stove when wearing loose-fitting clothing. Always tie back long hair.
- Salt, pepper, and other spices should not be stored on top of the stove where someone must reach across a flame for them.
- Always cover a frying pan with a frying screen to prevent a burn from spattered grease.
- When lighting a gas stove: always stand to the side; use long matches, if possible, to light the stove; when frying, always keep a lid cover and baking soda close at hand.
- If grease catches on fire and the flame is minimal, cover the frying pan with a lid and smother the flame. If the flame becomes bigger, throw baking soda on it, evacuate, and call for help!
- Always use pot holders to remove pots and pans. Do not store them over the stove where they may catch on fire.
- When cooking with only 1 or 2 burners on the stove, always use the back ones.
- Put a *child safety lock* on all cabinets which are used to store chemicals such as cleaning agents. *Chemicals can cause severe burns!*
- Hot water can cause very serious burns. If infants and small children are bathed in the sink: obtain all necessary equipment before beginning; test the temperature of the water before placing the child in it; and *do not leave the child alone for any amount of time.* If you must leave the sink, take the child with you. Left alone, children may burn themselves.
- With small children around, use placemats instead of table cloths.

Figure 12-9 Preventing burns (Reprinted by permission of The Burn Center at New York Hospital—Cornell Medical Center, 535 East 68th Street, New York, NY)

The kitchen is an important and busy workplace in the home. Children should not be allowed to play in the kitchen. It only takes a second to trip over a small child.

Living Room

- Wires should not be left running under a rug. Walking on the rug will eventually fray the wire and possibly cause the rug to catch on fire.
- Replace frayed wires immediately.
- Attachments added to an outlet to increase the number of plugs are potentially very hazardous.
- Outlets not in use should be covered with child safety covers to prevent children from putting their fingers in the openings.
- Fireplaces must be covered by a protective screen at all times. Magazines and newspapers should never be left near the fireplace as a spark can ignite them.
- Never allow small children to be left unattended in a room where a fireplace is in use.
- DO NOT CONSUME HOT LIQUIDS WHILE HOLDING A CHILD! Keep children at a safe distance from all hot liquids—they make very quick movements.

Bedroom

- NEVER SMOKE IN BED!
- If you must use a space heater be sure that it is a safety-approved model and in good working order. Do not leave small children or pets unattended in the room with a heater in use, and never place a space heater on a rug or near curtains or other flammable materials.
- Never drape clothing over lamps.

Holidays

Increased activity and excitement often make people less careful just when they should be most cautious. Please take care all the time, but especially during holidays.

- Remember that Christmas trees are cut early in the season and quickly dry out to become fire hazards. Never put the Christmas tree in front of *any* exit.
- Never decorate Christmas trees with candles even if you do not intend to light them. Don't tempt someone else.
- Only buy Christmas tree lights which have been inspected by the Underwriters Laboratory. Inspect and test them each year before putting them on the tree.
- Never leave the Christmas tree lights on when you go out at night. If a wire should short out you might return to find your home on fire!
- Never place a Christmas tree near a fireplace. If there is no other place to put it, do not use the fireplace until the tree has been removed and the needles cleaned up.
- Never leave religious or holiday candles burning while unattended.
- When using a barbeque, *never* apply additional lighter fluid once the fire has been lit.

Miscellaneous Hints

- All children become curious about fire and should be taught about matches and fire safety. Teach children that matches are tools, not toys. They should be instructed in the proper way to strike a match and told not to do so except under the supervision of an adult. Matches should be stored in unattractive containers out of children's sight or reach.

Figure 12-9   *(Continued)*

- Water heaters should be lowered to 120–130°F. Thermostatically-controlled faucets and shower heads should be installed particularly in the homes of elderly or handicapped people.
- Smoke detectors are a vital part of being *burn wise*. Experts recommend one per floor in *every* home or office.

First Aid—What to Do

If you catch on fire:
DON'T PANIC. DON'T RUN— RUNNING WILL INCREASE THE FLAMES. *Instead:*
1. **Stop**
2. **Drop** to the ground.
3. **Roll.** Continue to roll until you have completely put out the fire.
4. Remove clothing from the affected area. *Do not* attempt to remove clothing that sticks.
5. Flush area with cool water.
6. Cover with a sterile pad or a clean sheet.
7. *Seek immediate medical attention.*

If the burn is from a chemical:
1. Follow steps 4–7 and be sure to flush with cool water for 20–30 minutes.
2. If the eyes are involved, flush the eyes for at least 20 minutes or until medical attention arrives.
3. Remove contact lenses.

If the burn is electrical:
1. Turn off electrical source before touching victim.
2. Check for breathing and pulse. If absent, start Cardiopulmonary Resuscitation (C.P.R.), if qualified.
3. Follow steps 4–7.

Home Fire Escape Plan
- **Develop a Family Escape Plan**
- **Include 2 exits from each room**
- **Plan a meeting place outside the home**
- **Practice the plan**

Plan of Escape:
Evacuate!
Do not attempt to fight the fire.
1. If in bed, roll off onto floor.
2. Stay low! Crawl if necessary. Smoke rises, and oxygen will remain near the floor.
3. Cover your mouth and nose with some clothing or material to aid in breathing.
4. Place your hands on any closed door before opening it. If it is hot *do not open!* Find another exit. If it is not hot, open it slowly, standing to the side. *Do not use elevators.*
5. *If you are trapped in a room:*
   a. Roll a rug or other materials and place across the bottom of the door
   b. Open a window, both top and bottom, to allow air to enter and smoke to escape.
   c. Telephone for help, if possible.
   d. Attract attention and call for help.
(For further information call 212-472-6890)

Figure 12-9 *(Continued)*

1. Know the location of the nearest fire alarm box in the area.
2. Know how to phone for the fire department.
3. Remember the location of the nearest exits.
4. Close any door which will tend to confine the fire.
5. See that everyone is out of danger.
6. Know where a fire extinguisher is located and how to operate it. Check batteries of smoke alarms regularly.
7. Never try to fight a fire in a room filled with smoke; the fumes and lack of air are dangerous.
8. Never try to enter a room where much fire is in evidence.
9. Remember that a woolen blanket or other heavy covering will help to smother a small fire.
10. Keep pound boxes of inexpensive baking soda handy to extinguish kitchen fires. The boxes can be kept in the refrigerator so you will always be able to find them.
11. Use baking soda instead of water to extinguish small grease, oil, paint, varnish, and similar fires because water spreads such a fire. Dust the flames with baking soda; this smothers the flames physically and chemically with carbon dioxide gas.
12. Smother small grease fires in cooking utensils by covering them with a lid or long-handled pan, or by throwing baking soda on the blaze.
13. Extinguish small broiling pan fires by first turning off oven and then throwing handfuls of baking soda on the blaze.
14. Throw baking soda on small fires in ash trays, waste baskets or upholstered furniture.
15. Do not try to be a hero. If the small fire does not respond to your efforts to extinguish it immediately, remove the client and yourself from the house as quickly as possible. Call the fire department from a neighbor's house or flag down passing motorists and ask them to call.

Figure 12-10   Basic rules for the home health aide to follow in case of fire in the client's home

If an aide uses a fire extinguisher on a minor fire, the manufacturer's operating instructions must be carefully followed. Most extinguishers have a lock on the handle which must be unlocked before use, figure 12-12. The extinguisher should be held firmly and the nozzle aimed at the near edge of the fire. **Caution:** Do not aim toward the center of the fire. Discharge the extinguisher, using a slow, side-to-side motion, until the fire has been extinguished. Avoid contact with the chemical residues from the extinguisher. To prevent personal injury, the aide should always stay a safe distance from the fire.

Once an extinguisher has been used in a fire, it must be replaced or recharged. Notify your agency of the need for replacement.

If the fire extinguisher has a gauge, like the one shown in figure 12-12, check the gauge periodically to be sure the extinguisher is fully charged.

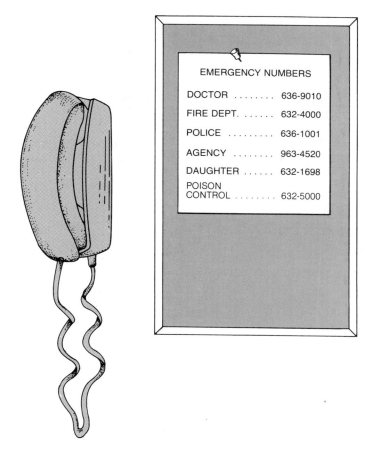

Figure 12-11 Important phone numbers posted next to the phone may save precious moments at the time of an emergency. Check your local directory for the correct numbers.

To review the prevention of common household hazards in every room of the house, see figures 12-13 to 12-20.

principles of good body mechanics

The way in which the body moves and keeps its balance through the use of all its parts is referred to as **body mechanics.** When the human body is used incorrectly, the bones, muscles, and organs are thrown out of alignment. Use of body mechanics means that each part of the body works together. Some muscles are better at pushing than pulling. The body organs are held in their cavities by the muscles surrounding them. When one part of the body is under strain, it may affect other parts of the body.

Good body mechanics are important in:
- providing safety and comfort for the client
- preventing muscle strain, fatigue, or personal injury to either the client or aide
- maintaining proper body alignment

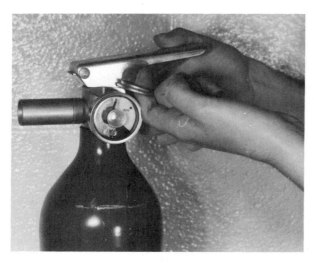

Figure 12-12 Most fire extinguishers have locks which must be released before the extinguisher can be discharged (courtesy of Louise Simmers, *Diversified Health Occupations*, Delmar Publishers, Albany, NY, 1983).

There are several key points to remember in order to use proper body mechanics:

- Maintain a broad base of support.
- Kneel or squat, bending from the hips and knees, instead of bending from the waist, figure 12-21 on page 165. The leg muscles are stronger than those in the lower back.
- Use the strongest muscles to do the job.
- Use the weight of your body to push, pull, or move objects.
- Avoid twisting your body when you work. Instead, move your entire body, including your feet.
- When moving or carrying heavy objects from one place to another, hold the objects close to the body. This causes the weight to be distributed more evenly over the entire body, rather than on the arms alone.

The lifting of heavy or awkwardly shaped objects can be accomplished by following a few simple rules:

RULES FOR LIFTING

1. TAKE A WIDE BASE OF SUPPORT.

2. KEEP THE LOAD CLOSE TO YOUR BODY.

3. BEND YOUR HIPS AND KNEES; KEEP YOUR BACK STRAIGHT.

4. SHIFT YOUR FEET TO TURN; DO NOT TWIST YOUR BODY.

5. DO NOT LIFT OVER YOUR HEAD.

applications to client care

Many client care procedures require moving and turning the client. To ensure the safety of the client and to avoid self-injury or injury to the client, the home health aide should apply the techniques of good body mechanics to the work situation. This means that the aide should do the following:

- Stand straight rather than slouch. Keep the back and shoulder muscles in a straight line.
- Push, pull, slide or roll the client whenever possible. Try to avoid lifting the client.
- When turning the client, try to make the movement smooth and fluid so that the entire body shifts at the same time.
- When repositioning the client in bed, turn the client toward you rather than away from you. This lessens the danger of the client falling out of bed, and keeps your weight more evenly distributed.
- When walking with the client remain on the client's weak side. Try to stay near chairs or a couch so you can quickly seat the client if the client tires.
- If the client becomes faint while walking, help the client to sit in a chair. If there is no chair nearby, help the client slide slowly to the floor. Call for assistance.

SAFETY IN THE LIVING AND DINING ROOMS

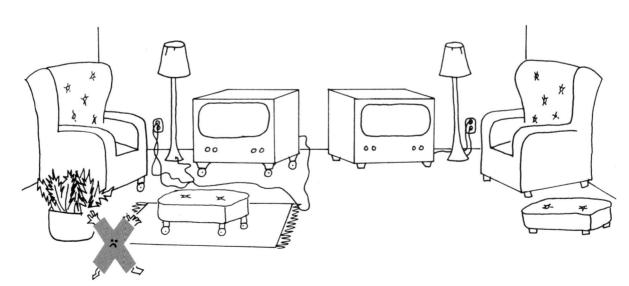

- Arrange furniture so that sharp edges are out of the way and the passageway is unobstructed.

- Do not use wheels under *any* piece of furniture.

- If furniture is to be rearranged, plans should be discussed with you beforehand so that you do not lose familiarity with your surroundings.

- Floors should be free of clutter and small objects, such as footstools, magazine racks, plants, etc.

- Door sills should be removed by a carpenter.

- Wipe dry any spilled water, grease or food.

- Keep all rugs and carpets in good repair. Scatter rugs should be either taped down or removed.

- Rough edges of carpeting should be taped in the same manner or tacked down. Frayed edges and loose strings could catch on toes or heels and cause a fall.

- Tack down telephone and electrical wires. Keep electrical equipment away from walking areas. Don't run electric cords under rugs or doors.

- Carry dishes on a tray or utility cart to and from the table. Always keep vision clear when carrying things.

- Keep the trash basket and garbage pail away from areas where people walk.

- Keep mops, brooms, vacuum cleaner and hoses, etc. stored in a closet.

- Always eat at the table.

Figure 12-13 Safety in the living and dining rooms (*courtesy of The Burke Rehabilitation Center, White Plains, NY, the Auxiliary and Sylvia Watkins, Ph.D.*)

SAFETY IN
THE KITCHEN

- Do not stand on chairs to reach objects on shelves. Always ask someone to reach for you or use reachers if the object is not heavy. Reachers, with magnets on the tips, should be kept in the kitchen to help pick up objects that fall to the floor.

- The kitchen should be kept well organized and uncluttered, especially if it is small. Frequently used items must be kept where they can be easily reached so that you need not bend.

- Do not wax your floors. Waxed floors are slippery, and the shine of the wax may cause glare.

- Always wipe up water, grease and food spills. A fall in a kitchen can be very bad. There is an added danger of burns and cuts happening during the fall.

- Keep floor tiles and linoleum repaired.

- Keep drawers and closet doors closed.

- Keep electric appliance cords up away from the edge of the counter.

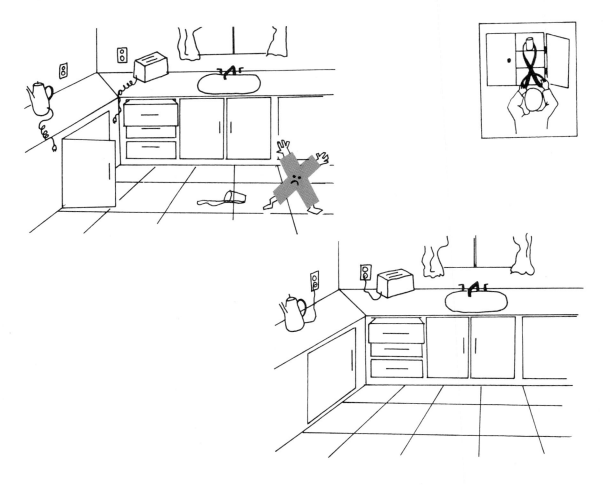

Figure 12-14   Safety in the kitchen (*courtesy of The Burke Rehabilitation Center, White Plains, NY, the Auxiliary and Sylvia Watkins, Ph.D.*)

SAFETY IN THE BEDROOM

• A chair with armrests and a firm seat should be part of the bedroom furniture. Dressing should be accomplished while seated in the chair, eliminating the risk of falling.

• Your bed must be low enough to allow you to get in and out with ease but should be no lower than knee height. If your bed is too high, a carpenter can adjust the height by cutting off part of the legs.

• Night lights should be installed in wall sockets near the bedroom door, in the hallway leading to the bathroom and in the bathroom. They help you avoid accidents.

• A urinal or bed pan may be kept within reach on the bed table, or commode placed by the bed for nighttime use to eliminate walks to the bathroom.

• Never get out of bed in the dark. Make sure that you have a night light or light switch within easy reach of your bed. Also keep a flashlight handy.

• Keep a clear path between the bed and the door.

• Do not wear loose-fitting slippers, night clothes and clothing. Always tie your robe and clothing with belts attached. Loose garments can cause a fall by catching on drawers, door knobs and other objects. Keep cuffs of trousers at proper length to avoid catching heel and tripping.

• Keep drawers and closets closed to avoid bumping into them.

• Before getting out of bed or standing, check your legs for numbness.

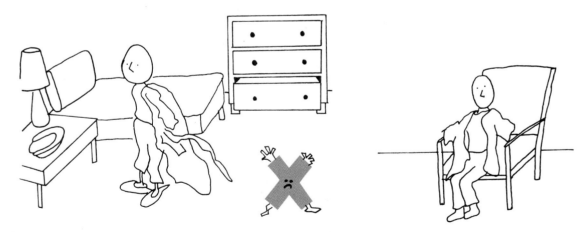

Figure 12-15 Safety in the bedroom (*courtesy of The Burke Rehabilitation Center, White Plains, NY, the Auxiliary and Sylvia Watkins, Ph.D.*)

SAFETY IN THE BATHROOM

- Do not use small bathroom scatter rugs on the floor. A large rug that covers all of the floor is best.

- Place non-skid decals, strips or rubber mats on the floor of the shower or tub to help eliminate falls.

- Do not use glass tumblers for drinking water in the bathroom. Paper or plastic cups are safe, inexpensive and disposable.

- Place grab bars in strategic locations around the bathtub, shower and toilet. Never support yourself on towel racks or wall soap holders, as they are not designed to bear weight and may break away from the wall under pressure. If standing tires you, a tub bench or bath chair may be useful.

- A raised toilet seat can be purchased from a surgical supply house and attached to the toilet. The raised seat increases the height of the toilet from the floor and it helps to make it easier to sit down and to rise from the toilet.

- Always step over the edge of the tub when getting in and out. You can easily lose your balance or slip on the edge of the tub.

- Do not keep clothes lines in the bathroom. Clothes may drop on the floor, and you might trip over them. Have a clothes hamper or basket for dirty clothes.

- Never use an electric appliance while in the bathtub or shower.

- Hang up towels and wash cloths. Place hooks clearly above or well below eye level.

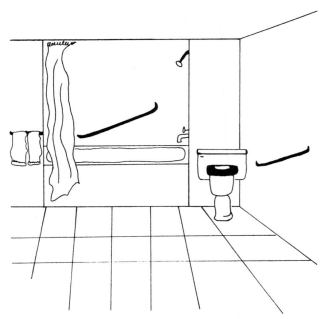

Figure 12-16 Safety in the bathroom (*courtesy of The Burke Rehabilitation Center, White Plains, NY, the Auxiliary and Sylvia Watkins, Ph.D.*)

SAFETY OUTSIDE

- Avoid using steps whenever possible. When steps must be used, make sure there are sturdy railings and USE THEM.

- When using an elevator, wait until it has leveled completely before stepping on.

- On the curbs, be aware of holes. Do use appliances prescribed. Do not attempt to cross the streets unless the "WALK" sign is lighted and you have checked for cars in both directions.

- If your vision is poor, do not hesitate to ask for help when crossing the street.

- If weather is inclement, consider postponing your outing until better weather. When you go out, wear supportive walking shoes with non-slippery leather soles. Tie shoes are more supportive than slip ons. Avoid wearing heels.

- When you go shopping, use the pushcart to hold your groceries and walking equipment. Do not attempt to hold a cane with one hand and a shopping bag with the other hand. You may lose your balance and fall. Ask for assistance when putting groceries in the car.

- Consider using catalogs for department store items and clothing, i.e., J.C. Penney or Sears Stores.

- Avoid going out at night; you may not see a dangerous spot.

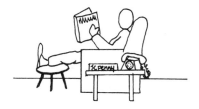

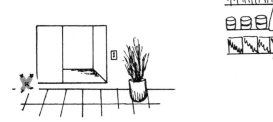

Figure 12-17 Safety outside (*courtesy of The Burke Rehabilitation Center, White Plains, NY, the Auxiliary and Sylvia Watkins, Ph.D.*)

SAFETY IN THE BASEMENT

- Keep the passageway unobstructed.

- Do not carry heavy or large piles of loose laundry. You may drop some of the clothes and trip over them.

- Keep clothes lines above head height.

- Do not use basement steps for storing things. Keep steps clean.

- Never accumulate junk in the basement. Get rid of trash, boxes, old newspapers, and anything else you don't need. In addition to causing falls, junk is responsible for spreading fires.

- Keep all tools put away when not in use.

Figure 12-18   Safety in the basement

SAFETY AT STAIRWAYS

- Stairways and hallways should be equipped with handrails on both sides.

- Keep stairways well lighted. There should be a light switch at the top and the bottom of stairs.

- Keep all objects off the stairs.

- Don't put scatter rugs at the bottom or top of the stairs.

- Wipe dry immediately all spilled water, food, etc.

- Watch your step when wearing loose-fitting slippers or shoes.

- Put a gate at the top and bottom of stairs to protect a confused or wandering family member.

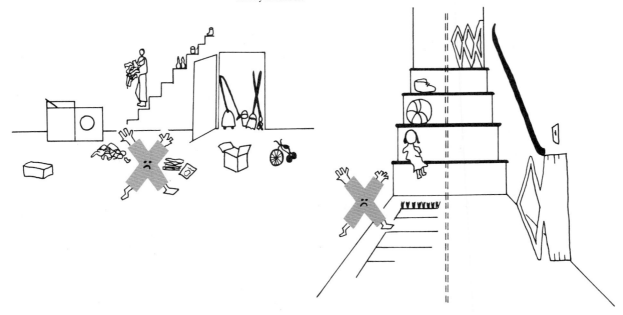

Figure 12-19   Safety at stairways (*courtesy of The Burke Rehabilitation Center, White Plains, NY, the Auxiliary and Sylvia Watkins, Ph.D.*)

SOURCES OF HELP IN THE COMMUNITY

- Self-help Groups

- Adult Day Care Programs

- County Health Department, Public Health Nursing Office

- County Office of the Aging

- Social Service Agencies
    Catholic Charities
    Family Service Bureau
    Jewish Family Service
    Protestant Welfare Agency

- Specialized Neurological Clinics

- Visiting Nurse Services

Figure 12-20 Sources of help in the community (*courtesy of The Burke Rehabilitation Center, White Plains, NY, the Auxiliary and Sylvia Watkins, Ph.D.*)

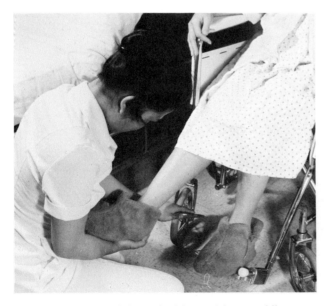

Figure 12-21 Bend from the hips and knees while performing procedures (courtesy of Louise Simmers, *Diversified Health Occupations*, Delmar Publishers, Albany, NY, 1983).

summary

- A practicing home health aide should do everything possible to ensure a safe environment.
- Hazardous items or conditions should be identified and measures taken to correct the situation.
- The home health aide should be aware of the types of accidents to which the client's age group is prone.
- The aide should make sure that emergency phone numbers are visible and are posted near the phone.
- It is also important for the aide to know what procedures to follow in the event of a fire.
- In performing all tasks, the aide should use proper body mechanics so as to avoid self-injury or injury to the client.

review

1. Name two ways to extinguish grease fires in cooking utensils.
2. How should a fire in an ash tray or upholstered furniture be extinguished?
3. Why should baking soda be used to extinguish grease, oil, and similar fires?
4. Name five common home accidents.
5. Name two physical conditions of the elderly that contribute to accidents.
6. What does the term *body mechanics* mean?

Unit 13
Understanding Illness

key terms

symptoms	tachycardia	apnea
cardinal signs	chronic	respiration
sign	rales	diastolic
rehabilitation	sphygmomanometer	contracture
acute	systolic	range of motion
pulse	dyspnea	exercises
bradycardia		blood pressure

learning objectives

After studying this unit, you should be able to:
- Identify the four cardinal signs and their normal values.
- Name three body sites where temperature is taken.
- Identify four signs that a client may be ill.
- Define rehabilitation.
- Explain the difference between a sign and a symptom.
- Describe the care given to the unconscious client.

Wellness is the normal state of the human body. Wellness is when all body systems are functioning normally. Illness occurs when the body machinery is not working properly. This may be caused by external factors or it may result from an internal disorder (abnormality). Internal problems occur when some part of the body is not working correctly. Accidents and environmental hazards are examples of external causes of illness.

Some external environmental factors which may affect people's health are air and water. There are particles or organisms in the air and water which can enter the body and cause illness. People who have asthma and lung disorders have great difficulty breathing when the air quality is poor. Men who work in coal mines breathe in coal dust which harms the lungs. These particles can seriously damage the respiratory system. Viruses are external organisms which are carried through the air in water droplets. When they enter the nose or mouth they can cause infectious diseases. Flu, the common cold, and measles are examples of virus infections.

Illnesses may be either acute or chronic. An **acute** illness is one that begins suddenly and usually is severe. A **chronic** illness is one that continues to affect a person for a long period of time.

Illness, an accidental injury, or a birth defect may be the cause of a disability (a physical, emotional, or mental handicap). Usually, a disability involves an impaired body function, such as eyesight or ambulation (walking).

Because the home health aide will be caring for clients who are ill or disabled or who are recovering from an illness, it is important for the aide to understand the basic principles and terms related to disorders and diseases as well as their treatment.

internal disorders

Internal disorders may happen at any age. However, they are more likely to occur as the body grows older and becomes more prone to break down. Usually young people recover more quickly from accidents and diseases because their body tissues and cells repair and grow at a faster rate. It takes much longer for recovery in older persons because the growth rate of new cells is slower. The circulatory system often becomes less efficient as people age. Heart diseases, strokes, diabetes, and hypertension are major physical disorders of the aged.

mental disorder

An internal disorder that can happen at any age is mental or emotional breakdown. Some mental disorders are so severe that the client must be hospitalized. Many times, a person who normally functions well suffers an emotional breakdown when outside stress becomes too great. Mental illness in the aged usually has other causes, however. Organic brain disorder (or senile brain atrophy) and Alzheimer's disease are caused by a change in the brain tissue. The client loses memory of recent events and is often confused. Another mental condition of the aged is caused by arteriosclerosis. In this condition, the blood vessels become narrow and do not permit enough blood flow into the brain. The resulting lack of oxygen going to the brain causes periods of confusion and irritable behavior from time to time. In either condition, clients often cannot remember when they have had their last meal. They forget that they just had a visit from close relatives. Often, early childhood memories are more real to them than the present. A home health aide must show patience with aged persons having these conditions. The aide must recognize that mentally ill clients, young or old, need just as much care and consideration as the ones with heart conditions or other physical disorders.

Emotional illness may sometimes cause a physical illness. For example, a client who believes that there is poison in the food will refuse to eat. This can lead to severe malnutrition. Physical illness can bring on emotional problems, too. Some clients seem more able to cope with illness than others. One person may become emotionally disturbed because of illness; another is able to take illness in stride. A home health aide must be able to recognize and deal with the emotional and psychological effects of an illness on both the client and the client's family.

observing signs and symptoms

In later chapters, individual medical conditions will be discussed. For each condition, the home health aide will be told the signs and symptoms which may arise during that illness. The aide must be able to recognize, record, and report significant signs and symptoms. A **sign** is a change which can be observed or measured. Signs of emotional stress might include wringing of the hands and unusual or sudden changes in behavior. Signs of a physical change which are common include changes in the client's appearance. For example, the client may become flushed, turn pale, break into a heavy sweat, or turn blue (cyanotic). With experience, the home health aide learns which signs should be reported to the supervisor. Irregular eating patterns, swelling of lower limbs (edema), and a deep yellow complexion (jaundice) are also physical signs which may be observed. **Caution:** Medical signs which should be reported at once are bleeding, vomiting, unusual coldness, flushing and heavy perspiration, or loss of consciousness.

A home health aide should also be alert to the client's symptoms. **Symptoms** are changes which cannot be observed but are experienced by the client. Examples of symptoms are pain and discomfort. A pain can be described as dull or sharp. It may be localized (in one area) or generalized (all over). The aide should have the client describe how the pain feels so that the pain can be reported accurately to the supervisor. As a home health aide becomes more familiar with a client, the aide can better observe signs of stress and recognize symptoms. After the aide has seen the normal reactions of the client, deviations (changes) which could be serious can be recognized.

cardinal signs

Cardinal signs are those signs which quickly indicate the status of a person's life functions. They include temperature, pulse, respiration rate, and blood pressure. Cardinal signs must be measured accurately and regularly. Changes out of the normal range must be reported to the supervisor. The home health aide will be given exact instructions as to when to take these measurements for each assigned case.

temperature

The difference between the heat produced and the heat lost is the body temperature. Temperature is measured with a thermometer. An oral thermometer is used to take oral and axillary temperatures. When the temperature must be taken in the rectum, a rectal thermometer with a rounded end is used. Figure 13-1 shows the normal body temperatures taken by various methods. The detailed procedure for taking temperatures is presented in a later unit. The instructor will demonstrate the correct procedure and the kinds of thermometers to be used. Each home health aide must be able to take and record temperature accurately.

pulse and respiration rate

Two other cardinal signs that a home health aide is required to take and record are the pulse and respirations. These two readings are usually taken one after the other. After taking the pulse, the client's arm is held in the same position and the respirations are counted. It is better if the client does not realize that respirations are being counted. The results are more accurate if the client thinks that only the pulse rate is being checked.

The **pulse** is the artery contracting. Arterial contractions are initiated by the heart. Thus, the pulse rate should be the same as the heart rate. The pulse may be taken at any of the sites shown in figure 13-2. The most common site for checking the pulse is the radial artery which can be felt inside the wrist. Pulse rates differ depending on age, sex, size and physical condition of the client, figure 13-3. An extremely slow heartbeat is called **bradycardia.** An extremely rapid heartbeat is called **tachycardia.** A sudden change to either condition must be reported immediately to the supervisor. Pulse readings show the rate, rhythm, and volume of blood pulsing through the artery. Rate is the times per minute. Rhythm is the evenness or regularity of the beat. Volume is the fullness of the beat. An

METHOD	AVERAGE NORMAL TEMPERATURE (Fahrenheit and Celsius readings)	USAGE
ORAL	98.6°F (37.0°C)	Most commonly used Most convenient Held in place 3 minutes
RECTAL	99.6°F (37.6°C)	Most accurate Used with infants Used with adults when ordered by a doctor Held in place 5 minutes
AXILLARY OR GROIN	97.6°F (36.2°C)	Least accurate Used only when oral and rectal methods cannot be used Held in place 10 minutes

Figure 13-1 Body temperature is measured with a thermometer by various methods.

example of how a normal pulse would be recorded is 70 (rate), regular (rhythm), and full (volume). An abnormal pulse for an adult might be 90 (rate), irregular (rhythm), and weak or thready (volume).

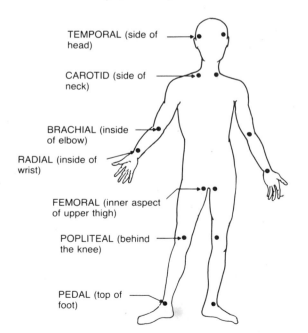

TEMPORAL (side of head)

CAROTID (side of neck)

BRACHIAL (inside of elbow)

RADIAL (inside of wrist)

FEMORAL (inner aspect of upper thigh)

POPLITEAL (behind the knee)

PEDAL (top of foot)

Figure 13-2 The pulse may be taken at any of the places shown.

Respiration is the sum total of processes which exchange oxygen and carbon dioxide in the body. However, respiration is most commonly known as breathing. The act of inhaling and exhaling once is counted as one respiration. Difficult or labored breathing is called **dyspnea.** Sometimes respirations stop for a few moments. This absence of breathing is called **apnea.** A bubbling sound may be heard when fluid or mucus gets caught in the air passages. This condition is called **rales,** and can often be heard in clients with pneumonia or emphysema. The normal rate of respirations for adults is 16–20 per minute. In adults, respiration rates of 25 or more are called accelerated. Weak respirations which are characterized by only slight chest movements are described as being **shallow.** Breathing characterized by many large breaths is described as being deep.

blood pressure

Blood pressure is measured in two parts—systolic and diastolic—by using an instrument called a **sphygmomanometer.** While

Age Group	Beats per Minute	Rhythm and Volume
Adult men	60-70	Regular and Full
Adult women	65-80	Regular and Full
Children over 7	72-90	Regular and Full
Children 1-7	80-120	Regular and Full
Infants	110-130	Regular and Full

Figure 13-3 Normal pulse readings

this procedure requires concentration and demands accuracy, the home health aide should become familiar with the technique. A new type of sphygmomanometer is now available that has a read-out which simplifies the procedure. This type of sphygmomanometer is not always available for individual home use.

As the heart beats, it relaxes and contracts much like the opening and closing of a fist. As the heart contracts, blood is forced into the arteries to travel through the body. When the heart relaxes, blood enters from the venous system, thus completing the cycle. The arterial measurement (as the blood is pushed out into the lungs to get oxygen) is the **systolic** pressure. This pressure rises during periods of hard activity or excitement and falls during times of rest. In the normal, relaxed, sitting adult, it may be as low as 100 and as high as 140 millimeters of mercury. The **diastolic** pressure is a measure of the pressure counted between beats of the heart when the heart muscle is relaxed. A normal measure is 60–85 millimeters of mercury.

Unusually high blood pressure readings can be extremely dangerous and are often life threatening. Studies to date link obesity and hypertension (high blood pressure) as common physiological problems. Careful attention must be given to this growing health condition. High blood pressure can lead to serious medical problems. Blood pressure varies with age, sex, race, altitude, muscular development, and according to the state of mind or tiredness. It is usually lower among women than men. It is also generally low in childhood, becoming higher with advancing age.

In some areas of the country, taking and recording blood pressure is considered to be too technical for the home health aide to perform. Other areas expect home health aides to be able to take and record blood pressure accurately. Home health aides should check with their particular agencies to determine if they are permitted or expected to obtain blood pressure readings.

conscious and unconscious clients

In most cases, a home health aide will be assigned to care for clients who are conscious. **Consciousness** is the normal state of awareness. Conscious people are responsive and know who and where they are. Normal consciousness varies in intensity throughout the day.

Have you had the experience of going to look for an item only to forget what it was when you got into the room? Have you ever been talking to someone and at some point lose the purpose of the conversation? These examples show that different levels of consciousness exist. While doing routine work, thoughts may wander and daydreaming may occur. At other times, a person may be extremely aware and sensitive of surroundings and events.

Just as there are varying levels of consciousness there are different levels of unconsciousness, figure 13-4. Sleep is a temporary

LEVEL	PHYSICAL SIGNS AND CLIENT REACTIONS
Somnolence	Client can answer questions but is confused and fades in and out of sleep. (Restraints may be ordered by the doctor).
Stupor	Client is restless and can only be aroused by continuous stimulation. Must be protected from falling out of bed. (Restraints may be needed.) Responds to bright lights, loud sounds and can locate painful site.
Semicoma	Client can only be aroused with difficulty. May groan or mutter, reacts to painful stimuli (when pinched or stuck with needle). Usually loses control of bowel and bladder (is incontinent).
Coma	Responds only to painful stimuli if at all. In a deep coma, all responses are lost. Must be turned and repositioned or will remain in one position. Client is incontinent.

Figure 13-4 Levels of unconsciousness

state of unconsciousness. Other types of unconsciousness are due to a body malfunction or an injury. Fainting is an example of a temporary loss of consciousness. The blood supply to the brain is decreased; the person feels dizzy and may black out. When the head is lowered, the blood rushes back to the brain and the faintness disappears.

The deeply unconscious client is totally helpless and the home health aide must follow doctor's instructions carefully. The client's bed should be comfortable and kept clean and dry. The client should also be given frequent mouth care. Two of the greatest problems for an unconscious client are the chance of developing bedsores and contractures. **Contracture** is the abnormal shortening of muscle tissue. When contractures occur, the muscles become in-

elastic and fixed. The hands may curl into tight fists and become locked into that position. The arms and legs also become stiff. In some cases, the entire body curls into the fetal position. Exercising the clients limbs can help prevent contractures. Exercises done to prevent contractures and the loss of motion in the joints are called **range of motion exercises.**

An unconscious client must have special care. Figure 13-5 indicates the special needs of the unconscious client and how to meet those needs.

diversion, recreation and rehabilitation

A care plan is developed to make the ill client comfortable and to bring about recovery. Several factors influence the care which is planned. The home health aide must consider the sex and age of the client and the type and severity of the illness. The personal habits and the client's personality also enter into the total care plan. Suitable foods must be given to the client and the physical environment must be maintained. In addition, the client must have diversion and some kind of recreation. The client's thoughts need to be taken off the illness. Illness often confines the client and this is rarely pleasant. The home health aide should make special efforts to give the client outside interests. It is not hard to plan small pleasures to ease the boredom of illness. Some clients like to read; books can be borrowed from the local library, figure 13-6. If the client is well enough, visits from friends may be enjoyable. A home health aide can suggest activities to a client. Even moving the bed so the client can look out the window and watch the sky and trees can be a diversion for the client. The client who is able should be taken out of doors in nice weather. This provides a change of scenery and makes the client feel better. Reading to the client may also be a pleasant diversion, figure

CARE REQUIRED	FREQUENCY	WHAT TO DO
Mouth care	Every 2 hours	Wipe tongue, lips, gums, and teeth with gauze pad or cotton swab moistened with water or mouthwash. Lubricate and moisten mouth tissues with glycerin or vegetable oil. Wipe away saliva as it dribbles from the mouth.
	When client vomits	Turn client to side at first sign of vomiting. Catch vomitus in a bowl or basin held to the side of the mouth. Wipe mouth with gauze pads or clean damp cloth.
Eye care	Wipe clean in A.M. and P.M.	Cover eyelids with soft cloth moistened in preboiled water. (Prevents eye cavity from becoming dry, since eyes may not close or blink).
Repositioning	At least every 2 hours	Turn from back to side, and side to front, etc. (This prevents decubiti (bedsores) from forming).
Range of motion (ROM) exercises	As ordered by doctor	Exercise all client's body parts if permitted by doctor. (Keeps blood circulating, prevents contractures, and prevents loss of motion in joints).
Body massage with lotion	At least daily	Rub skin firmly but gently. Rub in a circular motion around bony prominences.
Care of bowel and bladder drainage	At least every hour	Check perineal area and bed linens to see if they are clean and dry. If client has not voided for 8 hours, report it to the supervisor. If client has not had bowel movement for two days, report it to the supervisor.
Accident prevention	At all times	Put up guard rails or place chairs beside bed to prevent falls. Use wrist, leg, or halter restraints to protect client from harming self — *used only on order of doctor.* Observe for signs of vomiting and keep saliva wiped away; client may choke or inhale fluids into the lungs. Keep blankets and pillows away from the client's nose and mouth to avoid smothering.
Easy access to client	At all times	Safety and ease of working with client. Place the bed away from the wall so both sides of the bed are accessible.
Room ventilation	Open windows or vent daily	Keep temperature between 66–70°, keep drafts from client. Open windows or vents to circulate air.
Tender Loving Care (TLC)	At all times	Talk to the client as if the client were conscious. Client may be able to hear and understand. (Communication gives client link with reality).

Figure 13-5 Meeting the special needs of the unconscious client.

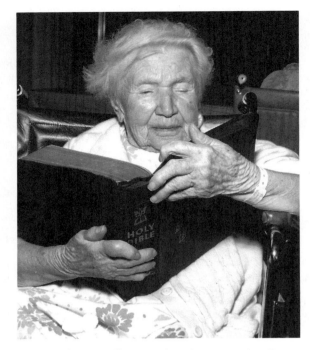

Figure 13-6 Reading can give pleasure to the client.

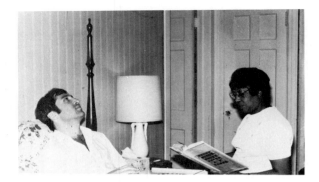

Figure 13-7 Reading to the client often creates a pleasant diversion.

13-7. The activities the client can participate in depend upon past interests, age, and present condition. The possibilities for activities are unlimited. A recreational therapist can recommend activities geared to the abilities and interests of the client, including:

bingo and playing cards
writing/taping oral history
clay sculpture
water colors
sketching
dictating poetry to a home health aide, or letters to family and friends
finger paints
handcrafts
needlecrafts
simple to advanced crossword puzzles
planting seeds for a window garden
making scrapbooks
couponing
bird watching and recording birds sighted

Diversion and recreation play an important part in lifting the spirits of a sick person.

Another part of the care plan intended to help a client may include **rehabilitation.** This is the restoring of physical abilities to the highest level possible. Most rehabilitation is planned and carried out by a specialist such as the physical or occupational therapist. When physical ability or skill has been lost, the client must relearn it or adjust to coping without it. A blind client must be taught self-feeding and learn how to become more independent. A stroke victim must learn again to use parts of the body which may be paralyzed. Range of motion exercises, speech therapy and other kinds of rehabilitation may be needed. In some cases the home health aide will be able to assist in the rehabilitation program.

summary

- The home health aide must learn to understand both the emotional and physical aspects of illness.
- Routine care requires the aide to accurately measure and record the cardinal signs: temperature, pulse, respiration, and blood pressure.

- An important duty is to report to the supervisor any unusual or significant changes in the client's appearance or behavior.
- The aide must also give the special care required by the unconscious client.
- A total care plan includes diversion for the client as well as recreation and rehabilitation.

review

1. a. List the four cardinal signs.
   b. Indicate the normal values of each cardinal sign.
2. What is the difference between a sign and a symptom?
3. a. Describe the mouth care given to an unconscious client.
   b. How often is mouth care given to the unconscious client?
4. How often should an unconscious client be repositioned?
5. What is rehabilitation?

Unit 14
Preventing the Spread of Disease

learning objectives

After studying this unit, you should be able to:
—— Name the best defense against pathogens.
—— Identify three medical aseptic techniques.
—— Give five examples of the ways germs can be carried.

The air is filled with tiny living plants and animals which cannot be seen with the naked eye. These living structures are called microorganisms. Most microorganisms are harmless to humans, but some are pathogenic. A pathogenic microorganism can cause a disease or infection in the human body; they are often called **pathogens** or **germs. Bacteria** are microscopic organisms. **Protozoa** are tiny one-celled animals. Bacteria and protozoa can live for a long time and continue to multiply in air and water. Most of these organisms like dark, damp, warm, and dirty places. Many types of bacteria and protozoa exist, but only a few cause disease.

Viruses are microorganisms which can only live by feeding on living cells. Most viruses can cause infections. The time between the entry of germs into the body and the appearance of the first sign of disease is called the **incubation period.** Infections only occur when the body cannot control the growth of germs. Strong, healthy people are more able to fight off pathogens than weak or unhealthy people.

Fungi include two groups of organisms—yeasts and molds—that live normally on the skin. Under optimum conditions they can cause diseases such as athlete's foot (*tinea pedis*), ringworm (*tinea capitis*), thrush or vulvovaginitis (*candida albicans*).

Most pathogens grow and reproduce very rapidly. They spread disease from one part of the body to another. They also may spread disease from one person to another. A home health aide must learn how to keep pathogenic organisms from spreading.

Cleanliness is the best defense against pathogens. When there are a great many germs present, the area is said to be **contaminated,** or dirty. The absence of germs is called **asepsis.** The methods used to destroy pathogens are known as aseptic techniques, figure 14-1. Medical asepsis is used to keep pathogens from spreading from person to person or place to place. When an object is absolutely free from all microorganisms, it is **sterile.** Pathogens are found most everywhere. Therefore, special procedures must be followed regularly to get rid of them.

cleanliness in the home

"Cleanliness is next to godliness," "Dirt breeds germs, and germs can make you sickly and weak," "Her house is so clean you could eat off the floor." These are all old sayings about cleanliness. Of course, one does not expect to eat off the floor. However, cleanliness can help stop the spread of germs and, therefore, limit the spread of disease. This is why it is so important to keep the environment clean.

In many homes, the kitchen is the center of family life. Most families eat three meals a day, and may raid the refrigerator for between meal snacks. This means that the traffic in and out of the kitchen is heavier than in any other room in the house. The kitchen probably offers the home health aide more challenge than any other room. Keeping the kitchen clean can be a time-consuming job. Good organization can lighten the work load a great deal. In some kitchens, the aide will see piles of dirty dishes and garbage. Floors may also be dirty and sticky. When dishes are washed as they are dirtied, spills wiped up at once, and garbage taken out regularly, this messy condition does not develop. Equipment should be kept clean

and supplies properly stored immediately after use. Kitchen tasks that are left until the end of the day cause unsanitary and unhealthy conditions. Hours are added to the work load because the dirt has hardened.

Much of the home health aide's job is to clean the kitchen and prepare meals. However, other important housekeeping duties are to clean the bathrooms and the client's room. The same need for cleanliness applies to these rooms as to the kitchen.

controlling the spread of illness

Most everyone practices aseptic techniques in daily living. Some of the most common practices are:

- Handwashing, bathing, brushing teeth
- Changing clothing regularly
- Using fresh towels and washcloths
- Sterilizing baby bottles
- Cleaning bathroom sink, tub, bowl and floor
- Cleaning kitchen, washing dishes
- Vacuuming and mopping floors
- Laundering clothing and linens

When illness is present, added care must be taken to prevent the spread of germs. An ill person's body is producing pathogens. At the same time, the person is weak and cannot resist other germs. The person's body is so busy fighting one illness that it cannot fight off other germs. The home health aide is responsible for controlling the spread of the client's germs so others in the home will not be harmed. The aide must also help protect the client from the germs carried into the home.

Germs can enter the body in many ways, figure 14-2. However, they are harmful or pathogenic only when they enter and settle in the particular part of the body that is most suited to their growth. For example, a germ that causes the common cold will not cause a

WAYS TO KILL MICROORGANISMS	DESCRIPTION	USE
DISINFECTION:	The use of chemical products to kill pathogens. Mouthwash, green soap, borax, commercial disinfectants, alcohol, boric acid, creosols, sulfur. Follow instructions.	Household items Clothes Hands Wounds Thermometers
STERILIZATION:	The application of dry or steam heat under controlled conditions. (Boiled or steamed in pressure cooker or covered pot at $212°$ — in oven 2–3 hours at $165–170°$ — aired in sunlight for 6–8 hours)	Baby bottles Dishes and utensils Hypodermic needles Contaminated clothing Bed linens
INCINERATION:	Burning contaminated items such as tissues, etc.	Used tissues Soiled dressings Disposable paper products
PEST CONTROL:	Use of chemicals and other means to rid area of pests. (Follow instructions carefully to avoid danger of accidental poisoning).	Rats, mice Flies, roaches Fleas, mosquitos

WAYS TO RESTRICT MICROORGANISMS	DESCRIPTION	USE
WASTE DISPOSAL:	Daily removal of nonburnable waste products, double bagging and discarding in covered garbage cans.	Food scraps Tin cans, bottles Contaminated dressings or tissues
ISOLATION TECHNIQUES:	Keeping client in controlled environment so germs won't spread or new ones enter. Of special importance if client has highly contagious disease, or is weakened and unable to resist added infections. Using special equipment and supplies such as rubber gloves, apron or coveralls, cap, mask and disposable paper products.	Restrict client's mobility Contaminated dishes Contaminated linen Body discharges Personal and household items
DAMP CLOTH DUSTING AND MOPPING	Use of wet cloth or sponge to remove germs and dust from surfaces. Prevents raising germs into the air where they can be spread easier.	Furniture surfaces Floors Walls and window sills

Figure 14-1 Microorganisms can be destroyed or restricted by applying aseptic techniques.

cold if that germ enters the skin. If the germ enters the respiratory system (the nose, the lungs, etc.) the person would develop a cold because the respiratory system provides just the right climate for the cold germ to grow.

Germs can be spread when others touch contaminated objects or surfaces. Tissues used by the client should be placed in a paper bag at the client's bedside, figure 14-3. Dressings or bandages from open cuts or wounds must

AIRBORNE	ANIMAL CARRIED	INSECT CARRIED
Colds Flu (influenza) Measles Chickenpox Smallpox	Rabies; occurs from bite of infected dog, squirrel, bat Trichinosis; occurs from eating poorly cooked pork of an infected pig Tularemia (rabbit fever); occurs from touching or eating contaminated rabbit	Bubonic or Black Plague; occurs from rat or flea bites Malaria; occurs from bite of Anopheles mosquito Sleeping sickness (narcolepsy); occurs from bite of a tsetse fly Dysentery; common fly may transfer microorganism
CONTACT	HUMAN CARRIED	PRENATAL
Mononucleosis Venereal diseases (syphilis, gonorrhea and AIDS) Infectious hepatitis Tuberculosis Conjunctivitis Poliomyelitis	Typhoid fever Mumps Impetigo Whooping cough (pertussis) Diphtheria Poliomyelitis Syphilis and gonorrhea	Syphilis may cause fetal blindness, deafness, malformation, or retardation Rubella (German measles); may lead to fetal blindness, deafness or malformation
FOOD CARRIED	WATER CARRIED	SOIL CARRIED
Dysentery Botulism Worms Salmonella	Typhoid fever Dysentery Poliomyelitis	Tetanus (lockjaw) Dysentery Worms

Figure 14-2   Most diseases may be carried in more than one way.

be double-bagged in paper and then discarded. Careful cleaning of the client's room is very important in stopping indirect spread of germs.

Contagious diseases are those which spread rapidly and easily from person to person or place to place. Many contagious diseases that once caused many deaths have been largely controlled. Today there are vaccines given to children to prevent polio, diphtheria, whooping cough, mumps and measles. Gamma globulin shots may be given to persons exposed to diseases such as hepatitis, measles, and mumps. While these shots do not always prevent the disease, they cause the client's reaction to be milder.

isolation

The client with an easily transmitted or contagious disease may be placed in **isolation**. This means that the client is kept away from others in the household. Isolation helps prevent family members from getting the client's germs. The home health aide will have to be especially careful in maintaining aseptic conditions. Isolation is more difficult to arrange in the home than it is in a hospital. Isolated clients should, ideally, have a bathroom which only they may use. However, when this is not possible, the home health aide will have to clean the sink and toilet area each time the client uses it. The

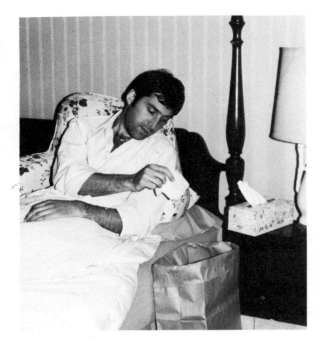

Figure 14-3 Tissues should be discarded immediately after use to prevent the spread of germs.

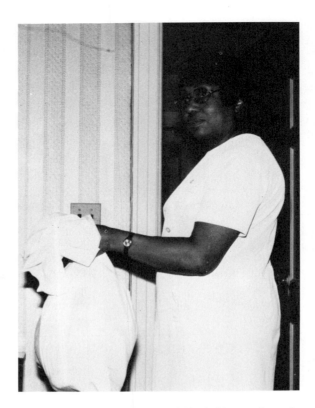

Figure 14-4 Soiled linens should be held away from the uniform.

aide's hands and the client's hands should be washed often. Handwashing destroys many germs. Disposable dishes, equipment or tissues should be used whenever possible. The client should use a separate set of dishes and utensils than is used by the family. Combs, brushes, toilet articles, towels and washcloths used by the client should not be used by others. Keeping these items separate helps prevent indirect spread of infection.

Aides should wear a bib apron or smock over the uniform while in the client's room. Before leaving the room, the cover garment should be placed into a laundry bag or hung inside the door of the client's room. When changing the bed linens, the soiled linens should be held away from the aide's garment, figure 14-4. Tongs or clothespins can be used to pick up soiled linens and transfer them to a laundry bag. Rubber gloves may also be used in special cases.

All contaminated materials from the client's room must be **disinfected** by washing in boiling water or discarded by placing in a paper or plastic bag and burned or placed in a covered garbage container. Disposable tissues, dishes or equipment should be burned. In some cases, linens must be boiled but most often hot water and soap is adequate. The client's linens and clothing must be washed separately from other family laundry. The client's dishes must be washed separately in hot, soapy water, rinsed with boiling water and air dried. After the isolation period is ended, any items used by the client should be sterilized or disinfected completely. It is important to destroy all germs on the items used before returning to general family use.

aseptic techniques

A home health aide has a duty to protect clients from unnecessary harm. In addition to keeping the home environment clean and following everyday aseptic practices, the aide should also be in good physical health. An aide who is ill risks carrying pathogens into the client's environment.

The home health aide's hands are the most common means of carrying infection. In order to control the spread of germs and to protect the aide and client, the aide's hands must be washed frequently. Just a quick rinse is not acceptable. The aide should use plenty of warm water and soap, and wash for two minutes. If, for any reason, there is no water available, commercially prepared washing pads may be used. To dry the hands, use of disposable paper towels is best. Cloth towels can spread germs when reused. If the hands are dry and chapped, lotion may be used after washing. Hands should be washed:

- before and after each client contact
- before preparing food
- before and after each meal
- after blowing the nose or sneezing
- after using the bathroom
- after handling soiled items such as linens, clothing, or garbage

THE AIDE SHOULD KEEP IN MIND THAT HANDWASHING IS THE MOST IMPORTANT PROCEDURE INVOLVED IN CONTROLLING THE SPREAD OF DISEASE.

Other aseptic procedures a home health aide should use include the following. Many of these procedures will be explained more fully in subsequent units.

- Rinse off the tops of cans before opening. After being stored on a grocery shelf or pantry, the tops of the cans may have been contaminated. Wash pots, pans, or dishes which have been unused for a long time. They may have been contaminated by roaches, ants, flies, or mice.
- Wash fruits and vegetables before eating or before storing them. If they are stored, rinse again just before use. Cook pork and chicken thoroughly. Animal carried pathogens are killed by proper cooking.
- If sterile water is needed, boil water for 20 minutes. Sterile water which is stored in the refrigerator in a sterile container usually remains sterile for a 36-hour period.
- When dusting, use a damp cloth and dust away from the body. When cleaning, start in the least soiled areas and then clean the more dirty areas. When pouring liquids into the drain, pour slowly and directly into drain. Avoid splashing. Do not pour oily liquids into the drain.

summary

- Many types of microorganisms exist but only a few cause disease.
- It is the aide's duty to help prevent the spread of disease.
- Many homemaking skills are actually aseptic techniques.
- The body has natural defenses against disease. However, the aide must help the client maintain these natural defenses.

review

1. What is the best defense against pathogens?
2. Name three aseptic techniques commonly practiced in daily living.
3. List the times when the home health aide's hands should be washed.
4. List five ways that disease can be carried.

Unit 15

Caring for the Client With an Infectious Disease

key terms

infection	AIDS	empathy
invasion	ARC	contagious
tuberculosis	hepatitis	homosexual
infectious disease	immune deficiency	

learning objectives

After studying this unit, you should be able to:

- Recognize, define and use key terms appropriately.
- List six contagious/infectious diseases.
- Recognize and discuss the reasons for special precautions when caring for AIDS clients: handwashing, use of gown and gloves.
- Describe the care plan for "night sweats", skin and mouth lesions.
- Discuss laundry handling for AIDS client.
- Refer to dishwashing procedure and determine how dishes of AIDS client should be cared for.

infectious diseases

An **infection** is the invasion of body tissue by disease-producing organisms. An **infectious disease** is one which is readily communicable or easily passed on to others, figure 15-1. Included in such diseases are infectious mononucleosis, sometimes called the "kissing disease." It is an acute communicable disease marked by fever, sore throat, swollen lymph glands, and extreme feelings of fatigue. Quite often this disease affects teenagers and young adults. The care recommended is bed rest and a nutritious diet.

Infectious **hepatitis** affects the liver. It, too, causes fever and tiredness and the patient's skin becomes yellow (jaundiced), the client may be nauseous, have respiratory disturbances, and, in some cases, the liver becomes enlarged. Persons who have been exposed to hepatitis may be given a gamma globulin shot to reduce their chance of becoming infected.

Tuberculosis is an infection caused by the tubercle bacillus which usually affects the respiratory system. Abscesses form in the lungs and the lung tissue may harden or become fibrous and calcify. Tuberculosis can

COMMON COMMUNICABLE DISEASES

DISEASE	HOW IT ENTERS BODY	HOW IT LEAVES BODY	HOW IT IS TRANSFERRED
Typhoid Fever	mouth to intestinal tract	urine/feces	hands, linens, and articles used by patient. Water polluted by feces, food grown in polluted water, food washed in polluted water
Diphtheria	mouth to nose and throat	sputum, nasal discharge, skin lesions	coughing, direct contact with sputum, articles used by and around patient, hands
Pneumonia	mouth to lungs	sputum, nasal discharge	direct contact, articles used by and around patient, hands
Influenza	mouth/nose to lungs	as above	as above
Tuberculosis	mouth/lungs/ intestines/lymph system	sputum, lesions, feces	kissing, coughing, sputum, soiled dressings, hands
Poliomyelitis	mouth/nose	nasal and throat discharges	direct contact hands
Measles (Rubella)	mouth/nose	nasal/throat discharges	direct contact, articles used by and around patients, hands
Gonorrhea	mucous membrane	body discharges, lesions	sexual intercourse, towels, linens, toilets, hands
Syphilis	blood and tissues through skin breaks	infected tissues, lesions placenta to fetus	direct contact, kissing, sexual intercourse
AIDS	mucous membrane, blood, any discharge containing blood	placenta to fetus, transfusion, body discharges, blood	sexual intercourse (anal, oral, and vaginal) needles and syringes

* A **communicable disease** is a disease which may be transmitted directly or indirectly from one individual to another and which is caused by an infectious agent.

Figure 15-1 Common communicable diseases

also affect the bones, gastrointestinal system, nervous system, and even the skin. AIDS patients may also develop tuberculosis. Tuberculosis is usually acquired through contact with an infected person or by drinking milk from an infected cow.

Advances in chemotherapy have made home care an alternative to hospital or sanitarium care. Bed rest, a well-balanced diet, and relief from emotional tension are included in the treatment plan.

There are many children's diseases which are communicable and which most individuals have experienced personally. Among these are measles, rubella, mumps, chicken pox, small pox, and whooping cough. There are immunizations which most children are given so that they will not get these diseases.

special precautions to take

Here are some precautions a home health aide should take so as to prevent transmission of an infection.

1. A gown should be worn if there is a possibility of the aide handling bloody discharges or body fluids. The gown should be removed following client contact and placed in a laundry bag as one leaves the client's room.
2. Disposable gloves should be worn when handling blood or body fluids.
3. Particular care should be given to handwashing procedures both before and after client contact for the protection of the aide as well as the client. (Even when gloves are used, hands must be thoroughly washed.)
4. Disposable items contaminated with blood or body fluids should be discarded and placed in a carefully sealed plastic bag. Sheets, towels, pillowcases, client's clothing and gowns should be placed in a special laundry bag and washed separately from

other laundry in hot water, disinfectant, and soap.
5. If the client is given medication by hypodermic needle and the aide is responsible for disposing of that needle, or if a swab stick or syringe has been used, care should be taken to avoid needle-stick injuries to the aide. Such items should be placed in a hard plastic container with household bleach, sealed, and discarded.

immune deficiencies

There have been some instances of children who are born without an immune system. That means that their bodies are unable to fight off any bacteria, virus, or other infectious disease. Perhaps you have read about the little boy who lives in a "bubble." This plastic container keeps him safe from germs that could cause serious illness or death.

AIDS (Acquired Immune Deficiency Syndrome) is a life-threatening disease which attacks a person's immune system and causes death by damaging the body's ability to ward off infectious diseases. It is estimated that by the end of 1991 (just ten years from the time it was first diagnosed) 270,000 individuals will have developed the disease and 179,000 will have died from it.

how AIDS is transmitted

AIDS is a viral disease that can be transmitted by intimate sexual contact—oral, vaginal, rectal—or by "dirty" hypodermic needles. When it was first diagnosed, it was found mainly among homosexuals and intravenous drug users. Later, it was discovered that it was also transmitted by contaminated blood transfusions. At this time it is considered to be the most dangerous of the sexually transmitted diseases. It has been found in persons of both sexes (male and female) and in homosexuals and heterosexuals from all walks of life. It has spread to over one hundred countries.

There is a great deal of fear as well as a lot of misinformation about this disease. With all of the publicity about the disease and the fact that a number of famous people have died from it, many people have become unreasonably fearful. In a town near Kokomo, Indiana, a large number of citizens grew alarmed because it was learned that a young boy suffering from hemophilia had developed AIDS from blood transfusions given to him at the hospital. They demanded that he not be allowed to go to the public school because he would spread the disease. For several months he was denied the right to attend school and some teachers refused to go to his home to give home-bound classes.

It has been found that AIDS can also be transmitted to newborn babies during delivery or through the mother's milk. A new mother infected by a blood transfusion can also pass the disease by breastfeeding her infant. However, diagnosis of an infant with AIDS is difficult during the first year of life. Nonetheless, every effort is being made to make an immediate diagnosis of the newborn since it is hoped that an experimental drug (AZT) may arrest the disease if given immediately after birth. Children with AIDS need special attention and care, figure 15-2.

The incubation time for the virus varies, but can be as long as 7–15 years. Thus, it is possible that individuals who received blood transfusions as far back as 1977 may be at risk for AIDS. Anyone who feels that he or she has been exposed because of sexual contact, transfusion, or drug use can be tested for AIDS. The results of such tests are kept confidential.

As more information has come to light about this dread disease, the public is more aware of what is and what is not true. According to Dr. C. Everett Koop, Surgeon General

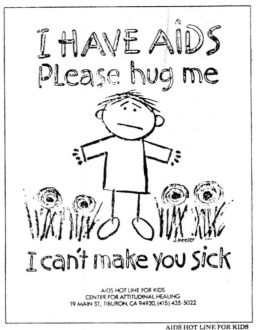

AIDS HOT LINE FOR KIDS

Love might be the hardest thing to get. (courtesy of the Center for Attitudinal Healing, 19 Main St., Tiburon, CA 94920 415-435-5022)

Figure 15-2

of the United States, we must come to terms with the fact that we are fighting a disease, not the people who have AIDS. He also said that those who are already afflicted are sick people who need to be cared for like any other sick patients.

how to protect against AIDS

At this time there is no vaccine to prevent AIDS and there is no cure for AIDS. There are experimental drugs being used for AIDS victims and a great deal of research is underway to isolate the virus and discover effective treatments.

The only way to lessen the impact of the AIDS virus is to avoid situations that are dangerous. For example, careful choice of sex partners, practicing safer sex by using condoms, establishing a monagamous relationship (staying with one partner), practicing abstinence, not "shooting" drugs intravenously, not using a "dirty" needle (best of all, not getting involved in drug use of any kind), making sure that blood used for transfusions is free from the AIDS virus, and using precautions when caring for an AIDS patient. Such precautions include wearing gloves when cleaning up vomitus or when changing a soiled bed.

AIDS-related complex

There are persons who test positive for the AIDS virus who do not have signs and symptoms of the disease. However, they can transmit the virus to others by sexual contact, by sharing drug needles, or by offering their blood for transfusion. Most hospitals and agencies providing blood for transfusions are extremely careful. Since the AIDS virus factor has been isolated, all blood samples are tested before acceptance for transfusion.

ARC (AIDS-Related Complex) occurs in an individual testing positive for the AIDS infection, but is often less severe than the physical deterioration of a person with classic AIDS. Signs and symptoms of ARC can include loss of appetite, weight loss, fever, night sweats, skin rashes, diarrhea, tiredness, swollen lymph nodes, and lack of resistance to infection. Those with ARC may recover and feel perfectly well until another infection comes along and causes a recurrence of symptoms. ARC patients may or may not develop classic AIDS.

By 1991 it is predicted that of the 270,000 people who develop AIDS and/or ARC, will require hospitalization at least once and that 179,000 will die of AIDS in the United States alone. This means that home health aides will probably be involved in caring for AIDS clients between hospital visits. The Surgeon General states that quarantine has no role in the management of AIDS because AIDS is not spread by casual contact, unless the AIDS victim deliberately exposes others by sexual contact and sharing drug equipment.

caring for the AIDS client

What does this information mean to a health care worker? One of the major concerns of the Department of Health is to provide proper care for the AIDS patient while protecting the health care workers. At this time the center for disease control indicates that one cannot get AIDS from casual social contact (shaking hands, hugging, coughing, sneezing, or kissing), contact with tears of an AIDS patient, or from their perspiration. AIDS probably is not spread by swimming in pools, bathing in hot tubs, or from eating food prepared or served by an AIDS victim, or from health team members working with AIDS patients. You will not get AIDS from handling bed linens, towels, cups, straws, dishes, or other eating utensils. You cannot get AIDS from toilet seats, telephones or household furnishings. However, until definitive answers are found, it is strongly recommended that health care workers take special precautions.

what an aide can and should do

First, it is essential that you be informed that your client has AIDS. You have the right to refuse to care for such a client. If you choose to take on an AIDS client then you must follow *all* instructions from the doctor and your supervisor. Always follow the client care plan, figure 15-3. A light but nutritious diet is recommended. Many AIDS clients suffer severe loss of appetite and may be better off with several small meals daily. Perhaps the client should suggest what foods might taste "good".

Please remember that, by word or action, you must not cause embarrassment or

SAMPLE CARE PLAN FOR CLIENT WITH AIDS

SIGN/SYMPTOM	CARE TO PROVIDE	PURPOSE
Weakness/tiredness	High calorie diet with in-between meal high protein snacks	To provide protein nutrition and it slows muscle deterioration
Fever	Sponge baths, give additional fluids by mouth; cover with blankets during chill periods	To lower the temperature and to prevent complications. To get client comfortable
Night Sweats	Sponge baths, frequent linen changes, give additional fluids to avoid dehydration	To provide comfort and to return skin to normal condition
Cough	Observe and record patterns and changes and report findings. Offer cough medicine if prescribed. Gloves required when working.	To make the client comfortable and to obtain relief from strain
Dyspnea	Note patterns and changes—record and report. Calm client and avoid exertion by client and help with breathing exercises	To provide breath control and relaxation
Skin lesions	Keep client from scratching—be sure nails are properly cut by nurse—wear gloves when working with client with lesions and wash hands carefully after contact with client	To prevent infections
Dry hair and hair loss	Avoid too frequent shampooing— use mild shampoo containing no alcohol. Use hair conditioner	To prevent further hair loss and to avoid scalp irritation
Mouth lesions	Provide saline or anesthetic mouthwashes; brush teeth gently. Check to be sure client can swallow without difficulty—observe, record and report to supervisor. Avoid spicy, acid foods and carbonated beverages. Gloves are required when giving mouth care.	To provide infection control, client comfort, and maintain adequate nutrition.
Diarrhea	Encourage fluid intake; change linens as needed; apply diaper if required; observe, record and report; gloves required	To maintain nutrition and fluid balance. To prevent decubitus ulcer formation

Figure 15-3   Sample care plan for client with AIDS

SIGN/SYMPTOM	CARE TO PROVIDE	PURPOSE
Impaired Immune System (when client picks up any infection around)	Give daily shower or bath; both client and HHA wash hands frequently; request nurse to apply sterile dressings as needed with gloves; do not allow visitors who have infections, such as colds; do not come to give client care if you are suffering from any infection	To prevent infection and to assist in client protection
Unstable emotional responses	Be aware of clients feelings as well as your own. Be honest with client and accept him as a person not as an AIDS victim. Offer emotional support, kindness. Communicate by touching client's hand, pat on back, etc.	To create an atmosphere of mutual trust

The possibility of a home health aide getting AIDS from a client is remote. However, if you are emotionally able to handle an AIDS client, you must take all possible precautions. Your supervisor and the medical team will tell you how to protect yourself.

THE FOLLOWING RULES ARE DESIGNED TO PREVENT TRANSMISSION OF THE INFECTION:

1. Wear a gown if there is a possibility of soiling your clothing with blood or body secretions of client.
2. Wear gloves when touching blood or body secretions.
3. Wash hands before and after client contact and immediately if they are potentially contaminated with blood or body secretions.
4. Discard articles contaminated with blood or body secretions and secure in plastic bag.
5. IF YOU HAVE AN OPEN CUT OR WOUND DO NOT CONTAMINATE THE WOUND WITH CLIENT'S BODY SECRETIONS.
6. Follow any additional instructions by your supervisor or health team member.

Figure 15-3 (*Continued*)

discomfort to the client. If you can't be comfortable around the client, you should not accept the assignment. An aide working with AIDS clients must also be sure that his or her family supports that decision. Otherwise, the home health aide's family may resent or be angry and feel that the aide is risking his/her own family's health.

AIDS clients are not guilty of any "crime" but are the victims of a serious disease. They are to be treated with kindness, compassion, and understanding. If at all possible, a home health aide working with AIDS clients should be given intensive training so that they can provide the highest quality of care possible, figure 15-4. Also, a home health aide must be prepared to accept the fact that the client will probably die within a year.

1. Be with the client. Listen to him/her. Do not lie or give false encouragement. Empathize rather than sympathize.
2. Get the client to participate in care plan. Allow him/her to be dependent, but encourage as much independence as possible.
3. Assist as necessary but allow the client to do as much as possible for himself/herself.
4. Encourage participation in social, recreational, and occupational activities. Don't allow client to become a "professional patient" and wallow in self-pity.
5. Encourage client to talk, but discourage self-pity or self-blame.
6. Do not start working with an AIDS client if you think you may not be able to handle it. If you take an AIDS client work with your supervisor and plan a regular rotation so that the client has consistent care.
7. Don't try to become the client's "best friend", but do try to establish a good relationship and develop mutual trust.
8. Allow your client to feel anger and frustration and recognize that he may take it out on you. Let the client vent the anger or frustration—but don't take it personally.
9. Do not condemn or blame yourself if you feel fear, anxiety, or discomfort. Working with terminally ill clients is very difficult. Such feelings are natural. Discuss your feelings with your supervisor. Learn as much as you can about the illness. Facts can fight fears!

Figure 15-4

AIDS clients should also be educated about prevention of the transmission of the disease. It is their responsibility to practice commonsense hygienic measures to protect others with whom they live in close contact, figure 15-5.

summary

- There are any number of infectious and contagious diseases.
- A home health aide may be assigned to care for a child with measles, mumps, chicken pox or rubella. These diseases last for a limited period of time. In the case of measles, bed rest is prescribed and it is recommended that the patient's eyes be protected.
- Rubella, or German measles, can be extremely dangerous if a pregnant woman should get the disease because of the possibility of birth defects including blindness, deafness, or retardation.
- Mumps are particularly dangerous to men and boys just entering puberty. Bed rest is prescribed and exercise is forbidden as mumps can affect the reproductive system causing sterility.
- Of all the infectious diseases, AIDS is the most serious. Death may occur within a year of diagnosis.
- Some of the rules an aide must follow when caring for an AIDS client include:

1. Wear disposable gloves when handling blood or other bloody body secretions—urine, vomitus, sputum, or fecal matter
2. If you have open cuts on your hands or face, make sure they do not come in contact with the client's blood.
3. Wash your hands thoroughly before and after all client care procedures and contact

- Just as it is important for a home health aide to protect his or her own health when caring for an AIDS or ARC client, it is equally important to consider the AIDS client. If, for example, an aide has a cold or other infection, it would be foolhardy to expose the AIDS client to further risk.

INFECTION PRECAUTIONS FOR PEOPLE WITH AIDS LIVING IN THE COMMUNITY

People with AIDS who are able to care for themselves at home can safely live with both individuals who do not have AIDS or with other persons with AIDS. Certain common sense hygienic measures protect both the person with AIDS as well as others in close contact.

• Principles of common-sense hygiene should be followed when working with a person who has AIDS. Sharing a bathroom or kitchen is fine. Dishes may be shared provided they are washed with soap and hot water after each use.

• Tissues, bandages or dressings should be discarded in a paper bag or lined garbage can. Other trash may be handled by normal means.

• Toothbrushes, razors, enema equipment and sexual toys **should not** be shared..

• Laundry should be washed in hot water. If linens or clothing are soiled with blood or bodily secretions, use a bleach solution (1 part bleach to 10 parts water).

• Floors should be mopped at least weekly. A bleach solution (1:10) can be used to disinfect floor, showers, tubs, sinks, sponges and mops. Full strength bleach can be poured into the toilet bowl for disinfection. Any spills of body fluids should be cleaned as they occur and the area then disinfected.

• People with AIDS can cook safely for others. Unpasteurized milk and milk products (associated with Salmonella infections)

should not be included in the diet. Organically grown food (if composted with human or animal feces) should be peeled and/or cooked.

• If there are pets in the house, the person with AIDS **should not** clean the fish tank, the cat litter box, or the bird cage. (Each may contain potentially dangerous bacteria.) Cat litter boxes should be changed daily.

• Disinfection procedures for human skin exposure to body fluids are:

Open cuts or wounds: wash exposed surface with a solution of 3% hydrogen peroxide in water or 10% bleach in water.

Skin: wash exposed surface with a **70%** solution of ethyl or isopropyl alcohol or 3% hydrogen peroxide.

This article is based on information prepared by:

Grace Lusby, MS, RN, Infection Control Co-ordinator, San Francisco General Hospital

Helen Scheiting, MA, RN, Director, Shanti AIDS Residence Program

Michael Helquist, San Francisco AIDS Foundation

Distributed by Gay Men's Health Crisis, Education Department

Figure 15-5 Infection precautions for people with AIDS living in the community (courtesy of Gay Men's Health Crisis, Inc., 132 W. 24th St., New York, NY 10011)

• Probably the most important rule to follow with an AIDS client is to treat him or her with respect and dignity. Do not make judgments about how the disease was transmitted.

• Many people are so fearful of getting AIDS that they will not go near an AIDS patient. This causes the victim to feel even more isolated. More than anything, an AIDS client needs to know that someone cares!

review

1. List four communicable diseases (include signs, symptoms, and transferrance).
2. Name two ways in which AIDS is spread.
3. Explain the difference between ARC and AIDS.
4. List three *safety practices* a Home Health Aide should follow when caring for an AIDS client. How are these practices different from those followed with other communicable diseases?
5. Discuss why you WOULD or WOULD NOT be willing to care for an AIDS Client.
6. Define *infection* and *communicable* disease.
7. Describe the nursing care needed for the AIDS client.
8. List six rules for the prevention of the spread of infections.

Caring for Clients with Acute and Chronic Disorders

Unit 16

Caring for Clients with Diabetes

---

key terms

diabetes	blood lancet	amputation
juvenile diabetes	subcutaneous	phantom pain
hormones	gas gangrene	prosthesis
glucose	diabetic complications	

---

learning objectives

After studying this unit, you should be able to:
— Name four symptoms of diabetes.
— Name three ways to control diabetes.
— List three ways to test for diabetes.
— Name three long-term complications of diabetes.
— Describe foot care given to the diabetic client.
— List symptoms of insulin shock and diabetic coma and the immediate care given for each.

The endocrine system is made up of ductless (tubeless) glands. There are other glands in the body which do have ducts, such as tear glands, sweat glands, salivary glands, and oil glands. Examples of ductless glands are the adrenal gland, thyroid gland and the islets of Langerhans in the pancreas.

Ductless glands secrete substances called hormones. **Hormones** are natural chemicals that the body secretes directly into the bloodstream. The hormones are carried through the bloodstream to regulate and control specific body functions. Each hormone does a specific job. Hormones are very powerful substances; only a small amount of a hormone is needed to trigger body reaction. The brain sends messages to the endocrine glands. This message stimulates the gland to secrete the hormone needed by the body.

diabetes

The islets of Langerhans is the ductless portion of the pancreas that secretes insulin. Insulin controls the use and distribution of sugar in the body. When insulin is not manufactured, or cannot be used correctly, a condition called **diabetes** develops. In diabetes, the blood is very high in sugar. This is because the sugar remains in the blood instead of being absorbed into the tissues and used for food. The unused sugar is excreted in the urine. The diet of a diabetic must be carefully watched because this disease disturbs the body's metabolism of nutrients such as fats and proteins as well as sugar.

The buildup of sugar in the blood is unhealthy for other reasons. It disturbs the fluid balance in the body because it causes kidney problems. Diabetes suppresses the immune system and this allows infections to flourish. Sugar buildup also causes damage to blood vessels thereby restricting circulation. The lack of a nourishing blood supply to certain body areas causes many problems.

Diabetes ranks third, after heart disease and cancer, as a cause of death in adults. There is no cure for it. However, it can be controlled by proper diet and regular exercise, usually combined with medication. There are 10 million people with diabetes in the United States today. At least one million of these are juvenile diabetics. People who acquire diabetes before the age of 30 are called *juvenile diabetics*. Diabetes is more difficult to control when it is acquired in childhood or young adulthood. Injections of insulin are often required for the young diabetic in addition to regular exercise and diet control. Diabetes is typed as:

1. Insulin dependent, or
2. Noninsulin dependent.

symptoms and diagnosis

Adult diabetes usually strikes after age 40, and commonly around the age of 55. Diabetes is less severe at this time and can often be controlled without medication. A controlled diet and regular exercise are necessary. An oral medication may be prescribed. The oral medication *is not* insulin; however, it does stimulate the pancreas to secrete insulin for the body's needs. Such patients are said to have the noninsulin-dependent type of diabetes. In some cases, insulin is necessary. This best describes the *insulin dependent* person who must obtain insulin by injection with an insulin syringe.

Every person should have a physical examination annually, as symptoms of diabetes may otherwise go unnoticed. Some of the symptoms to watch for are:

• weakness
• sudden weight loss
• unusual thirst
• frequent need to urinate
• excessive hunger
• crankiness

testing

Tests for diabetes are important for early detection and accurate diagnosis. Tests are necessary for adults since they often have no symptoms at all. The tests for diabetes are included in a complete physical exam. However, if any of the symptoms of diabetes are present, a person should go immediately for a physical. The tests for diabetes are:

- Blood Sample—usually taken from the arm; tested for blood **glucose** (type of sugar).
- Urinalysis—sample of urine tested by dipping a chemically treated stick in the urine. Both sugar and acetone readings are made.
- Glucose Tolerance Test—series of tests on blood and urine.

Diabetics must take responsibility for performing urine testing at home. There are special kits for this purpose available at any drugstore. These kits (Ketodiastix, Diastix®, Clinitest®, Tes-Tape®) include specially treated strips of paper to be dipped in urine specimens and read according to instructions on the product. Most recently, a home testing technique on the blood has been perfected, figure 16-1. All of these products require careful and correct performance to ensure accurate results. For example, the blood sample might have to be taken before the client has eaten, or after the client has exercised; the urine specimen may need to be a ''clean catch,'' or taken before meals. Accurate timing and careful attention to the color of the paper strip are very important to ensure accuracy. It is extremely important to follow the instructions on the product.

In some instances, a doctor will determine that a diabetic should be on a sliding scale of insulin instead of one or two injections daily of the same amount. This means that the client will take insulin based on the amount of sugar in the blood at a given time. In this test, a drop of blood is obtained by using a **blood lancet,** figure 16-2. The drop of blood is placed on the chemically-treated strip. Following a chart on the test kit, a determination is made as to the amount of insulin required.

Diabetics are instructed by their own doctors with regard to self-testing and reading

of results. **Caution:** These tests can only be done by someone who has been properly trained in these techniques.

The client should always be instructed to check the expiration date on the insulin bottle. The insulin should not be used if it is past the expiration date indicated because it might

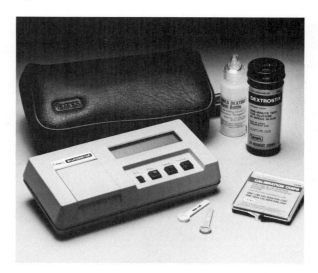

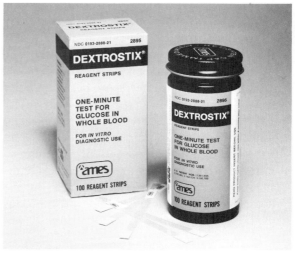

Figure 16-1 The Glucometer®/Dextrostix® test is just one test available for measuring blood glucose (courtesy of Ames Division, Miles Laboratories, Inc.).

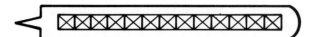

Figure 16-2 A blood lancet is used to obtain a blood sample for diabetic testing.

not be effective. It is no longer necessary to refrigerate insulin.

treatment

After a diagnosis of diabetes has been confirmed, treatment is started at once. In many cases, the person is hospitalized for a few days. This allows the doctor to keep a close watch on the results of a prescribed medication and diet. After the condition is stabilized (put in balance) by the medicine, diet, and recommended exercise, the person can be released from the hospital.

control of diabetes with medication

In diabetes, the body cannot regulate its own insulin production and usage. Therefore, one treatment used is to supply the body with insulin through medication. The amount of insulin needed for control varies greatly. The doctor, to some extent, can plan for the person's insulin needs. General needs are based on body weight, frequency and type of insulin injections, diet content, and the person's usual amount of exercise. However, needs may change throughout the day; vigorous exercise, emotional stress, illness, or changeable conditions in pregnancy increase demands on the body. Sometimes, changes cannot be controlled. At other times, controls on diet or activity are neglected.

insulin injections

Insulin is injected **subcutaneously** (under the skin). The diabetic is taught where,

when and how to inject the medication, figure 16-3. If a person is unable to give self-injections, another member of the family is taught how to give the injections. Some diabetics are too young to give themselves injections; other diabetics may have poor eyesight or coordination. Most diabetics, if instructed properly, are able to inject their own insulin. **Caution:** A home health aide is NOT permitted to inject insulin. The aide's responsibility is limited to bringing the medication to the client. The aide should assist as needed, and return the medication to storage. Children as young as five years old can be taught to inject their own insulin. The dosage must be carefully checked by a responsible adult.

Once insulin is prescribed, it will have to be used for the rest of the diabetic's life. The two most important factors to remember about insulin are:

1. The measurement must be accurate.
2. The drug must be taken at the same time each day.

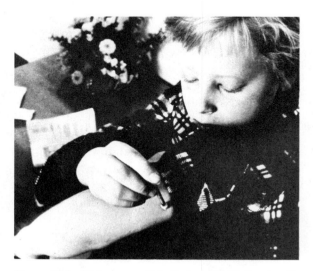

Figure 16-3 This young diabetic is self-injecting insulin into the upper arm (courtesy of Diabetes Education Center, Minneapolis, MN).

The doctor may prescribe different kinds of insulin. Some insulin is fast acting and some is slow acting. The doctor will prescribe the type of insulin needed. The frequency and time of day for injections are also specified by the doctor.

Current practice is to have the diabetic inject insulin at one location for a period of seven days, then use a different site for the next seven days. Injections can be made in the upper or lower arm, in the abdomen, or in the thigh. When someone other than the diabetic is giving the shots, other areas of the body can be used, such as the back or buttock.

The insulin pump is a recent development. A small needle is inserted in the abdomen. The needle is connected to a pump worn at the waist which holds the insulin supply. This device administers a continuous amount of insulin. A control button or switch allows the client to adjust the release of insulin. In the future this device may be implanted in diabetics just as a pacemaker is now implanted for the heart patient.

Experiments are now being conducted with a nasal spray to deliver insulin and another using an air jet to inject insulin.

dietary control of diabetes

In some cases, diet alone can control the diabetic condition. All diabetics must follow very strict diet rules. All foods must be measured and sugar intake limited. The doctor will give each diabetic a list of the foods and the amounts allowed each day. A measured amount of food is called an exchange. It is suggested that diabetics eat three regular meals each day plus snacks. Snacks should be eaten at midmorning, midafternoon and before bedtime. All foods used by a diabetic must be chosen from an exchange list.

The American Diabetes Association and the American Dietetic Association have grouped foods into six major lists:

List 1—Starch/Bread
List 2—Meat
List 3—Vegetable
List 4—Fruit
List 5—Milk
List 6—Fat

Each list includes measured amounts of foods containing nearly equal amounts of energy value (measured in kilocalories), carbohydrates, proteins and fats. Any one food in a list may be used in place of another food *on the same list* and still provide the client with the required amounts of nutrients and energy value.

Information about the exchange lists can be obtained from the local chapter of the American Diabetes Association or the national office: The American Diabetes Association, 1660 Duke Street, Alexandria, VA 22314. A publication "Exchange Lists for Meal Planning" is available from the Association for a small fee.

The diet for the diabetic client is planned in terms of the number of exchanges permitted from each list for each meal. The doctor will determine the number of food exchanges permitted. A diabetic can maintain a stable condition only by following the doctor's orders completely.

An important duty of the home health aide is to prepare meals using the doctor's prescribed diet and exchange lists. The aide must be sure the food selected for the meals include the Basic Four food groups and are allowable on the exchange lists and diet. The aide may need to help the diabetic adjust to using a carefully measured diet.

Excess weight and poor nutrition are two common problems in diabetes. Using the prescribed diet can limit these problems. Most diabetics who stick to a diet, take medication, and exercise moderately have fewer health problems. The diabetic who does not follow the doctor's orders risks serious problems.

care of the client with diabetic complications

Untreated or improperly treated diabetes can lead to many physical problems. Abnormal conditions which arise after a person develops diabetes are called **diabetic complications.** In some cases, even a well-cared for diabetic develops serious complications. The most common complications are described in figure 16-4. Insulin shock and diabetic coma are emergency conditions. The other conditions listed, such as vascular disease and risk of infection, are long-term disorders. Although many long-term disorders cannot be avoided, the aide can help the client deal with them.

neuropathy in the diabetic

Neuropathy is defined as a destructive disorder of the nerves. Diabetic neuropathy is the loss of sensation in nerves. Such persons may be unable to feel pain or hot or cold. This can be extremely dangerous. For example, a diabetic injures a foot or leg and, because no pain is felt, continues to use the limb. An infection can occur and the diabetic does not even realize there is a problem. Cuts or wounds not felt and thus not cared for can become infected. A home health aide must carefully observe his/her diabetic client's feet and legs for any sign of redness, any "warm" area, any swelling, or any open cuts.

giving good skin care

Good skin care includes washing the area, drying carefully, keeping bed linens dry, clean and wrinkle free, and turning the client regularly to avoid pressure spots leading to decubiti. Good skin care helps protect the skin from injury and infection. This is an important safety precaution for the diabetic client. Even minor cuts and skin injuries take a long time to heal. Slow healing is due in part to poor circulation. Breakdown of the blood vessels prevents nutrients from being carried to the injured tissue; this delays the healing process. The slow healing process leaves the skin open to infection. The risk of infection is also increased because of the extra sugar in the tissues. The extra sugar creates an ideal growing place for bacteria. Bacteria can multiply quickly before the body is able to defend itself. Poor circulation delays the transport of substances needed to fight off the bacteria.

When blood vessels are injured or diseased, the surrounding cells die from lack of nutrition. A large area of dead tissue is called gangrene. Gangrene is a serious condition because it is easily infected with certain bacteria. **Gas gangrene** is an infection. The bacteria causing tetanus and gas gangerene thrive in dead tissue. A person can be immunized against tetanus; however, no vaccine exists for gas gangrene. The bacteria spreads quickly, causing severe pain and greater tissue damage.

The aide and other health personnel should check the client's feet and broken skin areas for signs of gas gangrene infection. The first sign is a hot, red skin area. The area then becomes cold and bluish (cyanotic). After the tissues are dead, they flake off. Drainage from the area may bubble and will emit a strong, foul odor.

giving foot care

The home health aide should give special attention to the diabetic's feet every day. The feet should be bathed daily and thoroughly dried, especially between the toes. Lotion may

CONDITION	CAUSE	SYMPTOMS	TREATMENT	AIDE'S CARE
EMERGENCY CONDITIONS				
1. **Insulin Shock**	Too much insulin	Nervousness, dizziness, perspiration, headache, blurred vision, weakness, hunger, tremors, numbness of tongue and lips, stupor, unconsciousness	Hard candy, lump of sugar, or glass of orange juice with honey or sugar added.	Give the client candy, sugar, juice; call doctor
2. **Diabetic Coma**	Lack of insulin	Flushed dry skin, sweet odor on breath, nausea, vomiting, abdominal pain, dry tongue, senses dull, comatose	May require hospitalization to adjust insulin dosage	Call doctor; keep client warm
LONG-TERM DISORDERS				
3. **Blindness**	Cataracts, glaucoma, hemorrhage	Partial or total loss of sight, client drops items, stumbles or falls; develops tunnel vision	Surgery can remove cataracts; lost sight from glaucoma cannot be restored; save what sight remains	Assist in activities of daily living
4. **Gas Gangrene**	Poor circulation; skin breakdown; invasion of tissue by bacteria	Heat in area, skin reddened, formation of ulcers which don't clear up; foul odor and spread of infection and tissue destruction	Medication under doctor's order; may require amputation of limb	Assist with dressing changes and rehabilitation
5. **Kidney Disease**	Too much sugar free in urine; filtering system works inefficiently	Frequency, pain, burning while voiding; retention of urine may occur	Diet modification and medication	Observe and record Intake/Output; note color and composition of urine
6. **Vascular Disease and Nerve Degeneration**	High sugar level; poor fat metabolism; poor tissue repair; poor circulation	Open lesions form on skin tissue as vascular degeneration occurs; nervous system functions at decreased level—sight, sound, taste, touch, smell may be affected	Bedrest, moist heat/dressings, diet and medication	Give proper foot care. Assist in activities of daily living

Figure 16-4   Common complications of diabetes

be massaged into the feet. This helps stimulate the blood circulation to the feet. Bunions and corns should be treated by a podiatrist (foot doctor).

In the aged, the nails become thick and difficult to cut. Nail care (both fingernails and toenails) must be carefully done by a nurse or someone who has been taught to do it correctly. **Caution:** The home health aide may NOT cut the diabetic client's nails. There is danger of infection from skin cuts around the nails. In addition, improper cutting may cause ingrown toenails which easily leads to infection. If the client's feet are well cared for and examined daily, infection is unlikely to develop. The following foot care will help to reduce injury to the feet.

- Bathe the feet daily in warm, NOT hot water.
- Dry the feet completely.
- Massage the feet to increase circulation.
- Wear clean, white cotton socks, changed daily.
- Wear comfortable, well-fitting shoes.
- Avoid applying iodine, creosol or carbolic acid to cuts on foot.
- Avoid walking barefoot.
- Avoid using commercial corn pads.
- Avoid using garters or tight bandages.
- Avoid using a heating pad on the feet.

See Figure 16-5 for an example of a footcare checklist.

assisting the amputee

In some cases an injured foot that does not heal becomes infected with gas gangrene. When gas gangrene cannot be stopped, the foot and sometimes the leg must be amputated. An **amputation** is a surgical procedure in which a limb or a portion of a limb is removed.

The amputee is not released from the hospital until the surgical wound is fairly well healed. One of the aide's duties is to apply clean dressings to the stump. The client will have some pain for which medication is prescribed. The doctor's orders indicate the type of pain-killing medication which is best. The aide should be sure the client takes the medicine according to the doctor's orders. Even if the client pleads for more medication, these orders must be followed. Frequent use of strong pain killers can cause the client to become dependent on the drug. There are many drug addicts who can trace their addiction to prescribed medications.

Physical therapy is planned for most amputees. In some cases, a **prosthesis** is fitted after the stump is healed, figure 16-6. It is necessary for amputees to regain a feeling of independence. Amputees must develop pride in being able to help themselves. A therapist instructs the amputee in use of walking aids. The home health aide should follow safety precautions. Using safety measures helps the client avoid injury when using these devices.

Following the amputation of a limb, special care must be given to the surgical site or "stump".

stump care. Cleanliness is the first concern. Clean skin is less likely to become infected. When the stump is healed, the daily care plan should include:

1. Wash with mild soap and warm water to remove dirt and perspiration built up during the day.
2. Rinse well with warm water, removing all soap to avoid irritation.
3. Pat dry thoroughly with a towel; *do not rub*.
4. When skin is dry, apply mild lotion.
5. Rinse the stump with rubbing alcohol each morning if ordered by the doctor.

After surgery there is usually some swelling and pain. Edema is the accumulation of normal body fluids at the site of the amputation. Normally, movements of the foot and ankle keep fluids from settling in one location. When the foot or ankle are removed, other ways must be found to circulate the fluid away from the stump area. Ace or elastic bandages may be applied to the stump. They act as an external pump, pushing the fluids away from the stump. Elevating the stump while sitting may also prevent further edema.

ace wrapping. An ace wrap *cannot* be worn while a temporary prosthesis is in place as it could cause added swelling. Besides being painful, swelling can slow the rate the wound

DAILY FOOTCARE CHECKLIST

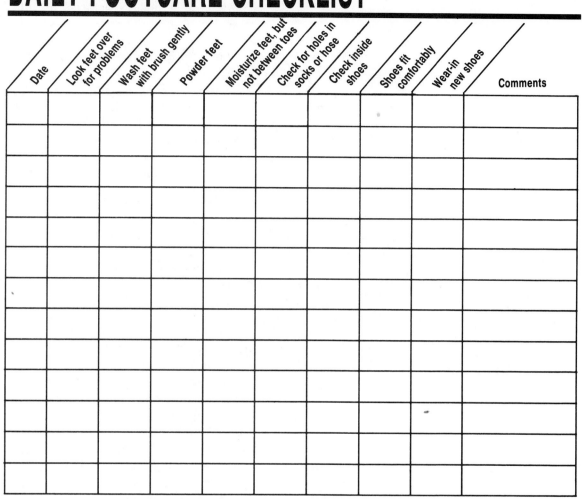

Date	Look feet over for problems	Wash feet with brush gently	Powder feet	Moisturize feet, but not between toes	Check for holes in socks or hose	Check inside shoes	Shoes fit comfortably	Wear-in new shoes	Comments

Contact your doctor about any foot problems.

Figure 16-5 Daily footcare checklist

heals. Ace wrapping is used after surgery to *shape* the stump in preparation for a prosthesis.

Stump bandages should be rewrapped every 4–6 hours to maintain firm support and retain the pumping action. However, if a bandage is wrapped too tightly, it can inhibit circulation causing severe pain, numbness, tingling or a cold sensation. At the first sign of these symptoms, the bandage should be rewrapped. (You will be instructed on the proper techniques of applying ace bandages.)

Elastic (ACE) bandages come in various widths and lengths. The proper size will be determined by the physician or therapist. Use tape to fasten the bandage. *DO NOT* secure the ace bandage with clips or pins as they could puncture the skin.

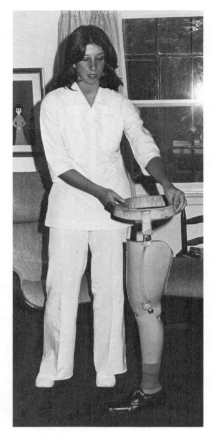

Figure 16-6 A prosthesis is usually made for an amputee.

tinues, suggest that he/she think about wiggling all toes or fingers to relieve the discomfort or stretch both legs or arms as fully as possible. Sometimes the amputee is so sure the leg is still there that he may try to walk normally. Phantom pain diminishes (fades away) in time.

There is actual pain and tenderness at the stump or along the suture lines even after the surgical wound is healed. This, too, should fade in time. If the client complains of intense pain or a different kind of sensation, report this to the supervisor immediately.

contractures. A contracture is the result of tightened muscles across the front of the hip or the back of the knee, making it difficult to straighten the joint. This can make fitting a prosthesis more difficult and cause pain while walking.

to avoid getting contractures

1. For below-knee amputations, keep the knee straight, especially while sitting. When in bed, keep hip and knee straight.
2. For above-knee amputations, remind the client to avoid bending the hip while in bed by holding the leg straight and flat against the bed. Where possible, sleeping on the stomach instead of on the side or back is recommended. Range of motion exercises are, of course, helpful in the prevention of contractures, see figures 16-7 to 16-10.

assisting the blind diabetic

Blindness is another long-term complication which some diabetics suffer. The person who has been blind since birth makes adjustments to the handicap early in life. A diabetic who becomes blind later in life may have a slow and difficult period of adjustment. One of the hardest tasks is learning to move around freely. The blind client has to practice even a

ace care. Bandages should be washed in warm water using mild soap. They should be carefully rinsed and laid flat to dry. Machine washing and drying can reduce their elasticity. Do not dry in direct sunlight or near direct heat. Allow the bandage to dry thoroughly before re-using. A damp bandage can irritate the skin or lead to an infection.

phantom sensation. Phantom sensation or phantom pain may occur after an amputation. An amputee may state he feels an itch or pain in the missing limb. When that happens, suggest that the client look at the stump and apply pressure to the area. If the pain con-

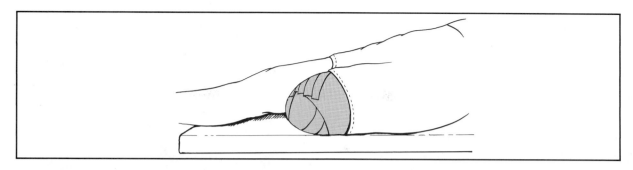

Figure 16-7 Proper positioning while lying on back (always keep leg straight)

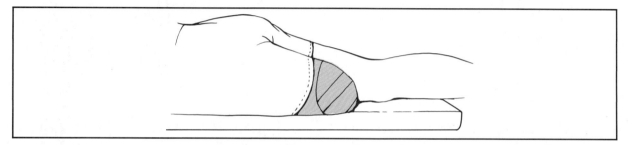

Figure 16-8 Proper positioning while lying on stomach (keep hip and leg straight)

simple task such as sitting down. Practice is also needed for getting in and out of bed, brushing teeth and going to the bathroom.

Loss of sight causes many people to lose their sense of direction and time. They become disoriented. They do not know where they are or whether it is day or night. These clients will have to be led from room to room until they have learned their way around. The home health aide should keep the furniture in exactly the same place so the person will not bump into it.

When walking with a blind client, the aide should gently hold the client's arm and walk slightly ahead and to the side of the client. If preferred, the client can grasp the aide's arm. A great deal of practice is necessary for the newly blind person to become accustomed to moving about comfortably.

Aides may have to help clients to learn how to feed themselves. One type of food should always be arranged on the plate in the same spot. By doing this, the client knows where a particular food is placed and can make the desired selection. Explain to the client that the food is arranged on the plate according to the face of a clock, figure 16-11. Then always remember to arrange food in the same pattern. Meat might be placed at 6 o'clock, vegetables at 9 o'clock, salad at 12 o'clock, and bread at 3 o'clock. The more blind people can help themselves, the better they will feel.

Arranging the client's clothing in a certain order will help the client in dressing. Most people like to feel neat and properly dressed. The aide can help by keeping clothes and personal items in order.

The aide should talk with the blind client and describe what is happening. This will help the client feel more a part of things. The

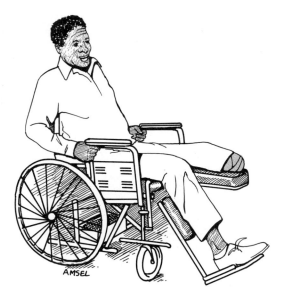

Figure 16-9 Proper positioning while sitting in a wheelchair (knee straight)

aide should encourage the client to be independent. However, the aide must be willing to lend a hand whenever the client needs it. During the early stages of blindness, it is natural for the person to feel self-pity. The aide can be of great help while the client works through the adjustment period.

identification tags

All diabetics should wear a Medic Alert ID. The ID is a labeled tag worn as a bracelet or necklace, figure 16-12. The ID tag should be worn by the diabetic at all times. The label indicates the person's:

- name
- address
- telephone number
- medical condition
- physician's name

In emergencies, the Medic Alert ID informs health personnel, police officers and others of the diabetic's medical condition. A dia-

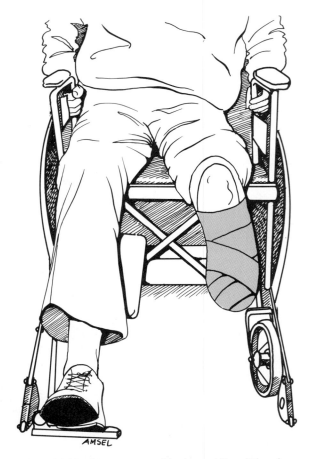

Figure 16-10 Improper positioning while sitting in a wheelchair (knee bent)

betic who develops acidosis or insulin shock needs immediate help. The ID tag notifies health personnel that the person's emergency is possibly a diabetic condition. If the person is unconscious, the tag may provide information necessary to save the person's life. Medic Alert tags are also worn by persons with epilepsy and with allergies to certain drugs.

summary

- Almost any illness or infection can cause added problems for a diabetic.
- Nausea and vomiting from a simple case of flu can upset the insulin balance in the body.

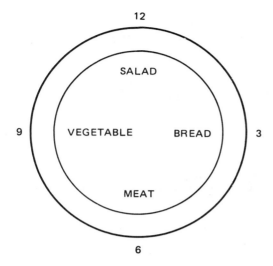

Figure 16-11 Food for the blind client should be arranged on the plate according to numbers on the face of a clock.

The doctor should be called in at once in order to correct the insulin deficiency.

• At the first sign of open sores on the client the home health aide should call the doctor. Proper care at once may save the client needless pain and suffering.

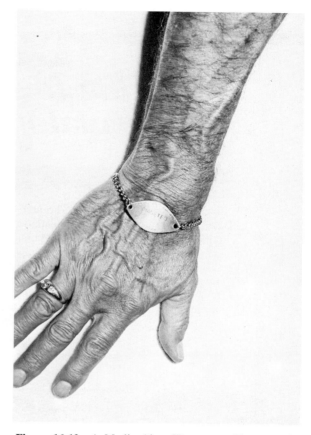

Figure 16-12 A Medic Alert ID tag provides essential information in case of an emergency.

review

1. What are the symptoms of diabetes?
2. Describe the foot care given to the diabetic client.
3. What three methods are used to control diabetes?
4. a. What are the symptoms of insulin shock?
   b. What is the immediate care given?
5. a. List the symptoms of diabetic coma.
   b. What should the home health aide do if these symptoms appear in the client?

Unit 17

Caring for Clients with Circulatory Problems

key terms

angina pectoris
sublingually
topically
coronary occlusion
anticoagulant
nitro-patch
congestive heart failure
edema
arteriosclerosis

thrombus
hemiplegia
automatic speech
cerebral vascular
   accident
atherosclerosis
cerebral infarction
intracerebral
   hemorrhage
euphoria

constrictive
collateral circulation
cognitive
spasticity
transient ischemic
   attack (TIA)
hypertension
hypotension
vasoconstriction
vasodilation

learning objectives

After studying this unit, you should be able to:
■ Identify symptoms of four heart conditions.
■ Describe care given for clients with heart conditions.
■ Explain the effect nitroglycerin has on the blood vessels.
■ Give two other names for a CVA.

disorders of the heart and circulatory system

In many cases, disorders of the heart and circulatory system force people to change their life-styles. Many people become very frightened when a heart or circulatory condition is diagnosed. The psychological effects can be almost as crippling as the illness itself. People may think they will be permanently disabled or wonder how they can support themselves and their families. People who have had one heart attack are usually afraid of having another heart attack. As a result, they often avoid moving about or doing any exercise. Inactivity usually leads to boredom; people may become short-tempered and hard to get along with.

The aide may be assigned to help people with heart problems. Certain conditions require clients to reduce their activity. Clients may need relief from household duties or child care. The aide may need to remind clients to avoid vigorous exercise or heavy lifting. The doctor's orders explain a safe range of activity. Helping the client adjust to the necessary changes may be the focus of the aide's care plan.

angina pectoris

Angina pectoris is a severe pain in the chest sometimes going to the left arm and up the neck area. This condition results from lack of oxygen in the heart muscle due to constricted blood vessels. Angina pectoris generally strikes men of middle age. An attack can last from a few seconds to several minutes. It may occur after physical exertion or during times of stress and anxiety. The person becomes pale and ashen and the body stiffens. Blood pressure increases dramatically (hypertension). The client becomes flushed and perspires heavily.

Immediate treatment for angina is physical rest. If this is not the first angina attack, the client will likely have medication on hand. A common emergency medication used for angina is nitroglycerin. Nitroglycerin may be taken **sublingually,** in which case the tablet is placed under the tongue. It can also be applied **topically** in the form of a **nitro-patch** placed on the skin, figure 17-1. The nitroglycerin is absorbed through the skin; a patch provides 24 hours of medication.

Nitroglycerin opens the blood vessels to ease the blood flow. The effects of the drug occur within two to three minutes. The pain from the angina is usually relieved in 5 to 10 minutes. Nitroglycerin is one of the medications that can only be used for a specified period of time because it loses its potency and effectiveness. The aide should check the expiration date carefully to be sure the medicine is still effective. Amyl nitrite is another emergency drug the doctor may prescribe for angina pectoris. This drug is inhaled and is effective within 30 to 60 seconds.

When angina pectoris has been diag-

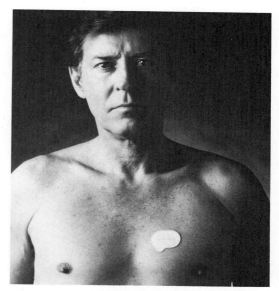

Figure 17-1 The client may receive nitroglycerin through the skin by means of a nitro-patch (courtesy of CIBA Pharmaceutical Co., Division of CIBA, GEIGY, Summit, NJ).

nosed, the client should avoid emotional stress, exercise after heavy meals, exposure to sudden cold, or overexertion. Medication should be placed near the client for immediate use during an attack. If there is no relief in 15 minutes, emergency care is required. Call an ambulance, family physician, family members, and nurse supervisor. Rest, limited activities and no smoking are commonly ordered by the doctor. The home health aide helps enforce these orders. The client often has a headache after taking the medication due to vasodilation.

acute coronary occlusion or myocardial infarction

Acute coronary occlusion or myocardial infarction is more commonly known as a coronary or a heart attack. A **coronary occlusion** is a condition in which a blood vessel of the

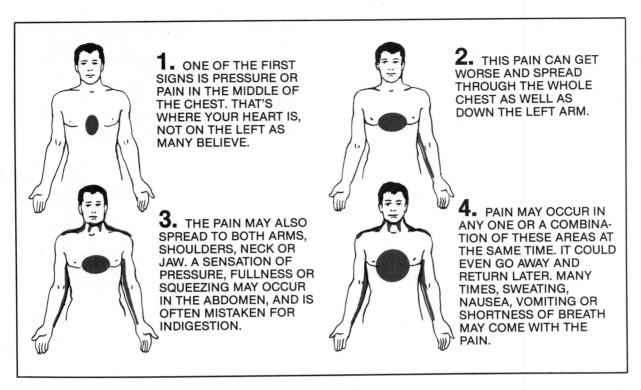

1. ONE OF THE FIRST SIGNS IS PRESSURE OR PAIN IN THE MIDDLE OF THE CHEST. THAT'S WHERE YOUR HEART IS, NOT ON THE LEFT AS MANY BELIEVE.

2. THIS PAIN CAN GET WORSE AND SPREAD THROUGH THE WHOLE CHEST AS WELL AS DOWN THE LEFT ARM.

3. THE PAIN MAY ALSO SPREAD TO BOTH ARMS, SHOULDERS, NECK OR JAW. A SENSATION OF PRESSURE, FULLNESS OR SQUEEZING MAY OCCUR IN THE ABDOMEN, AND IS OFTEN MISTAKEN FOR INDIGESTION.

4. PAIN MAY OCCUR IN ANY ONE OR A COMBINATION OF THESE AREAS AT THE SAME TIME. IT COULD EVEN GO AWAY AND RETURN LATER. MANY TIMES, SWEATING, NAUSEA, VOMITING OR SHORTNESS OF BREATH MAY COME WITH THE PAIN.

Figure 17-2   The symptoms of a heart attack (Reprinted with permission of the American Heart Association/New York City Affiliate, © 1987)

heart muscle closes or is blocked by a blood clot. The size and location of the incident determines the seriousness of the attack. There can be permanent damage to the heart. In the case of permanent damage, parts of the heart muscle die and *collateral circulation* may develop. This means that other small blood vessels take over the job of bringing blood to the heart muscle. These smaller vessels actually become enlarged so they can carry the required amount of fresh, oxygenated blood to the heart muscle. The symptoms of a heart attack are shown in figure 17-2.

The person may go into shock and collapse. Prompt emergency treatment is needed and is begun in the ambulance and continued in the hospital. In the hospital the client will be treated for a heart attack. The need for special-

ized treatment or surgery will be determined. One common operation is called coronary artery bypass grafting, or CABG. After release from the hospital, treatment at home may include bedrest, reduced activity, and diet control.

Anticoagulants and other drugs may be part of the treatment when a person has had a coronary attack. **Anticoagulants** are drugs which reduces the ability of the blood to clot. A home health aide should observe and report any signs of side effects from the use of anticoagulants. These may include bleeding from the gums, pinpoint hemorrhages, or bruising of the skin. The home health aide *never* massages the legs. This could loosen a blood clot and send it directly to the lungs, causing pain and severe breathing problems.

congestive heart failure

Congestive heart failure is a condition in which the heart cannot pump enough blood to the body. This condition can affect the right or left side of the heart, or even both sides at the same time. This is most often caused by heart muscle damage. Thus, the heart's pumping action is weakened. A victim of congestive heart failure may have one acute attack and then develop a chronic condition. The symptoms include a cough, dyspnea, cyanosis, and retention of fluid **(edema).** Fluid (frothy pink sputum) may accumulate in the lungs causing pneumonia. Congestive heart failure can lead to chronic invalidism.

Treatment for congestive heart failure usually includes two types of drugs. One is digitalis which slows and strengthens the heartbeat. The other is a diuretic which reduces fluid accumulation in the body. A diuretic medication causes the client to urinate frequently to help rid the body of excess fluids. The aide should help the client remember to take medications that have been prescribed.

Diet control is an important part of the treatment for congestive heart failure. Diets usually are low in sodium and fat. A diet high in bulk helps the client avoid constipation. A person who is constipated must strain to have a bowel movement; this strain can be dangerous for any person with a heart condition. People who are overweight should restrict their calorie intake as well. The doctor provides exact orders for diet preparation. Exercise and rest must be balanced. The correct amount of each is determined by the doctor.

Clients with congestive heart failure must stay in an upright or semiupright position (head higher than feet). They will need frequent position changes, elastic stockings or Ace bandages on their legs, bedside commode or bedpan, and a partial bed bath. A partial bed bath is needed since a full bath may prove too tiring

for the client. Because clients with congestive heart failure usually breathe through the mouth, they will need special mouth care.

The aide must help clients limit their activities. Clients with congestive heart failure usually cannot go up and down stairs. They must lead very quiet lives because they tire easily. Such clients get depressed because they must be dependent on others. To help reduce this feeling of dependence, the aide should give the client as much control over personal care and selection of activities as possible. Refer to figure 17-3 for a summary of the affects of congestive heart failure.

arteriosclerosis

Arteriosclerosis is a condition in which the arteries become hard and lose their soft,

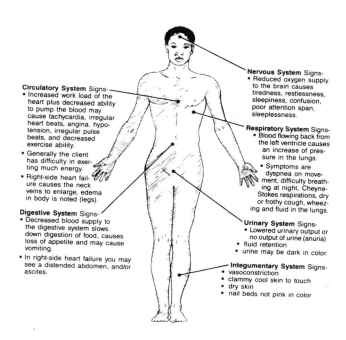

Figure 17-3 Congestive Heart Failure—Systems Involved

rubberlike stretchiness. It is caused by a buildup of fatty deposits on the inside walls of the blood vessels. It is thought that this condition is the result of cholesterol caused by the body being unable to properly digest fatty meats and foods high in fat content.

An important aspect of client care is to increase the client's circulation. A bath not only cleans the skin but also helps to increase circulation. Even if a client does not need a complete bath daily, the aide must wash the client's feet and massage them with lotion each day. After the feet are cleaned, a pair of cotton or wool socks may be needed. Arteriosclerosis clients often complain of cold feet. **Caution:** the home health aide must NEVER apply a hot water bottle or heating pad even if requested by the client. To warm the client's feet, the aide should give the client a second pair of socks or put a blanket over the client's legs. The socks should not fit tightly. Socks or other items of clothing which are tight further restrict circulation.

Decubitus ulcers (bed sores) are caused by poor circulation in particular areas of the body. Decubitus ulcers cause worry because the healing process is so slow. As a result of worry and discomfort, clients can be short-tempered. Loneliness is often a companion to illness. A home health aide should communicate with the client. Recreation and diversions should be planned to keep the client's mind off the illness.

contractures. If confined to bed, the client must be protected from deformities. Weight from the bedcovers can press against the feet. Bedcovers should be kept loose around the feet. Bed cradles may be used in holding bedcovers off the feet. Footboards may be placed against the soles of the feet so that the foot will not drop into an unnatural position. A contracture is a condition in which muscles become short-

ened and stiff. The muscles freeze in an uncomfortable position. Foot drop is a kind of contracture. The client who is confined to bed should be repositioned regularly as ordered by the nurse supervisor. This increases circulation, bringing more oxygen to the cells. It also has a warming effect. Prescribed exercise and repositioning helps prevent decubitus ulcers from forming.

diet. Some foods should not be given to people with arteriosclerosis. These foods include: butter or foods cooked in butter, fatty meats, chocolate, ice cream, whole milk, tea, coffee, cream, cheese and eggs. An arteriosclerosis diet is low in fat and high in protein. Vitamins may also be prescribed. The home health aide should make sure the prescribed diet is followed at all times. In most cases, a weight loss is desirable. In addition to using diet control, clients with arteriosclerosis should not smoke.

cerebral vascular accidents

what is a stroke? The word "stroke" was originally used to indicate any sudden catastrophic illness. Now the term is almost exclusively used to name a sudden paralysis caused by brain damage.

There are two types of stroke. The most common is caused by interruption or blocking of the circulation to a part of the brain, and the other is associated with sudden bleeding into the substance of the brain. Brain tissue deprived of circulation for even a few seconds stops functioning. If the circulation stops for a few minutes, brain tissue dies. This causes loss of voluntary motion and results in paralysis, often in one half of the body.

Brain cells die when they are without oxygen for four minutes. Once brain cells are destroyed, they cannot be brought back to life.

Unlike other cells in the body, new brain cells do not form to replace damaged ones. The most common cause of a CVA is high blood pressure. A CVA does not necessarily destroy all the brain cells. Some strokes are more damaging then others. Healthy brain cells can be trained to take over the duties of those destroyed by a CVA. For that reason, rehabilitation is of vital importance.

The following material is reprinted with permission from a booklet prepared for in-service training. Courtesy of The Burke Rehabilitation Center, White Plains, NY, the Auxiliary and Fletcher H. McDowell, M.D., Executive Medical Director:

risk factors in stroke: Often, long before a stroke occurs, there are conditions or symptoms which are now recognized as associated with an increased risk of stroke. These are:

Hypertension—sustained elevated blood pressure

Atherosclerosis (often called hardening of the arteries)—a disease in which fatty materials containing cholesterol platelets and calcium accumulate on the interior walls of the arteries. These accumulations can build up to the point where the vessel becomes obstructed. This condition is called atherosclerosis.

Heart Disease—(coronary artery disease, damaged heart valves)

Diabetes

Family history of heart disease and/or stroke

Illnesses such as sickle cell anemia, rheumatic fever, aneurysm

Consumption of birth control pills

In addition, there are several conditions which also may be risk factors. Among these are high blood fat levels, obesity, and cigarette smoking.

An individual who has one or more of these conditions or habits has a greater risk of developing a stroke than those without them. The risk increases with an increase in the number of factors found in a particular individual.

Statistics indicate that although stroke can happen at any age, strokes are more common in people who are 60 years or older. Men have more strokes than women, blacks have more strokes than whites.

what causes stroke? A stroke can begin in several ways: with transient ischemic attacks; gradual onset; or sudden onset of symptoms.

Transient ischemic attack, (T.I.A.), consists of a brief period of weakness, loss of speech or loss of feeling which lasts from minutes to hours and then goes completely away. These attacks are due to a sudden but temporary decrease or stoppage of blood flow to a part of the brain. These attacks are important because they are a reliable warning of possible permanent stroke.

Usually a person with T.I.A. reports one or more of the following: the sudden onset of numbness, tingling or weakness on one side of the body, or in the hand and face on one side; temporary blindness in one or both eyes; difficulty understanding words and using them correctly; dizziness; nausea; vomiting; staggering; fuzzy speech; or a combination of these symptoms. During an attack, people do not lose consciousness, and recover with no after-effect.

Whenever the symptoms described above occur, it is very important that a physician be notified, even if the episode seems to pass as quickly as it came. Knowing and heeding these symptoms can help to avoid a completed stroke since treatment of the underlying conditions which caused the attack often is possible, either with medications or with surgery.

When T.I.A.'s have occurred, an individual with them should receive a careful neurologic examination to determine if the condition causing the T.I.A. can be corrected. Most T.I.A.'s are caused by atherosclerosis which may build up and block an artery, or may break up and release bits of debris which travel through larger arteries and may block small arteries in the brain, stopping blood flow transiently to a part of the brain. Most commonly, the site of arterial disease is in the carotid artery where it divides into two large vessels—one going to the brain the other to the face, jaw and eye. This site is important because it is accessible to surgery and often the obstruction or plaque can be removed. Also, medications which reduce blood clotting or prevent blood platelets from clumping together can help stop T.I.A. and reduce the chance of stroke.

Clinical evaluation of T.I.A. usually includes an examination by a neurologist, examination of blood vessels in the arms, legs and neck; ultra-sound examination of the arteries in the neck; and often an arteriogram. The arteriogram is a series of x-ray pictures which show the flow of blood in the arteries, in the neck and head taken after the injection of 'dye' or contrast substance into the artery. The 'dye' causes the arteries to stand out clearly in the X-ray picture, allowing the physician to identify sites of vessel disease and obstructions. This allows the physician to determine whether surgical correction of an obstruction is possible.

Cerebral Infarction is the term used to describe the condition in which a portion of the brain dies when an artery becomes blocked and blood is prevented from reaching that part of the brain. The blockage can be the result of hardening and eventual blockage of the artery (atherosclerosis), or be caused by a blood clot in the vessel, or other substances plugging a vessel (emboli). The portions of the brain which are thus starved of blood, die and cannot function. The effects of the stroke, weakness, paralysis and loss of feeling, become evident in those parts of the body controlled by the affected part of the brain. When a person has a completed stroke, which means that the paralysis or loss of sensation does not go away rapidly, that person should be hospitalized to be given needed care and to be sure that there is no further progression of the stroke. Treatment of a patient after a completed stroke is difficult as there are no known remedies which can reverse the brain damage or cause nervous system tissue to regenerate. If improvement occurs in nerve function, it happens naturally. Function in a person with stroke can be adapted and improved by rehabilitation.

Risk factors which, singly or in combination, increase the chances of stroke caused by the interruption of blood flow to the brain, resulting in cerebral infarction, are the same as for T.I.A. Frequently, a person may have a stroke with no recognized underlying cause. Cerebral infarction is the most common form of stroke and is responsible for the majority of partially or completely disabling strokes. The most desirable form of management of this condition is prevention.

Intracerebral Hemorrhage means there is bleeding into the brain which destroys or disrupts brain tissue. Normally, blood flows to the brain through arteries under high pressure. In vessels with weakened walls, the pressure may cause a rupture and blood will escape into the brain. Under high pressure, blood can spread rapidly in all directions from the point of rupture and may disrupt or damage a large area of the brain causing weakness, paralysis, loss of sensation and frequently loss of consciousness. Intracerebral hemorrhage has a high risk of being fatal.

High blood pressure is the main risk factor for hemorrhage into the brain, as almost all cerebral hemorrhages occur in patients with high blood pressure. Treatment of high blood pressure is the only satisfactory means to deal with cerebral hemorrhage. Survivors usually have severe physical disability.

possible after effects of stroke: Stroke can affect an individual in many different ways, depending on which part of the brain has been damaged. Among the possible consequences are:

Physical Deficits
   Paralysis or complete loss of strength or mobility in a part of the body usually the arm, leg and face on one side
   Weakness in a part of the body. Usually weakness is more marked in the hand than in the arm, and the arm is more affected than the leg
   Spasticity (stiffness)-a loss of muscular control with automatic muscle contraction
   Loss of sensation (feeling) in parts of the body, usually on one side
   Loss of bladder and bowel control
   Speech and language disability. Difficulty thinking of and saying words or difficulty using or understanding words
   Difficulty in swallowing
   Loss of coordination, such as unsteady gait

Perceptual/Cognitive (thinking) Problems
   Loss of awareness
   Denial or neglect of the right or left part of the environment
   Inability to understand time
   Difficulty performing tasks in proper sequence
   Disrupted sleep-wake cycles
   Uncontrolled laughter or crying
   Confusion, forgetfulness, memory loss, impaired judgment

Personal/Family Problems
   Loss of job
   Inadequate financial resources
   Loss of independence. Dependence on others who may or may not be willing or capable of accepting the new responsibility for continuing care.
   Loss of sexual capacity
   Loss of self esteem

Psychological Problems (mood)
   Depression, apathy
   Anger, hostility
   Euphoria

Environmental Problems
   Architectural barriers in the home
   Lack of accessible transportation

Not all of these problems happen to each individual. When any of them do happen, there are degrees of difficulty. Most of these problems can be improved. However, after a completed stroke, there will always be limitations. Those with paralysis, those whose perceptual capacities are affected, or whose memory and orientation are diminished, have the greatest difficulties.

signs and symptoms. The person who suffers a stroke usually loses consciousness and becomes incontinent of urine and feces. In addition, breathing becomes labored or difficult. If consciousness is not lost, the client may complain of a severe headache, slurred speech, and blurred vision. After a CVA there is usually a weakness or paralysis on one side of the body. This one-sided weakness or paralysis is known as **hemiplegia.** The use of muscles is temporarily or permanently lost when paralysis occurs. Thus, there may be difficulty in speaking, eating, swallowing, and even hearing. The client may take a long time to eat his/her meals. The home health aide must be patient and permit the client to be as independent as possible. That means *assisting* with eating, *not force feeding,* in order to finish the meal. Remember, the client is the most important person and you are in the home to *assist* that client.

By the time the home health aide sees a CVA client in the home, the client will probably be past the acute stage. However, this does not mean that recovery is complete. Some clients have more than one stroke. Before or after the first major stroke the client may have several small CVAs. A small stroke is characterized by periods of nausea, vomiting, or dizziness. In some cases the client becomes disoriented. Disoriented clients lose track of time, forget names, or forget where they are.

rehabilitation after stroke. Under the supervision of a nurse or a physical therapist, exercises will be planned for a CVA client. Exercise is important for bringing back strength to the paralyzed or affected parts of the body, figure 17-4. Through exercise, the client is retrained to use the body. Breathing exercises may be needed so the client will not develop pneumonia. Exercises will also be used to prevent contractures. Active range of motion (ROM) exercises which the client does without help should be supervised by the physical therapist, figure 17-5. Passive ROM exercises are those in which the client moves, but exerts no effort. Passive exercises usually require the help of another person. A nurse or physical therapist can train the aide in helping the client with these exercises. Passive ROM exercises are carried out about four times a day.

Many clients who are learning to walk after a stroke use braces, figure 17-6. While the client gains muscle strength and balance, the braces provide support. If the client is using braces, the aide is expected to assist in putting them on. The aide will be expected to help the client into and out of bed, figure 17-7.

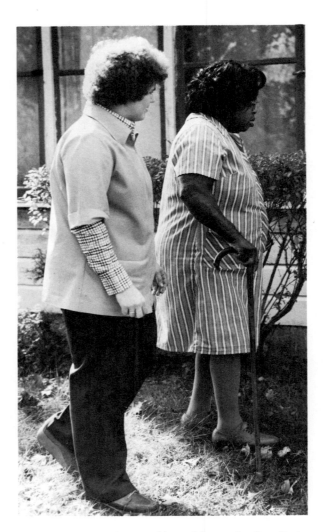

Figure 17-4 Walking provides mild exercise for clients regaining their strength after a stroke.

Mouth care is of special importance for the CVA client. One-sided paralysis (hemiplegia) often causes food to stay in the weakened side of the mouth. Special facial exercises to strengthen these muscles may be suggested by the therapist. Food particles left in the client's mouth could cause choking and suffocation. After a client finishes a meal or snack, the home health aide must check the client's mouth. The aide should remove food still in the mouth to

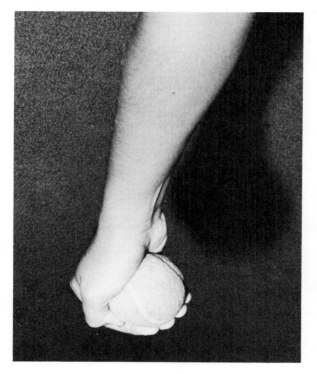

Figure 17-5 Curling the fingers around a tennis ball is an active range of motion exercise for the fingers.

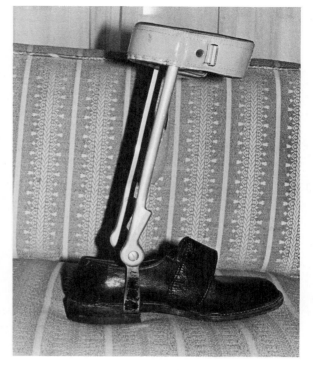

Figure 17-6 A brace can be used to support weakened leg muscles.

prevent it from blocking the air passage. In addition to food particles, the client may be unable to swallow saliva and may have excess saliva dribbling from the corner of the mouth. The aide should wipe the client's mouth as often as necessary. The mouth should also be checked for saliva which can collect and block the airway.

Bowel and bladder retraining may also be part of the rehabilitation of a stroke client. The aide should follow a schedule suggested by the doctor or nurse. The urinal, bedpan or commode should be presented at specific times during the day. For example, the client who is given the bedpan after each meal and before bedtime eventually becomes adjusted to using it at that time. The body becomes regulated. Before the client adapts to a schedule, the aide should be sure to keep the client's bed dry and clean.

communication problems. The CVA victim often has a great deal of trouble communicating. The home health aide must be patient and understanding of the speech problems. Aphasia is a condition in which the ability to speak is impaired. Aphasia is a frequent complication of the CVA. Some clients have no useful speech and may be very depressed. The home health aide must remember that even if the client cannot speak properly, hearing is not impaired. Therefore, the aide should not shout or speak in angry commands. The client may be unable to read, write, or speak. Other CVA clients may retain some speaking skill but misuse words and numbers. Sometimes the only

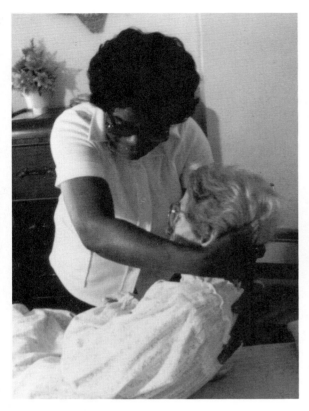

Figure 17-7 At home, the client who has had a CVA may require assistance into and out of bed because of paralysis or weakness of the affected side.

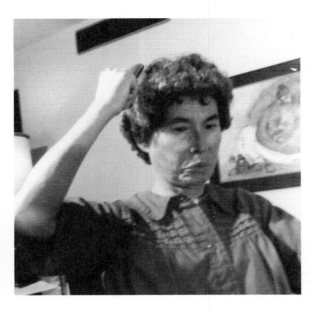

Figure 17-8 This client has had a CVA. Note the sagging facial muscles which is characteristic of paralysis following a CVA. The client is exercising the affected side by using the motions of combing her hair.

words a CVA client uses are curse words or nonsense syllables. This is called **automatic speech** (involuntary speech). The home health aide should avoid treating the client as a child. In speaking to a stroke client, the aide should use simple sentences that require only short and simple answers from the client. Speaking clearly and simply aids the client's understanding. Stroke clients usually need a great deal of encouragement and reassurance.

Clients who normally wear glasses should continue to wear them even if their sight has been affected by the stroke. This makes the client feel less changed in outward appearance. The same is true if the client wears den-

tures or a hearing aide. These courtesies show that the aide respects the client.

An important fact to remember is that the home health aide should encourage clients to help themselves as much as possible. This may take more of the aide's time, but it is a form of rehabilitation. The more the clients help themselves, the more progress they will make, figure 17-8.

summary

- A home health aide should have a basic knowledge of the common heart conditions. This knowledge increases the aide's awareness of the signs of distress and potential dangers to the client.
- The aide should be able to tell when the client's condition has changed for the worse and contact someone for help.
- The home health aide is responsible for making the client as comfortable and content as

possible. The client must always be treated with concern and respect.

- The disorders of the heart and circulatory system demand unusual care in the following areas:

  1. Diet is of utmost importance in most heart conditions. A diet prescribed by the doctor must be followed very carefully.

  2. For clients on bedrest, the home health aide must remain alert to signs of decubitus ulcers, contractures, and poor alignment.

  3. Suitable exercise and rest periods are to be given as ordered by the doctor.

  4. Medications should be taken when prescribed.

review

1. Describe an angina attack.
2. What effect does nitroglycerin have on the blood vessels?
3. What are the symptoms of an acute coronary occlusion?
4. Describe the care given for a client with congestive heart failure.
5. What are two other names for cerebral vascular accident?

Caring for Clients with Arthritis

learning objectives

After studying this unit, you should be able to:
- describe the care given to clients with arthritis.
- define the terms relating to arthritis.
- discuss the exercises related to arthritis.

definition of arthritis

Arthritis means inflammation of a joint. Many people complain of rheumatism in relationship to their many aches and pains. The Arthritis Foundation states that arthritis is the number one crippler in the United States. It affects one in seven people. There are several types of arthritis. The two main ones are rheumatoid arthritis and osteoarthritis. A comparison of the two types is shown in figure 18-1.

Other infections such as gonorrhea, tuberculosis, syphilis, typhoid fever, streptococcal infection, and staphylococcal can also cause arthritis. Gout may even lead to arthritis.

rheumatoid arthritis

Rheumatoid arthritis starts slowly with a general feeling of weakness and stiffness. Sometimes an individual may have a sudden severe illness which is followed by arthritis. The symptoms include loss of appetite, feeling of tiredness, and fever. The joints involved become painful, swollen, and stiff. This is especially noticeable after the client has been in the same position (sitting, for example) for an extended period of time. Some clients complain of coldness and "funny" feelings in their hands and feet. Joint deformities appear, figure 18-2. The victim may become disabled, losing mobility and the ability to function independently. Unfortunately, the cause is un-

RHEUMATOID ARTHRITIS	OSTEOARTHRITIS
affects the lubricating fluid in the joints	affects cartilage-connective tissue
inflammation	wearing down condition
system disease (total body)	health not generally affected
good and bad periods of pain	no particular good periods without pain
results in deformity	limits motion only
affects any joint	affects weight-bearing joints
affects all ages—even young people	affects older age group

Figure 18-1 Comparison of rheumatoid arthritis and osteoarthritis

known and there is no known cure. Treatment may involve medication, paraffin (wax) baths, rest, special exercises, walking aids such as a cane or walker to prevent falls, application of heat, and sometimes surgery. The inflammation is treated and efforts are made to prevent or limit deformities as much as possible.

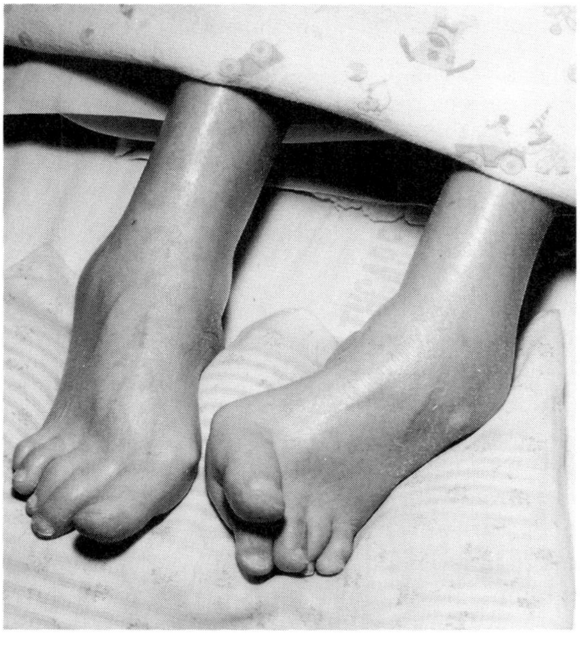

Figure 18-2 Deformity resulting from rheumatoid arthritis

osteoarthritis

Degenerative joint disease, osteoarthritis, is a chronic disease which affects the joints. Women are more often affected than men and one indication of the disease is the enlargement of the finger joints. Although the cause is unknown, it appears to be hereditary. Very often the victims show signs of stress and appear to react strongly to traumatic experiences. Many who have osteoarthritis are obese. Whether the obesity and stress factors have any bearing on the illness has not been determined. The affected joints become larger and stiffen. Changes in the weather appear to cause an increase in pain. Drugs, such as salicylates (aspirin), may be prescribed along with an anti-inflammatory medication. Physical therapy can be effective and a low-calorie diet may be prescribed to reduce obesity. Nonweight bearing exercises and limited activity may be recommended. Surgery may become necessary.

role of the home health aide

A home health aide can play a vital role in limiting deformities by assisting the client with prescribed exercises. The exercises are shown in figures 18-3 to 18-17, including a description of how each exercise is to be per-

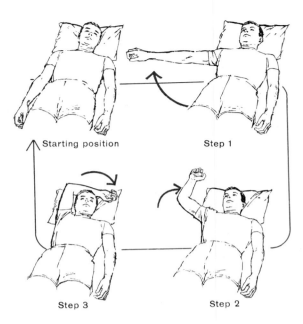

exercise 2 | Shoulder Abduction

STARTING POSITION: Lying on the back, arm at side.

STEP 1. Keep the elbow straight and move the arm out to the side away from the body.

STEPS 2, 3. Turn the arm so that the palm faces up, and continue the arm back until it rests on the bed next to the head. The arm may be bent at the elbow if the headboard of the bed will not permit the arm to be carried all the way back.

Return to the starting position, rest, then repeat the exercise.

Figure 18-4 Exercise 2—shoulder abduction (Courtesy of the Burke Rehabilitation Center, White Plains, NY, and the Burke Auxiliary)

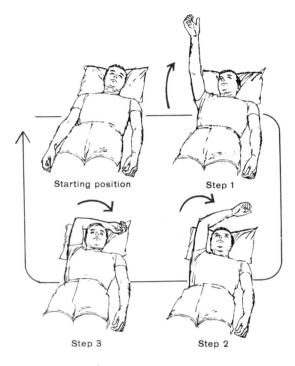

exercise 1 | Shoulder Flexion

STARTING POSITION: Lying on back, arm at side, palm facing body.

STEP 1. Keep elbow straight and lift arm until hand points to the ceiling.

STEPS 2, 3. Continue to move the arm back until it rests on the bed next to the head. The arm may be bent at the elbow if the headboard of the bed will not permit the arm to be carried all the way back.

Return to the starting position, rest, then repeat the exercise.

Figure 18-3 Exercise 1—shoulder flexion (Courtesy of the Burke Rehabilitation Center, White Plains, NY, and the Burke Auxiliary)

formed. These range of motion exercises are commonly ordered by the physician for any client whose physical condition prevents adequate movement and exercise. These range of motion or movement exercises are not limited to those with arthritis, however. Any client whose movement is limited because of confinement, such as bed rest, or who has limited

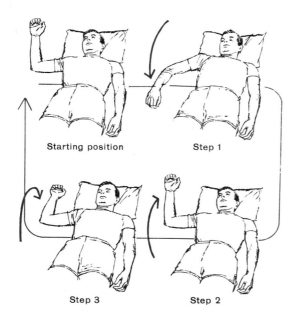

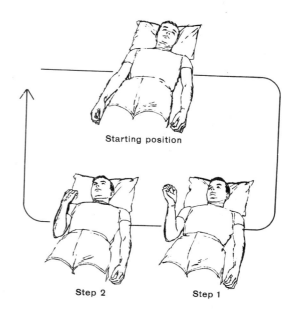

exercise 3 | Shoulder Rotation

STARTING POSITION: Lying on the back, arm out from side at shoulder height, elbow bent, hand pointing toward the ceiling.

STEP 1. Keep the upper arm against the bed and move the forearm down until it rests on the bed, palm down.

STEP 2. Return to the starting position.

STEP 3. Continue to hold the upper arm against the bed, and move the forearm back until it rests on the bed, palm up.

Return to the starting position, rest, then repeat the exercise.

Figure 18-5 Exercise 3—shoulder rotation (Courtesy of the Burke Rehabilitation Center, White Plains, NY, and the Burke Auxiliary)

physical activity, can benefit from range of motion exercises.

If the client is confined to bed, the aide must frequently reposition the client to prevent decubitus ulcers. Exercise periods and periods of rest must be carefully balanced. Usually the arthritic client is referred to a rehabilitation center for planning a special exer-

exercise 4 | Elbow Flexion and Extension

STARTING POSITION: Lying on the back, arm at side, palm facing body.

STEPS 1, 2. Bend the elbow and bring the hand as close to the shoulder as possible.

Return to the starting position, rest, then repeat the exercise.

Figure 18-6 Exercise 4—elbow flexion and extension (Courtesy of the Burke Rehabilitation Center, White Plains, NY, and the Burke Auxiliary)

cise regime. The exercises are most effective when done just following a warm bath.

Surgical joint replacements are available for elbow, shoulder, ankle, hip, knee, and finger joints.

One who suffers from arthritis can become frustrated, irritable, impatient and depressed. If an individual has lost a job as a result of the crippling effects of the disease, he or she will worry over loss of income and costs of treatment. Sexual relationships may fail due to the pain and discomfort of the victim.

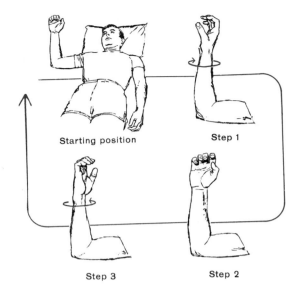

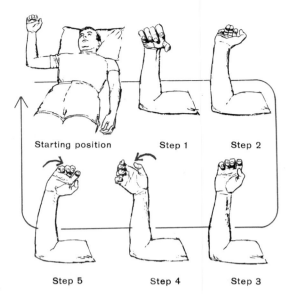

exercise 5 | Forearm Pronation and Supination

STARTING POSITION: Lying on the back, arm out from side, elbow bent, hand pointing toward the ceiling, fingers relaxed with thumb side of hand toward the face.

STEP 1. Turn the forearm so that palm faces away from the body.

STEP 2. Return to starting position.

STEP 3. Turn your forearm so that palm faces the body.

Return to the starting position, rest, then repeat the exercise.

Figure 18-7 Exercise 5—forearm pronation and supination (Courtesy of the Burke Rehabilitation Center, White Plains, NY, and the Burke Auxiliary)

exercise 6 | Wrist Flexion and Extension; Ulnar and Radial Deviation

STARTING POSITION: Lying on the back, arm out from side, elbow bent, hand pointing toward the ceiling.

STEP 1. Bend the wrist forward as far as possible.

STEP 2. Bend the wrist back as far as possible.

STEP 3. Return to starting position.

STEP 4. Bend the wrist sidewise as far as possible in the direction of the little finger.

STEP 5. Bend the wrist sidewise as far as possible in the direction of the thumb.

Return to the starting position, rest, then repeat the exercise.

NOTE: The tendency of the wrist to become fixed in the bent forward position and also to bend toward the little finger side of the hand is a common problem. When this problem exists, Steps 1 and 4 are usually omitted and Steps 2 and 5 are emphasized. The doctor will prescribe the wrist exercises you should do.

Figure 18-8 Exercise 6—wrist flexion and extension; ulnar and radial deviation (Courtesy of the Burke Rehabilitation Center, White Plains, NY, and the Burke Auxiliary)

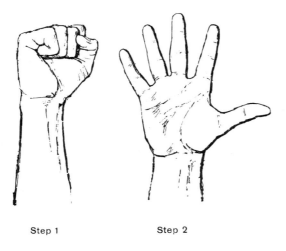

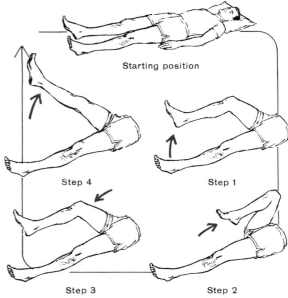

exercise 7 | Finger Flexion and Extension

STEP 1. Curl the fingers, beginning at the tips, and make a fist.

STEP 2. Uncurl the fingers, completely straightening and spreading them.

Look at Step 1, you will see that the fingers when closed in a fist normally tend to form right angles to the joints.

When the fist is opened and all fingers are stretched out, as in Step 2, you will see that they form fairly straight lines.

Figure 18-9 Exercise 7—finger flexion and extension (Courtesy of the Burke Rehabilitation Center, White Plains, NY, and the Burke Auxiliary)

exercise 8 | Hip and Knee Flexion and Extension

STARTING POSITION: Lying on the back, leg straight.

STEP 1. Lift the leg, bending it at the knee and at the hip.

STEP 2. Continue to move the leg, bringing the knee toward the chest so that the hip and knee are bent as far as they will go. (Keep other leg flat on the bed.)

STEPS 3, 4. Lower the leg, then straighten the knee by lifting the foot upward.

Return to the starting position, rest, then repeat the exercise.

Figure 18-10 Exercise 8—hip and knee flexion and extension (Courtesy of the Burke Rehabilitation Center, White Plains, NY, and the Burke Auxiliary)

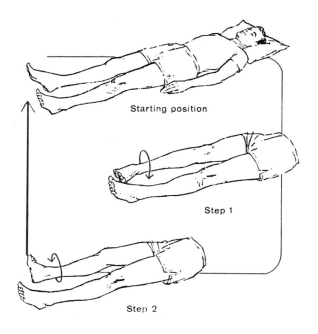

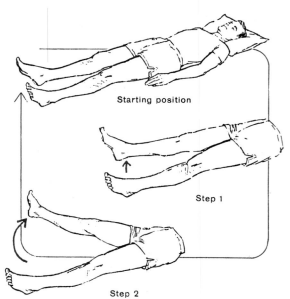

exercise 9 | Hip Rotation

STARTING POSITION: Lying on the back, leg straight.

STEP 1. Roll the entire leg in.

STEP 2. Roll the entire leg out.

Return to the starting position, rest, then repeat the exercise.

Figure 18-11 Exercise 9—hip rotation (Courtesy of the Burke Rehabilitation Center, White Plains, NY, and the Burke Auxiliary)

exercise 10 | Hip Abduction

STARTING POSITION: Lying on the back, leg straight.

STEP 1. Keep the knee straight and lift the leg so that the heel is about 4 inches from the bed.

STEP 2. Move the leg out to the side.

Return to the starting position, rest, then repeat the exercise.

Figure 18-12 Exercise 10—hip abduction (Courtesy of the Burke Rehabilitation Center, White Plains, NY, and the Burke Auxiliary)

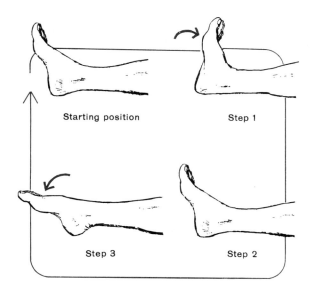

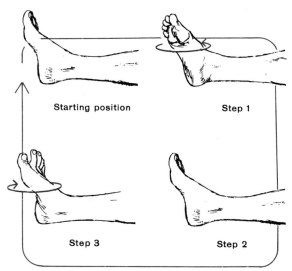

exercise 11 | Ankle Dorsi and Plantar Flexion

STARTING POSITION: Lying on the back, leg straight, foot relaxed.

STEP 1. Keep the leg straight. Bend the ankle, pointing the toes toward you.

STEP 2. Relax the foot — Tell client.

STEP 3. Bend the ankle, ponting the toes away from the body.

Return to the starting position, rest, then repeat the exercise.

Figure 18-13 Exercise 11—ankle dorsal and plantar flexion (Courtesy of the Burke Rehabilitation Center, White Plains, NY, and the Burke Auxiliary)

exercise 12 | Foot Inversion and Eversion

STARTING POSITION: Lying on the back, leg straight.

STEP 1. Turn the foot in so that the sole faces toward the other foot.

STEP 2. Return to the starting position.

STEP 3. Turn the foot out so that the sole faces away from the other foot.

Return to the starting position, rest, then repeat the exercise.

Figure 18-14 Exercise 12—foot inversion and eversion (Courtesy of the Burke Rehabilitation Center, White Plains, NY, and the Burke Auxiliary)

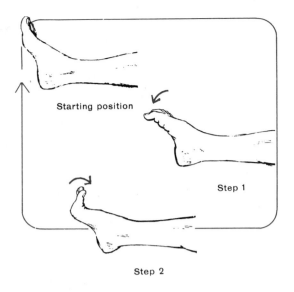

Starting position

Step 1

Step 2

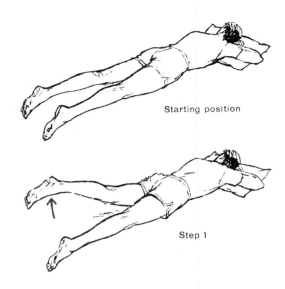

Starting position

Step 1

exercise 13 | Toe Flexion and Extension

STARTING POSITION: Lying on the back, leg straight.

STEP 1. Curl the toes down.

STEP 2. Straighten the toes and then pull them back.

Return to the starting position, rest, then repeat the exercise.

Figure 18-15 Exercise 13—toe flexion and extension (Courtesy of the Burke Rehabilitation Center, White Plains, NY, and the Burke Auxiliary)

exercise 14 | Hip Extension

STARTING POSITION: Lying on the stomach, leg straight.

STEP 1. Keep the knee straight and lift the leg straight up so that the knee is about 4-6 inches above the mattress.

Return to the starting position, rest, then repeat the exercise.

Figure 18-16 Exercise 14—hip extension (Courtesy of the Burke Rehabilitation Center, White Plains, NY, and the Burke Auxiliary)

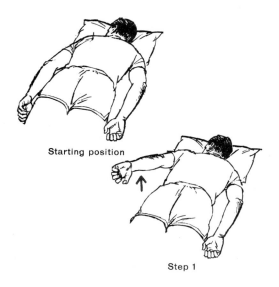

Starting position

Step 1

exercise 15 | Shoulder Extension

STARTING POSITION: Lying on the stomach, arm straight at side with palm facing body.

STEP 1. Lift the arm straight up, so that the elbow is about 4-6 inches above the mattress.

Return to the starting position, rest, then repeat the exercise.

Figure 18-17 Exercise 15—shoulder extension (Courtesy of the Burke Rehabilitation Center, White Plains, NY, and the Burke Auxiliary)

review

1. Define the vocabulary words.
2. What are the differences between rheumatoid and osteoarthritis.
3. Make a care plan for a disabled individual.

Unit 19
Caring for Clients with Cancer

key terms

cancer	ileostomy	laryngectomy
carcinogen	colostomy	tracheostomy
remission	irrigation	trachea
chemotherapy	benign	articulates
biopsy	mammography	lobectomy
hysterectomy	metastasize	pneumonectomy
mastectomy	larynx	jejunostomy

learning objectives

After studying this unit, you should be able to:
■ Identify three diagnostic tests for cancer.
■ Identify six surgical procedures used in cancer treatment.
■ List nine warning signs of cancer.
■ Define metastasis, benign tumor, and remission.
■ Name three types of treatment for cancer.
■ Describe the care given to a client with cancer.

Cancer is the uncontrolled growth of abnormal tissue. In healthy tissue, body cells grow, die, and are replaced by new cells. This is a normal process that goes on day after day. Sometimes cells do not follow the rules of the body; they begin to grow quickly, steal nourishment from surrounding cells, and push normal cells out of the way. They prevent normal cells from doing their regular jobs. Finally, these cells cause changes in the body which produce signs that indicate something is wrong. Any one of the warning signs listed in figure 19-1

should be called to the doctor's attention as soon as possible.

The exact cause of cancer is unknown. However, studies are beginning to show some factors which lead to the formation of cancer cells. A substance or agent which produces cancer is called a **carcinogen.** The general groups of carcinogens are chemicals, environmental factors, hormones and viruses. A chemical could be ingested with food such as red dye #2. The chemical could be inhaled as is tar and asbestos. Environmental factors in-

```
╔══════════════════════════════════════════╗
║            WARNING SIGNALS               ║
║  1.  Unusual bleeding or body discharge  ║
║  2.  A lump or thickening in an area of the body  ║
║  3.  A sore that does not heal           ║
║  4.  A change in bowel or bladder habits ║
║  5.  Hoarseness or a chronic cough       ║
║  6.  Indigestion or difficulty in swallowing  ║
║  7.  A change in size, shape or appearance of a  ║
║      wart or mole                        ║
║  8.  Sudden and unexplained weight loss  ║
║  9.  Unusual tiredness that lasts for a long period  ║
╚══════════════════════════════════════════╝
```

Figure 19-1 Warning signs of cancer

clude such physical agents as x-rays, sunlight or trauma. Hormones may be cancer-causing because of their excess, deficiency, or imbalance. Viruses seem to upset the functions within a cell.

The way that carcinogens change normal cells into cancer cells is unclear. Therefore, prevention is not yet possible. Most physicians agree, however, that the sooner cancer is detected, the less chance it has of spreading to other parts of the body, figure 19-2. When cancer is treated early and does not reappear for five years, the cancer is considered to be cured or in remission. **Remission** means no longer growing or spreading.

It has been estimated that in the United States alone over one thousand people a day die from some form of cancer. Since 1949 there has been a sharp rise in the number of men who develop cancer. Cancer of the lung has risen sharply in women also. Cancer of the breast, colon and rectum occur most often among women. There are over 100 types of cancer. Cancer is second only to heart disease as the leading cause of death each year. However, statistics also show that deaths due to cancer are increasing whereas those due to

heart conditions are decreasing. Research continues into the cause and cure for cancer.

cancer treatments

There are several kinds of treatment which may slow or stop the growth of cancer cells. Surgery is used to remove tumors and organs of the body which have become cancerous. Sometimes surgical techniques alone are used. At other times, x-ray or cobalt therapy may be used following surgery to kill any cancer cells around the surgical area. X-ray and cobalt therapy are sometimes the only treatments used. The rays are aimed deep in the body to reach cells which cannot be removed surgically. Very often, however, surrounding cells are destroyed by the rays. The site of the therapy is marked in ink on the body. The home health aide must be careful not to remove these marks when bathing the client. The marked area should not be touched by the home health aide.

Side effects of radiation treatment may include nausea, skin damage, itching of the area, and loss of hair. Some people wear wigs to cover bald heads caused by radiation.

Chemotherapy is the use of one or a combination of chemicals to attack cancer cells. Chemotherapy may be used after surgery or in combination with x-ray therapy. In some cases chemotherapy works only for a short time after which it no longer kills cancer cells. New combinations of chemicals are then prescribed. This treatment, too, can cause unpleasant side effects. All of the cancer treatments cause damage to healthy cells around the cancer site.

So-called miracle cures for cancer are sold in many forms. Most people who market these products are only interested in making a profit from the misfortune of others. Some people with cancer choose to take experimental drugs. However, a person is wiser and safer to follow the advice of a trustworthy physician.

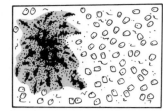

MALIGNANT CANCER GROWTH
(NO CAPSULE WITH RANDOM GROWTH)

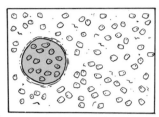

BENIGN TUMOR GROWTH
(WITH CAPSULE AROUND IT)

Figure 19-2 Growth of cancer cells

The best treatment plans are based on sound research.

caring for the client with cancer

Studies of people with cancer show that proper nutrition and special diets are a very important part of cancer care. Clients should be given foods they like unless otherwise ordered by the doctor. Four to six small meals are usually preferred. If meals look attractive and are served nicely they may stimulate the client's appetite. Usually these diets are high in calories—as much as 2000 calories per day. Foods high in protein are most often suggested.

Clients who are confined to bed should be protected from the hazards of prolonged bedrest. Repositioning and skin massage increase circulation and help prevent bedsores. The soap used for the client's bath should be mild and not perfumed. A mild soap keeps the skin soft and naturally oiled. The skin should also be protected from the irritation of rough clothes or bedcovers. Bed cradles may be used

to hold the bedclothes away from the body parts affected by cancer. Bedding should be lightweight.

Pain-killing medications may be ordered. The home health aide may assist the client by bringing medications to the client at the times ordered by the doctor. **Caution:** The aide should NEVER help the client with medications not prescribed by the doctor. The client should not be allowed to take extra medicine for pain, even when the pain is severe. However, gentleness, kindness and concern are very important at all times. Be sure to tell the client that you understand and will report the problem to the supervisor.

cancer of the female reproductive system

Among women in the middle years, problems may occur in the reproductive system. All women should have an annual physical examination which includes a Pap smear. A Pap smear detects early cellular change. In this test, a microscopic examination is made of cells scraped from the uterus. If repeated Pap smears show cellular changes, the doctor takes a biopsy. A *biopsy* is a sample of tissue cut from the area where cellular change is present. The biopsy determines the seriousness of the cell changes. Sometimes a cone-shaped section is cut out for examination. If cancerous cells are found, a partial or complete hysterectomy may be performed. A **hysterectomy** is a major surgical technique in which the uterus, and sometimes the ovaries and fallopian tubes are removed.

Some women develop fibroid tumors in the uterus. These tumors are **benign** or noncancerous. They can become large or cause unusual bleeding during menstruation or cause pain. When these problems exist, a hysterec-

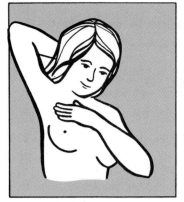 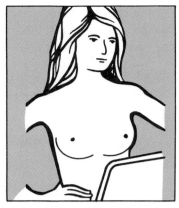 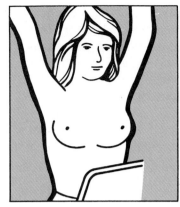

A. With the fingers, flat, check for a knot, lump or thickening.

B. Flex your chest muscles and compare breast shape.

C. Raise your arms and compare breast shape.

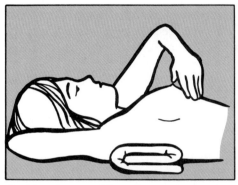 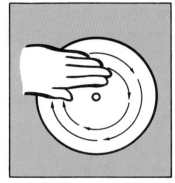 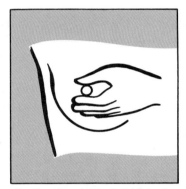

D. Lie down with a towel under the shoulder and one arm behind the head. Check again for any knot, lump or thickening.

E. Move fingers in a circular motion, inward toward the nipple.

F. Gently squeeze the nipple to check for a clear or bloody discharge.

Figure 19-3 Self-examination helps to detect breast cancer at an early stage.

tomy may also be needed. After any major surgery it may take from nine to twelve months for full health to return. Very often women are depressed following a hysterectomy. For some women there is a feeling that they have lost the ability to enjoy sex. If the ovaries have been removed, hormones are usually prescribed to replace those normally produced. The hormone pills help the body to adjust physically and help restore a sense of well-being. Although a hysterectomy prevents further childbearing, it does not prevent enjoyment of sex.

cancer of the breast

Another area in which women develop cancer is the breast. The best method of detecting breast cancer is self-examination, figure 19-3. Each woman should self-examine her breasts monthly about one week after each period. A woman checks for changes in the shape of each breast, a swelling, dimpling of the skin, or changes in the nipple. She checks for lumps while lying on her back. Using flat fingers, she presses in a clockwise motion around the breast. If a lump is noticed, she should go to her gynecologist for further examination. All lumps are not malignant (cancerous). Many women have simple, benign breast tumors. Sometimes it is necessary to remove the benign tumors through surgery.

One diagnostic technique used in suspected breast cancer is an x-ray called a **mammography.** Special x-ray studies can detect unhealthy or cancerous cells. In some cases, a biopsy is ordered if there is a chance of cancer of the breast. An incision (cut) is made in the breast and a microscopic examination of tissue is made at once. If cancer is diagnosed, some doctors remove only the growth itself. This can only be done when the diagnosis is made early. This procedure is sometimes known as a lumpectomy. Sometimes it is necessary to remove the entire breast tissue, underlying muscles and the lymph glands under the arm. This procedure is called a radical **mastectomy.** If there is any sign that the cancer cells have **metastasized** (spread), both breasts may need to be removed. Women are often ashamed and embarrassed after a mastectomy. They see the altered shape of their body as a deformity. However, an increasing number of women who have had this surgery can talk about it quite openly. Because they have talked about their own surgery, other women have become more aware of the need to examine themselves. As a result, many breast cancers were discovered early enough for successful treatment.

Following a radical mastectomy, there is often a time of mental depression. It is very important that a mastectomy patient has the support of her loved ones. She must understand that her life can continue as before. Part of this is accepting that she is just as much a woman as she was before surgery. Because the surgery may involve the underarm glands and muscles of the chest and underarms, rehabilitation is very important. Special exercises are prescribed by the doctor. After a mastectomy pa-tient returns home, these exercises must be continued regularly. After the incision is healed, most patients are encouraged to have a prosthesis made. In some cases, the prosthesis may be surgically fitted under a flap of skin. Other prosthetic devices shaped as cups are fitted into a special bra.

volunteer groups. The American Cancer Society has been very active in sending volunteers who have had cancer surgery into hospitals to work with cancer patients. A rehabilitated mastectomy patient can demonstrate how the prosthesis restores her shape. She talks about the need for exercises and tells how she has adjusted to the special problems of her mastectomy. This has been a very successful program and has given many women the courage to face the loss of a breast.

cancer of the respiratory system

The respiratory system is on duty 24 hours a day from birth to death. Fresh air is breathed into the body and carried to the lungs. The oxygen from the air is carried to all parts of the body by the circulatory system. As oxygen is delivered to the cells of the body, waste gases are picked up and carried back to the lungs. Carbon dioxide is exhaled and thereby expelled from the body.

There are many infections and disorders that can affect the respiratory system. Everyone has had a common cold. Flu, pneumonia, bronchitis and other upper respiratory infections are some of the illnesses affecting this system. Cancer, too, can start to grow in the lungs. Signs of lung cancer are:

• a persistent, hacking cough
• pains in the chest area
• tiredness
• a low-grade fever
• sudden weight loss
• coughing up blood.

If a biopsy (microscopic examination of tissue) shows cancer cells, surgery can sometimes be done to remove all or part of a lung. Removal of part of the lung is called a *lobectomy*. Removal of the entire lung is called a *pneumonectomy*. Lung cancer grows slowly at first. However by the time it is diagnosed, seven out of ten cases are not helped by surgery. A person with lung cancer must be kept as comfortable as possible. In some cases the person can be cared for in the home; however, most are hospitalized as the pain becomes severe or when special equipment is needed for care.

cancer of the larynx

The **larynx** is the part of the trachea called the voice box. Cancer of the larynx occurs in men more often than in women. In addition, 75 percent of the people who develop cancer of the larynx have been heavy smokers. A common treatment for cancer of the larynx is surgical removal of the larynx, called a **laryngectomy.** In order to remove the larynx, a tracheostomy must be performed. A **tracheostomy** is a surgical opening made into the trachea below the larynx. The **trachea** is the airway between the nasal passages and the lungs. The tracheostomy is an artificial airway that can be used to supply oxygen to the lungs. A tracheostomy tube is placed into the artificial airway in order to keep it open, figure 19-4. In some instances the tracheostomy tube is no longer being used. Instead a stoma is created surgically. A small dressing called a bib is placed over the stoma. This should be kept damp so that the patient doesn't inhale dust or other foreign particles.

After the tracheostomy has been done, the second part of the surgery is completed and the cancerous larynx is removed. The tracheostomy tube remains in place permanently in a laryngectomy patient. After the patient has recovered from surgery, rehabilitation starts.

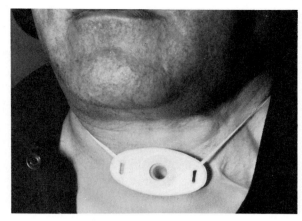

Figure 19-4 A tracheostomy tube provides an airway (courtesy of Dow Corning Medical Products).

Speech therapy is needed to teach the patient how to talk. One of the methods is to gulp air in through the tracheostomy tube, swallow it and then burp out words. It takes a great deal of practice to relearn speaking. Another method the laryngectomy patient may use to aid speech is an artificial larynx. A battery-powered vibrator is one type of artificial larynx. When wishing to speak, the patient places the vibrator against the side of the neck,

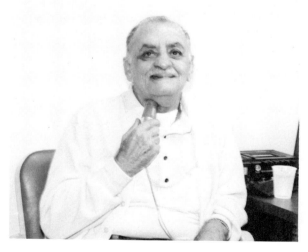

Figure 19-5 A vibrator is often used to aid the laryngectomy patient's speech.

figure 19-5. The vibrator vibrates the air inside the patient's mouth as the patient **articulates.**

A home health aide must be tactful when caring for such clients. It may be hard to understand what the client is saying. The aide should report to the doctor or supervisor immediately if the client has any difficulty breathing. Crusting or bloody discharge from the tracheostomy also must be reported immediately. A home health aide must be specially trained in order to clean and care for the tracheostomy. Most clients are taught how to care for a tracheostomy before leaving the hospital.

gastrointestinal cancer

Gastrointestinal cancer can lead to a long and painful illness. In cases too advanced to be helped by surgery, the person actually dies of starvation. One of the most common types of gastrointestinal cancer occurs in the large intestine. Early detection of such cancer is an important factor in survival. One treatment for this type of cancer is to remove the diseased part of the large intestine. An opening, called a **colostomy,** is made through the wall of the abdomen. The cancerous portion of the intestine is removed. The end of the intestine remaining is pulled to the outside of the abdo-

men, figure 19-6. The body wastes are expelled through this opening into a colostomy bag attached to the abdomen. The area where the intestine opens to the outside is called the stoma.

After surgery, the patient is taught how to care for the stoma. Care is important since drainage from the intestine can irritate it. The patient is also taught how to irrigate the colostomy. **Irrigation** is the use of water to clean out the colon. Family members are also instructed on how to help the patient care for the colostomy.

In some cases, a colostomy is temporary. It may be possible to reconstruct and reconnect the intestine after several months. When this is not possible, the patient's rectum

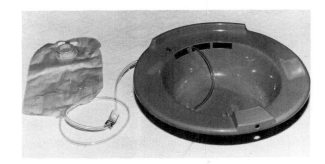

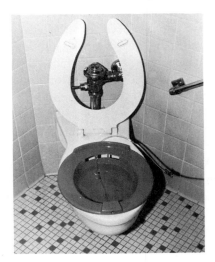

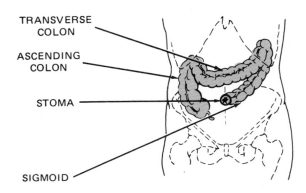

TRANSVERSE
COLON

ASCENDING
COLON

STOMA

SIGMOID

Figure 19-6 The cut end of the intestine is brought to the outside of the abdomen to form a stoma.

is surgically closed and the colostomy becomes permanent. The discharge from a colostomy is fairly solid. The kind of diet prescribed for these patients helps control the type of discharge. Each patient needs to experiment with diet and bowel habits until the best balance is found. Some people with a colostomy may be able to regulate bowel movements very well. They may only need to keep a gauze pad over the stoma. Some people are able to go swimming. Sitz baths are ordered to relieve any soreness around the rectum due to surgery, figure 19-7.

Cancer can destroy the functioning of the entire large intestine. When this occurs, the small intestine is cut and brought to the outside through the abdomen. This procedure is called an **ileostomy** or jejeunostomy, depending upon the location of the opening in the small intestine. Most ileostomies are permanent. The waste discharge from an ileostomy remains liquid and drains constantly. The drainage irritates the skin. Therefore, the stoma must be well cared for.

Odors from the bag may be controlled by oral medications taken by the client or a deodorizer put into the container bag.

client care

The home health aide should assist the client in cleaning around the stoma and changing the dressings and stoma bags. The aide can also help with colostomy irrigations and sitz baths. Clients are sometimes embarrassed or ashamed of the odor and the appearance of the stoma. A home health aide must be careful not to offend the client. Aides should never show disgust at the odor or shy away from helping the client.

summary

- In most cases a home health aide will only be sent to care for a client with cancer after a diagnosis has been made. Usually some form of cancer treatment has been started. The client may have had surgery. In some cases the client receives chemotherapy or x-ray treatments.
- When caring for a cancer client, a home health aide is given specific instructions.
- It is important that the client be kept as cheerful and comfortable as possible.
- Cancer not only causes physical pain and discomfort, but it also brings on depression and sadness.
- When caring for a client with cancer, a home health aide must be understanding and kind.
- Clients need to talk and to be listened to. Often cancer clients know that they are dying. They must be helped to feel that they are still contributing members of society.
- These clients should be kept clean and comfortable. They need large doses of tender loving care.

review

1. List nine warning signs of cancer.
2. What considerations should be given to meals for the client with cancer.
3. Name three types of treatments for cancer.
4. What is a colostomy?

Unit 20
Handling Emergencies

key terms

crisis	emergency
first aid	crisis intervention center

learning objectives

After studying this unit, you should be able to:
- Define emergency.
- Explain the purpose of a crisis intervention center.
- Identify two basic first aid techniques.
- Describe at least two family crisis situations which can arise.
- Name at least five emergency telephone numbers which should be posted near the telephone.

Some people consider any unusual happening an emergency. However, the best definition of an **emergency** is a sudden and unexpected (usually serious) happening. There are those who become overexcited when an emergency occurs. They expect the worst when they are placed in any unusual situation. With experience, a home health aide will recognize a real emergency and know the best action to take. Sometimes, the aide can handle the situation alone. At other times, the aide will need the help of others. Most emergencies can be avoided by practicing simple rules of safety.

family crisis situations

There are some events that may bring about sudden and/or unhappy changes in peo-

ple's lives. A home health aide should be able to recognize such events and have some understanding of why a person reacts in a certain way to these events. A **crisis** can best be described as a critical period. The time period required to readjust from a crisis varies greatly.

A crisis is not always negative or bad. A marriage can cause a crisis in a family. Everyone in the family may be very happy about the wedding. However, the pressure of getting out invitations, planning, organizing and buying special clothing can upset the family's routine and cause financial problems, more physical work, and mental strain. The parents may experience a sense of loss when their child moves out of the home.

Illness itself brings about a crisis in a family. The life-style of the ill person may have to be totally changed. The head of the household may lose a job because of illness. These crisis situations create added problems within a household. A home health aide may enter a home with a family crisis. The aide must be prepared to keep the household running smoothly during the crisis period.

In many large city areas, **crisis intervention centers** have been set up. These centers provide telephone hot lines so that troubled individuals can call for advice or receive information as to where they should turn for help. Some crisis situations which are handled at crisis intervention centers are attempted suicide, alcoholism, child abuse, wife beating or mental breakdowns. A home health aide should see if such centers are available locally.

giving first aid

In spite of all the precautions or care taken, accidents do happen. A home health aide is frequently the first person at the scene of a

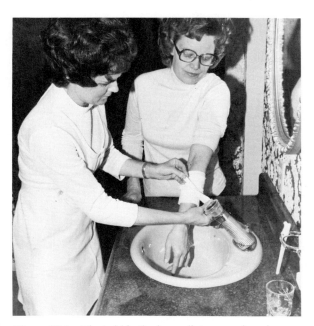

Figure 20-1 First aid is the immediate care given in case of injury.

home accident. What are the limits of the aide's responsibilities? What should be done at once? What should not be done?

First aid is the immediate care given in case of injury or accident, figure 20-1. The word **first** suggests that there is more to follow. After first aid has been given, the home health aide should contact a doctor or nurse. Aides must recognize their limitations. They must know who to call after first aid has been given. Each home health aide should prepare and post a list of emergency phone numbers and know the location of the nearest telephone. These numbers should include:

- the agency (supervisor's extension)
- family doctor
- police department
- fire department
- ambulance service
- hospital
- crisis intervention center
- poison control center
- member of the client's family

Fortunately, most of the accidents in the home are minor ones—simple bruises, small burns, a bloody nose or cuts and splinters. They need only simple first aid.

What if the injury is severe? There are certain injuries that must be recognized as a real emergency. The way a home health aide behaves during an emergency is important for the client. If the aide panics, the injured victim, who is already scared, will become more afraid. The confidence and calmness of the home health aide can make the victim less frightened and more relaxed. A calm, soothing manner is the initial step in giving any first aid.

Figure 20-2, lists first aid techniques for emergency conditions; the most serious conditions are listed first. The aide must use good judgment to determine whether danger exists. **Caution:** In most emergencies, the client should not be moved unless absolutely necessary. Cer-

INJURY OR EMERGENCY CONDITION	RECOMMENDED FIRST AID TECHNIQUE
Breathing stopped completely	Clear the airway if it is blocked. Give rescue breathing or cardiopulmonary resuscitation.
Uncontrolled bleeding	Apply pressure bandage or direct pressure on wound; use clean or sterile dressing; elevate area
Sucking chest wound	Place palm of hand, cloth or dressing tightly over wound.
Choking.	Heimlich Maneuver (abdominal thrust) Turn small child upside down to dislodge object; give four sharp blows between the shoulder blades.
Electric shock.	Separate victim from electric source using loop of rubber, cloth, dry wood, or leather belt. Give cardiopulmonary resuscitation.
Poison swallowed	Call for help immediately! Read label of the suspected poison and follow instructions. Sometimes, the victim should drink milk or water to dilute the poison.
Shock	Keep the victim warm and lying down; elevate legs
Heart attack.	Give cardiopulmonary resuscitation.
Severe heat burns	Cover with clean or sterile dressing.
Convulsions (seizures)	Protect client from injury. DO NOT restrain. Let convulsion run its course. Turn client on side if possible.
Fractures.	Keep client still. Do not move broken part. Get medical help.
Heat exhaustion	If client is conscious, give fluids and salt.
Chemical burns.	Flush with cold water.
Small heat burns	Flush with cold water or apply ice.
Animal bites.	Clean wound with warm water and soap. Take victim to hospital for a tetanus shot.
Insect bites/stings	Apply ice or baking soda. Apply meat tenderizer to a sting.
Cuts, punctures, skin wounds.	Wash with warm water and soap. For deep cuts, transport victim to Emergency Room for tetanus shot and stitches.
Eye injuries	If object is imbedded, cover eye with soft dressing; keep client still. Get medical help at once.
Fainting.	Have the client lie down; elevate feet somewhat.
Bruises (contusions).	Apply ice to area.

Figure 20-2 First aid for emergency conditions

tain emergencies can endanger a person's life. A second saved in starting first aid may mean the difference between life and death.

What should be done if the home health aide is the only person on the scene? If the aide knows what to do and is qualified to do it, first aid should be given immediately and then medical help called for. In most cases, the police and fire department are the first to respond to a call for help. Give the address and the nature of the emergency and then return to the client.

Special instructions for first aid procedures are outlined in any first aid manual. However, more advanced techniques should not be performed until a home health aide has been taught and has been certified to perform them.

cardiopulmonary resuscitation

Cardiopulmonary resuscitation is a procedure followed when an individual has stopped breathing. In order for the body to function, it must receive oxygen. When breathing stops or fails, brain cells begin to die within four to six minutes. If breathing is not restored quickly, permanent brain damage can occur. Damage may also be done to the heart, lungs, liver and kidneys.

The heart operates the circulatory system; the lungs operate the respiratory system. Between these two systems oxygen is brought into the body, carried to body cells, and released from the body as carbon dioxide (waste). The lungs require heart action in order to function, but the heart can pump for several minutes without the lungs working. When breathing has stopped because of choking, suffocation, drowning, poisoning, medication overdose, inhalation of toxic fumes, electric shock or crib death (Sudden Death Syndrome), cardiopulmonary resuscitation may revive the person.

Only an individual who has been through a special training program can perform CPR. Usually a course lasts for 8 hours. Theory and a review of anatomy are studied and a written test must be passed. In addition, students work under supervision with manikins to practice the lifesaving techniques until proficiency is attained. The American Heart Association, American Red Cross, and local hospitals usually offer this course. The home health aide should enroll for this course and become certified. Certification is usually good for one year at which time, a refresher course must be taken to maintain certification. The procedure for cardiopulmonary resuscitation is included in the Appendix as a reference to use after the home health aide has completed CPR training. Refer to the Appendix.

summary

- A practicing home health aide may come in contact with a number of emergency situations.
- The aide who has thought about what should be done and planned ahead will be better able to handle emergencies.
- Home health aides should recognize the limits of their knowledge and abilities.
- In giving first aid, the aide should not do anything that would cause greater harm to the client.
- In serious emergencies, the most important duty of the aide is to reach the person best qualified to take over.
- The home health aide can prevent many emergencies by making the home environment safe.

review

1. What is the first aid given for a client who may be choking due to food lodged in the trachea?
2. What should the home health aide do if the client falls and a fracture is suspected?
3. What should the home health aide do if the client has a convulsion?
4. What is the term used to indicate a critical period?
5. Define emergency.

Unit 21
Caring for the Dying Client

learning objectives

After studying this unit, you should be able to:
- Identify some cultural influences surrounding practices related to death.
- Identify the five stages of dying as described by Dr. Kübler-Ross.
- Identify the home health aide's responsibilities when the client dies.
- Identify ways in which a person may react to the death of a family member or friend.

Most people in our society feel uncomfortable talking or thinking about death. This is more true today than in earlier times in history. Gathering in the room of a dying relative was a custom practiced no more than 40 years ago. Death was accepted as the natural end to life. Children openly shared the final moments of life with a dying grandparent, parent or sibling. As the nation changed from an agricultural to an industrial society, and then into the Age of Information, life-styles changed. Families became separated in distant parts of the country. This brought about a change in the attitudes about death.

cultural differences

Indians and Eskimos followed customs that today may be thought of as uncivilized. The aged, ill members of Eskimo tribes were taken to an iceberg and left alone with a small amount of food. This was the accepted way to die. In certain Indian tribes, people who were ill and unable to do their share of work were taken to an isolated spot to await death. These customs were accepted as a natural and respectable way for life to end. They felt that it was good to allow life to end naturally. When human power to cure with herbs and medicines was not effective, it was time for death to come.

Medical science today has made treatments more available and more effective. In addition, advances have been made in living conditions. Clothing is warmer. Housing is better. Foods are more plentiful. Working conditions have improved. Because of these and other changes, people can expect to live for many years. Diseases which were once incurable have been conquered. New medicines and surgical techniques have been developed that save thousands of lives daily. Most of these medical advances improve the quality of life. However, some of the medical advances prolong life but do not always improve life. The value of life support systems is being questioned today. There are times when a patient is kept alive by machines but has no awareness of being alive. These machines take over the vital functions for the patient. In several states, laws have been passed which let the patient or family refuse the **mechanical life support** systems.

Changing attitudes toward death have appeared partly as a result of increased life expectancy. People seem to fear death as never before. They want to hold on to life and try not to think about death. Children are usually protected from the facts of death. When a beloved grandparent dies, children may be told that the grandparent has gone away. Since families are often separated by great distances, many children believe that their grandparents have just moved. How a family deals with death is a very personal matter, figure 21-1. A home health aide must respect the wishes of the family in dealing with the death of a family member. The aide must be aware of the needs of the dying person and the family.

psychological adjustments

Dr. Elisabeth Kübler-Ross has made careful studies of dying persons and their families. She has described a general pattern common to persons facing death. The pattern may apply to both the dying person and the person's family. Dr. Kübler-Ross has noted five stages of psychological adjustment to death.

1. **Denial**—This can't be happening to me; perhaps someone else, but not me.
2. **Anger**—An extension of denial; feeling that this death is unfair; bitterness and loss of faith in God; fighting against death or loss of a loved one.
3. **Bargaining**—"Dear God, I'll be good. Please, not yet—some other time, it's too soon.
4. **Depression**—Brooding, withdrawal, lack of communication; thoughts of suicide—"I'd rather kill myself than die from this disease" or, "I can't go on living if Mama dies."
5. **Acceptance**—Calmly facing what is to be or feeling a sense of peace; looking forward to release from pain and sorrow; hoping for the release of a loved one to a better world.

A home health aide who is in an environment of expected death may see these patterns develop. The aide should not offer advice to the family or client. The aide should be understanding and kind but not lose control emotionally. By knowing what to expect in the way of reactions, the home health aide is better prepared to adjust to the situation.

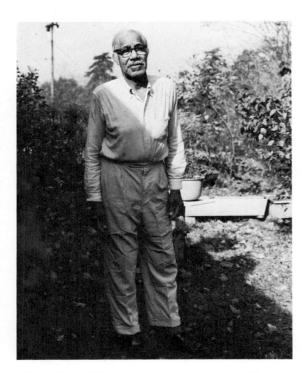

Figure 21-1 Working in his garden helps this man adjust to the death of his wife.

Sometimes a client may die suddenly and unexpectedly. Other times death is preceded by a long illness. Some people are relieved that life is ending. Some clients become unconscious just before death. Of the five senses (hearing, taste, touch, sight, smell) the last to go is hearing. For this reason when working with an unconscious client, the home health aide should be careful what is said in the client's presence. It would be cruel if the last words a client heard were, "Well, she's almost gone; she'll be dead by morning." The home health aide's first duty is to keep the client clean and as comfortable as possible. The client should be treated with kindness and dignity at all times. In addition, the aide should provide emotional support to the client and the family. Good communication skills are needed when dealing with the dying client and the family.

When death occurs, family members may be highly emotional. The home health aide must remain calm as there are many details to be taken care of. Figure 21-2 lists the duties of a home health aide when the client dies. A home health aide may be asked to remain on duty to help the family prepare for the funeral.

1. Call the family doctor and your agency at once. A death certificate must be filed by the doctor. Write down the time of death.

2. Do not touch the client until the doctor tells you to.

3. Call a family member after the doctor has been called.

4. Follow the doctor's instructions and clean the client's body. At death, all body functions stop. Relaxed muscles cause the bowel and bladder to empty.

5. Call the agency and ask for further instructions.

Figure 21-2 What to do if a client dies.

religious and cultural influences

Among some Jewish families, burial takes place within 24 hours after death. Religious practice forbids **embalming** the body and requires the casket remain closed. After the funeral the family may have a period of formal mourning. During this time, friends and relatives come to the home to comfort each other.

In other Jewish families and in Catholic or Protestant families, the body is usually taken to a funeral home. Friends and family meet at the funeral home during the two or three days before the body is buried. Religious practices differ from one group to another and even from family to family. Most people do recognize the need of sharing grief. This is part of the final acceptance of death. Some people weep, others are angry. Some are very quiet. As people work through their emotions, they come to accept the loss.

Death is usually a cause of crisis within a family. Some people may need special help to face the crisis of death. It usually takes several months to readjust to the loss of a loved one. The most difficult adjustment period is the first two or three months.

summary

- Dying is not accepted by everyone in the same manner. Many cultural influences affect the client's and family's concept of death. Besides the cultural differences, personal differences exist.
- Dr. Elisabeth Kübler-Ross has done research which shows five stages of adjustment to death: denial, anger, bargaining, depression and acceptance. People commonly pass through these five stages.
- The aide must be calm and perform the necessary duties when a client dies.

review

1. List the five stages of psychological adjustment to death.
2. What should the home health aide do if the client dies while the aide is on duty?
3. In what culture does burial follow within 24 hours of death?

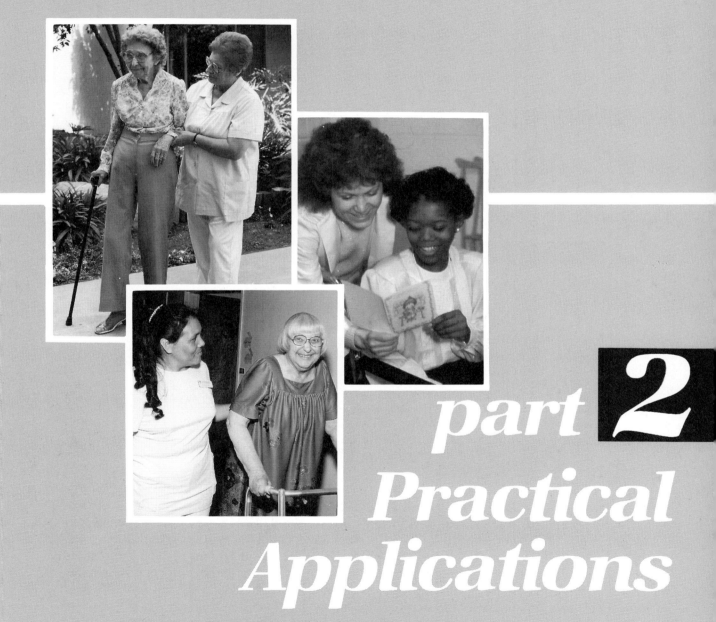

part 2

Practical Applications

Homemaking Services

Principles of Household Management

key terms
instinct   myth

learning objectives
After studying this unit, you should be able to: ▬ List at least four tips used to plan and organize tasks. ▬ Explain how to care for major home appliances. ▬ State some ways to combine client care and household tasks.

Managing a household is considered by many to be a mindless routine that requires no special ability. It has often been assumed that a person (especially females in the traditional role of wife, mother and homemaker) was born with the talent and **instinct** (inborn knowledge) to care for a home. In fact, one of the most foolish **myths** is the belief that anyone can run a home.

Actually, managing a household is like operating a daily 24-hour business. Homemakers raise children, manage a budget, provide a clean and livable house, prepare and serve meals and handle home accidents. It requires intelligence, understanding and real physical labor.

Home health aides not only run their own homes but take on a second job of assisting others to run their homes. Many home health aides have a basic knowledge of keeping up a house. However, the habits developed in their own homes may not be suitable to all working situations.

The units covering homemaking skills are presented to introduce homemaking techniques to the beginner. However, even the experienced homemaker may learn some helpful new tips.

The aide should realize that each home situation may offer different challenges. A professional home health aide must adapt to the physical surroundings of each job. This adjustment requires the aide to use whatever appliances and supplies the client has available. The aide must remember to show as much care for the property of others as is shown for personal property. The equipment and furnishings used by the home health aide belong to the employer. Reasonable care must be used, figure 22-1. The aide should read directions and ask questions before using unfamiliar equipment. If there is equipment with frayed cords, or appliances which do not work, they should be repaired. The aide should notify the supervisor or family so that repairs can be made. When using any cleaning product or appliance, the labels and directions should be read carefully. This not only makes for proper use, but can limit the number of accidents which might happen. Using rubber gloves helps avoid skin irritation caused by soaps or household chemical products. When performing regular household duties, the aide should make a list of any items in short supply. Toilet paper, laundry products, food or other necessities should be purchased before the house supply runs out.

Sometimes a home health aide handles the client's money. Honesty in money matters is an absolute necessity. When performing household chores, the aide should follow the rules of good body mechanics to avoid injury.

tips on planning and organization

No house takes care of itself. In a home where everything seems neat, the homemaker has probably used a set of well-organized plans. An important duty of the aide is to plan, organize, and carry out the tasks completely. The homemaker who plans the work, organizes the tasks and starts doing them will find the work load lightened. A home health aide will be given instructions for each assignment. The care of the client is of primary importance, but the household tasks cannot be ignored, figure 22-2 on page 250. The aide should take a few minutes each morning to plan the tasks that should be completed by the day's end. This can save time and energy.

- Carry a pad and pencil in the pocket of the uniform. Make a note of household supplies that may be needed in each room.
- Post a list of needed supplies on a kitchen bulletin board, or use a small magnet and put the list on the refrigerator door. Remind family members that if they use the last bar of soap or roll of bathroom tissue they should add the item to the list.
- Before starting to clean a room, the aide should stop to think which cleaning supplies may be needed. All the supplies needed to complete the work in a particular room should be taken to the room at one time.
- Carry cleaning supplies from room to room in a shopping bag or basket.
- Prevent buildup of dirt by tidying rooms, dusting, wiping surfaces and sponging up spots as soon as possible.
- Keep a sponge in the kitchen and bathroom for quick wipe-ups.
- Use a tray to carry dishes to and from the table.
- Schedule major jobs for a certain day of the week. For example, vacuum and wash floors

APPLIANCE	PURPOSE AND USE	CARE AND CLEANING
REFRIGERATOR	To retard spoilage of perishable foods. Door should be kept closed when not in use. Temperature control should be set so as to keep foods fresh but not to freeze them. Most refrigerators have zoned cooling. Store foods in a specific area. Meats to be used within two or three days belong in the meat storage compartment. Fruits and vegetables are kept in the bottom area, milk and dairy products on top shelves. Store leftovers in small airtight containers and use as soon as possible.	Discard leftovers if unused in three days. Wipe interior with warm water and baking soda to remove stale odors. At least every three or four weeks remove shelves and drawers. Wash them in water and detergent. Rinse thoroughly.
FREEZER COMPARTMENT OF REFRIGERATOR	Store frozen foods and weekly meat supply. Mark date of storage and use older products first. Frost-free refrigerators have a tray at the bottom. This tray should be pulled out and cleaned every two or three months. Persons with lung disorders may be sensitive to the dust and vapors from this area.	To defrost, put pan of hot water in emptied compartment. Turn control knob to defrost. Empty pan under freezer so water does not flood rest of refrigerator or floor. DO NOT USE SHARP KNIFE TO PRY ICE LOOSE. THIS COULD DAMAGE FREEZER COILS. When defrosting is completed, wipe inside with warm water and baking soda. Turn control on and replace foods. If any food has thawed completely, use it at once—do not refreeze foods.
FREEZER	Offers large, cold storage area and maintains a constant temperature. Foods may be stored for long periods of time. Some foods cannot be stored longer than 6 months. Instructions on care and wrapping foods for the freezer appear later in the text.	Defrost twice a year. If frost-free model, remove foods and wipe inner surfaces with damp cloth and baking soda.
STOVE	Heats food for boiling, broiling or baking. Uses gas or electricity as a fuel source. Keep pot holders and dish towels away from flame or heat unit. Never use the oven when it is greasy—FIRE HAZARD. Turn off stove when finished cooking. When using gas stoves, be sure the pilot light is burning before turning on gas jet of the burner. When lighting the oven, first light match, then turn on gas jet and put flame to it. Keep body turned away from open oven door for safety. If oven does not light, turn off jet and try again in a few minutes. Make sure gas jet is turned OFF when through using oven.	Wipe up spilled foods at once. Wipe off stove surface once a day. Scour burners and burner pans once a week. When cleaning the oven, follow instructions on cleaner can. Clean as often as needed. When daily spills and grease are cleaned up, a full oven cleaning is not needed as often. Self-cleaning ovens—follow manufacturer's instructions.

Figure 22-1 Proper use and care of household appliances reduces the need for repairs and the risk of personal injury.

APPLIANCE	PURPOSE AND USE	CARE AND CLEANING
MICROWAVE OVEN	Read instructions before using. Used for rapid food defrosting, quick heating of left-overs, baking, and cooking. Use only the recommended dishes or supplies (paper, plastic) in the microwave. Never use metal containers.	Wipe clean with damp cloth, following instructions in operator's manual. Soap may be used; rinse well and dry interior. If you are unsure about care and cleaning, ask a family member for a demonstration.
DISHWASHER	Washes dishes at a high water temperature; most dishwashers sterilize dishes. Rinse plates and utensils before placing in dishwasher—or turn on prewash cycle immediately after loading. Use *only* the dishwashing detergent. Wait until there is a full load before putting on wash cycle. (Saves water and electricity). Do not put plastic, cast iron or wooden items in dishwasher.	Clean filter once a week and wash interior with water and mild soap, rinse with damp cloth. **Caution:** Do not touch coils in dishwasher.
GARBAGE DISPOSAL	Appliance in sink which cuts up discarded food and disposes of it. Follow instructions in manufacturer's guide. Be careful to dispose only the food items listed, not bones or paper. **Caution:** Keep hands away from unit while in operation.	**Caution:** Do not try to repair; call for plumber if it breaks down. After using, rinse drain with hot water.
GARBAGE COMPACTER	Crushes garbage to save storage space. Follow instructions in manufacturer's guide. Use it only for those items recommended by manufacturer.	Call professional repairman.
WASHING MACHINE	Soaks and agitates clothing. Load as instructed—use correct water temperature for type of clothing. Use soap and bleach as needed according to instructions. Do not overload.	Clean out lint trap. About once a week wipe out inside with soap and water to get rid of grit. Take off agitator and clean carefully. Wipe outer surface after use.
DRYER	Tumbles and heats clothing to dry them. Load according to instructions, using temperature recommended for type of clothes.	Clean lint trap after each use. Wipe outer surface after use. Call repairman if machine works poorly.
SMALL APPLIANCES Automatic Blender Mixer Electric Fry Pan Slicing Machine Electric Knife Percolator Automatic Coffee Maker	Follow operating instructions. If you are unsure how to use it, do not use it. Pay special attention to all safety precautions provided by the manufacturer with the appliance.	Wash surface and store conveniently and carefully. Make sure the electric unit does not come in contact with water. Wash coffee maker with soap and water after using. Rinse thoroughly. Once in a while run a cycle of water and baking soda through pot to clean coffee oils away.

Figure 22-1 (*Continued*)

on Friday so the house will be ready for week-end use; launder and iron one day; plan weekly marketing on Monday or Wednesday; defrost refrigerator, clean oven, or straighten drawers or cabinets on a day when nothing big is planned.

- Arrange to do two or three tasks at one time. A load of laundry can be put in the machine just before lunch time. While the machine is running, lunch can be prepared and served to the client. If the laundry has to be done in the Laundromat, it can be planned for the same day as the weekly marketing. While hand laundry is soaking, the ironing could be done.

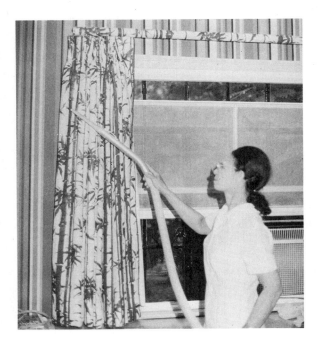

Figure 22-2 Vacuuming can be done at a time when the client does not require the aide's full attention.

- Learn how to use and care for the equipment in the home. Most appliances have an instruction manual. Read it before using the equipment. After using equipment, clean it so it will be ready for the next use. Store small appliances close to where they are used.

combining client care and household tasks

The order in which tasks are done is not always important. If one knows just what should be completed by the end of the day the work can be arranged around the client's needs. After the client's bath and after the bed linens are changed, the aide may decide to clean the client's room. The kitchen could be cleaned after the breakfast meal. The client's bathroom cleaning could be done after the bedpan has been used and emptied into the toilet bowl. These examples show how to pair client care procedures with homemaking duties. This technique saves time and energy by avoiding many extra steps a day.

summary

- Caring for the client's home is an important part of a home health aide's job. This requires learning how to use and care for equipment and organizing time effectively.
- While the physical care of the client is of primary importance, providing a clean and safe environment is also necessary.

Unit 23
Maintaining a Clean Environment in the Home

key terms

sanitary   incinerator   pathogens
mildew

learning objectives

After studying this unit, you should be able to:
- Name three factors which determine the aide's cleaning plan.
- List five cleaning tasks done daily.
- List five cleaning tasks done weekly.
- List five cleaning tasks which are only done periodically.
- Describe the correct method for disposing of garbage.
- Identify at least four steps used in cleaning a kitchen.
- Identify daily bathroom care which family members should perform.
- Identify two bathroom cleaning tasks the aide does daily.
- Identify the correct way to handle outdated or unlabeled medications.

The aide is expected to do general cleaning in the living room, dining room, family room and bedrooms. Home health aides set up their own routines for completing daily household tasks. There is no one pattern to be followed. The factors to be considered include:

- the needs of the client
- the size of the home
- the ages of people living in the home
- the number of people living in the home

When taking on the responsibilities for home care it is good to have a master plan. Some tasks must be done several times a day. Some should be done daily or weekly. Others need only be done on an occasional basis.

Home furnishings represent a costly expenditure for most families. Furniture and carpets should last for many years. The life of furniture and upholstery can be increased by proper care and attention. The home health aide should remember that the furnishings were expensive to buy, but would be even more expensive to replace. Cleaning has been made easier with modern electrical equipment and new cleaning products. These factors make it possible to clean quickly on a day-to-day basis. Big jobs done weekly or several times a year are also done much easier than in the past.

daily cleaning tasks

Certain tasks should be done every day in order to keep the home neat and clean. Some daily duties need to be done whether or not they have been assigned. The aide is expected to tidy rooms and clean up spills when they occur. Daily cleaning should not require longer than an hour or an hour and a half. The following duties should be done every day.

- Pick up toys, magazines, newspapers, and clothing, figure 23-1. **Caution:** Do not discard any of these items without the permission of a family member.

- Fluff cushions and pillows, make the beds or change linens when necessary.
- Dry dust furniture, lamps, and knickknacks, figure 23-2.
- Wipe off windowsills and radiators.
- Sweep or lightly vacuum carpets and floors. Hard floors can be dust mopped.
- Empty ash trays and wastebaskets.
- Remove spots and stains using a suitable cleaning product. Test the product first by trying it on a hidden spot. See whether the carpet bleeds or fades. After cleaning a difficult spot, cover it with a clean white cloth until the area dries. Never use soap on carpet stains. Dried soap attracts dirt and can cause permanent damage. To avoid spreading the stain, work from the outside of the stain toward the center (clean to dirty).

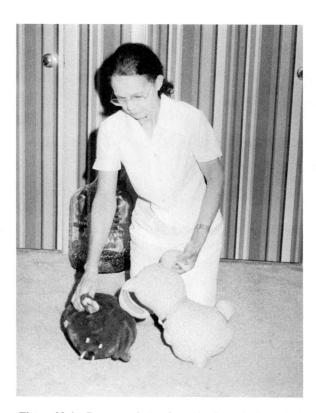

Figure 23-1 Remove clutter from the floors before starting general cleaning.

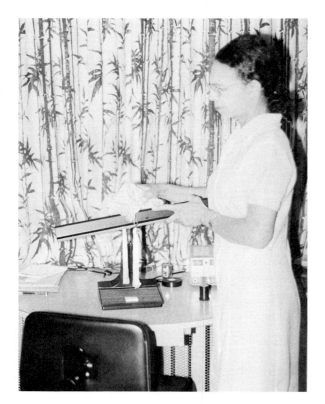

Figure 23-2 Dust daily with a soft, dry cloth.

weekly cleaning tasks

Weekly care can be done in more than one way. The aide may want to change the bed linens in every bedroom on the same day. On the other hand, the aide may prefer to completely clean and arrange one bedroom at a time. The aide's decision can vary with each assignment. The aide should always consider the needs of the client before making out a schedule.

- Change bed linens throughout the house. The client's bed may need to be changed more often.
- Vacuum floors and carpets, getting under furniture where dirt may lodge, figure 23-3. Change or empty the vacuum cleaner bag as required, figure 23-4; discard the dirt in a large paper bag. Avoid bumping the furniture and woodwork with the vacuum cleaner.
- Wipe windowsills and frames.

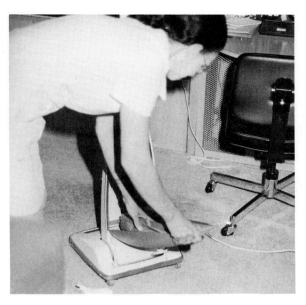

Figure 23-4 Change or empty the vacuum cleaner bag as often as needed.

- Vacuum upholstery and under seat cushions, figure 23-5. Vacuum lampshades and wipe away cobwebs.
- Damp or wet mop floors. Oiled dust mops are preferred by some people.
- Polish the furniture. Handle knickknacks carefully when dusting, figure 23-6. Use a flannel cloth, old diaper or cheesecloth. Use one cloth for dry dusting, another for polishing. Do not dust and polish until vacuuming and dry mopping have been completed. Pour polish onto the polishing cloth. **Caution:** Do not pour polish directly onto the furniture. Use long strokes along the grain of the wood. Refold cloth and add more polish as needed. Be careful not to spill polish on upholstery or carpets.

periodic cleaning tasks

Certain areas in the home do not require frequent cleaning. However, the aide should check these areas to be sure that dust and dirt

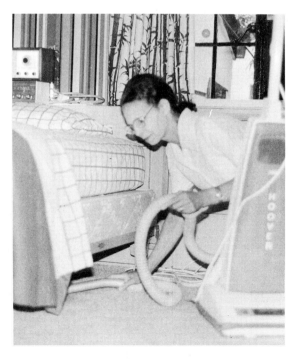

Figure 23-3 Be sure to vacuum under the furniture.

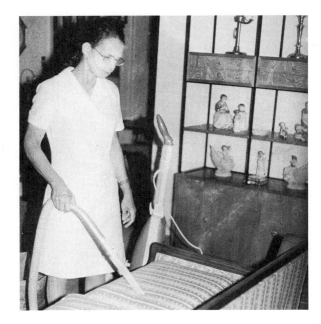

Figure 23-5 Be sure to vacuum under seat cushions when vacuuming upholstery.

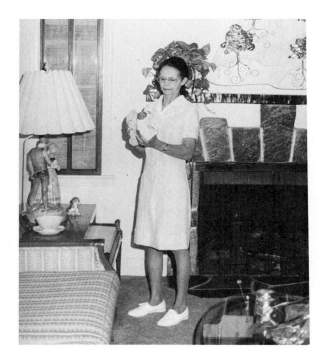

Figure 23-6 Handle knickknacks carefully to prevent breakage.

do not collect. The following tasks can be done on an occasional basis.

- Remove cobwebs from the ceilings, walls, curtains and shades. Use a long-handled dust mop covered with a clean cloth.
- Remove small pictures from the wall and dust behind them. Dust the frames and glass.
- Wipe mirrors or use glass cleaner on them as needed.
- Remove books from shelves and dust both books and shelves, figure 23-7.
- Clean lamp bases. Replace burned out bulbs as needed.
- Damp wipe lighting fixtures on walls or ceilings.
- Hand wash decorative plates and table ornaments in mild soapsuds.
- Vacuum draperies and window shades.

kitchen maintenance and cleaning

In many homes, the kitchen is the center of family life. For this reason, keeping the

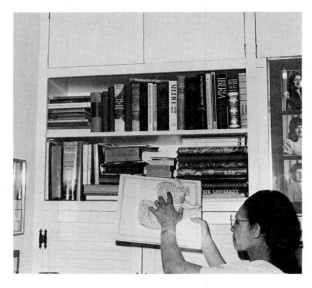

Figure 23-7 Remove books from shelves and dust both books and shelves.

kitchen in order probably requires more organization than any other room in the home. Not only must the aide prepare and clean up after each meal, but products must be replaced as they are used. Wastes must be discarded, leftovers stored for future use, and special menus and snacks prepared for the client. Kitchen work may seem to be an endless cycle, figure 23-8. With the right attitude it can be challenging and satisfying when it is done well. With a little effort, attractive and nutritious meals can be made. These meals can improve the client's physical condition; however, they must be made in a clean and healthful environment.

Following are some reasons for keeping a kitchen clean and neat:

- germs are less likely to grow in a clean kitchen
- it is easier to prepare meals in a neat area
- it is quicker to find equipment and supplies that have been properly stored, figure 23-9
- there are always clean dishes, utensils and pots ready for use

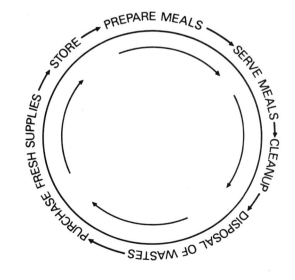

Figure 23-8 Because of the endless cycle of kitchen chores, keeping the kitchen in order requires organization.

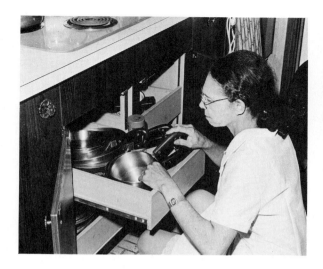

Figure 23-9 When equipment and supplies are properly stored, they are easier to find.

- accidents are less likely to happen when floors are free of spills
- insects (flies, roaches, ants) and rodents (mice or rats) are less likely to appear when food and garbage are properly put away.

Maintaining order is an easier task when the kitchen area is clean. The aide who keeps up with small cleanup jobs will find that this practice makes work easier. When these tasks are left undone, kitchen work becomes overwhelming. Routine cleanup procedures usually take no more that 15 to 20 minutes after each meal. Major tasks such as cleaning drawers and cabinets require more time. The aide should schedule these duties to be done at times when routine tasks are light and client is resting or has visitors.

disposing of garbage

Place a brown paper bag in a waste container or garbage can. Put dry wastes, cartons and tin cans in this container; for food wastes use a separate container lined with a plastic bag. All scraps of food and garbage which are damp should be placed in the container lined

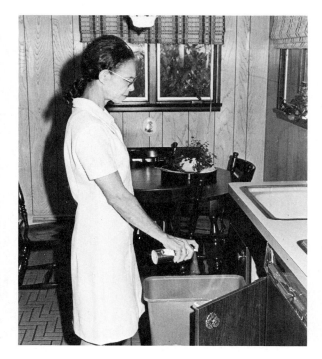

Figure 23-10 Odors and germs may be eliminated by spraying disinfectant into the garbage container.

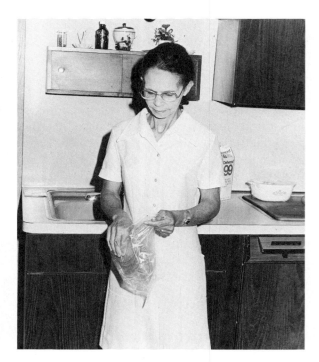

Figure 23-11 Leftovers may be preserved in a plastic bag or in a tightly covered container.

with plastic. Empty it as often as necessary, but at least once a day. This will prevent odors from forming and helps to prevent ants, roaches and mice from being attracted to the area. Spray the garbage container with a disinfectant, figure 23-10.

storing leftovers

Transfer usable leftovers to small containers, figure 23-11. Cover leftovers so that they do not dry out. Leftovers should be refrigerated as soon as possible.

dishwashing

If the client has an infectious disease, wash the client's dishes and utensils separately from the other family dishes. Rinse these dishes and utensils in boiling water. This is an aseptic technique used to prevent the spread of **patho-**

gens to other members of the family. When washing the family's dishes by hand, use hot water and liquid detergent. Wash the dishes in the following order: cups and glassware, utensils, plates and bowls, pots and pans. If the water becomes greasy, drain the sink and add fresh water and detergent. After washing them with detergent, rinse the dishes completely with hot water. Place the dishes in a drainer. Air drying is more **sanitary** then drying with a dish towel. Lay a clean dish towel over the dishes as the rest of the kitchen is cleaned. After the dishes are dry, put them away in cabinets.

Some homes are equipped with automatic dishwashers. Before placing dishes in the dishwasher, scrape and rinse them well. Some machines have a rinse cycle prior to the wash cycle. When using these machines, hand rinsing the dishes may not be necessary before loading. Pour dishwasher detergent into the correct area labeled on the machine. **Caution:** Do not use soap powder or liquid detergent. Run dishwasher only when it is fully loaded. Water and electricity are wasted when the dishwasher is half empty. Pots and pans should be hand washed and stored when dry.

wiping surfaces

Use a cloth or sponge, warm water and detergent to wipe the table, countertops, wall behind the stove, stove top, and outside surfaces of the refrigerator and microwave oven. Be sure to remove grease or splashes caused from cooking foods.

Use a cloth or sponge and vinegar to wipe out the inside of the refrigerator, figure 23-12. The inside of the microwave oven should be wiped with warm water and carefully dried.

Wipe the sink; use scouring powder if necessary. Scouring powder helps remove stains and marks left by pans or food wastes. After scouring, be sure to rinse the sink completely.

cleaning the floors

Wipe up any spills with a cloth, sponge, or paper towel as soon as they occur. Do not wipe with a sponge or cloth that is used for other surfaces; keep a separate cloth or sponge for floors only. For general sweeping, use a dust mop or broom. Gather crumbs and dirt on a dustpan and empty the dustpan into a garbage container. Damp mop floors at least once a week, figure 23-13.

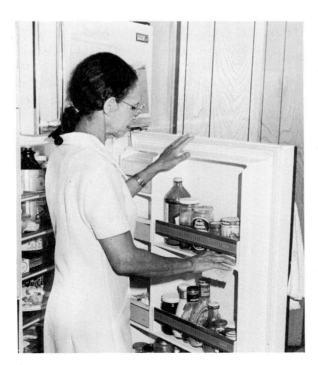

Figure 23-12 Shelves in the refrigerator are wiped clean with a sponge and vinegar.

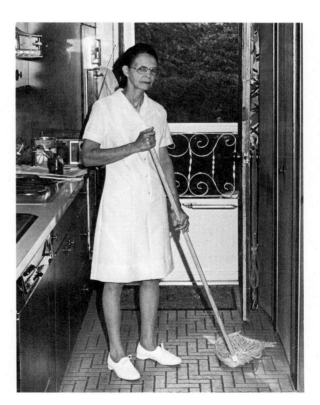

Figure 23-13 Floor areas should be cleaned with a damp mop.

cleaning cabinets and drawers

Dishes, glassware, and utensils should be stored in clean cabinets and drawers. Water vapor, smoke, and grease from cooking cause a buildup of oily film on kitchen surfaces. The film collects on both the inside and the outside of closed cabinets. The outside of cabinets should be cleaned at least once a week. The inside should be cleaned several times a year. The cleaning product used will depend on the type of cabinet being cleaned. Metal, formica and wood require different types of cleaning products. Drawers will remain neat if kitchen items are put away in order. Drawers should also be cleaned out several times a year.

storing cleaning supplies

Cleaning products should be stored in a place that children cannot reach. **Caution:** Many cleaning products are poisonous. Swallowing even a small amount of a poison can be fatal. In a home where children are living, do not store products under the sink. A high cabinet with a door is the best place to store cleaning products. Brooms, mops and rags should be put away after use.

bathroom maintenance and cleaning

Bathrooms must be given special care in homes where there is illness. The natural dampness in a bathroom causes the growth of **molds** and **mildew** which are unsightly and cause odors, figure 23-14. Moisture provides an environment ideally suited for the growth of microorganisms which may be present in the home. For this reason, the home health aide must be particularly concerned with cleaning techniques.

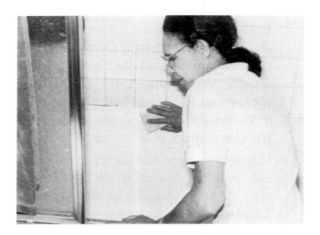

Figure 23-14 Daily cleaning of the bathroom is necessary to reduce the growth of molds and mildew.

daily care by family members

If more than one family member uses the same bathroom, each must assume certain responsibilities as a matter of courtesy to the rest of the family. After shaving, brushing the teeth and washing, the sink should be rinsed out. After bathing or showering, the tub or shower should be wiped out. Instruct family members to remove loose hair from the tub or shower floor. This practice helps avoid drain clogs. The toilet must be flushed after each use. Combing or brushing hair while standing over the wash basin should be avoided. Loose hairs are unpleasant to look at and can clog the drain. Towels should be hung neatly or put into the laundry hamper after use. Each person should replace the toothpaste or shaving cream cap after use. If these practices are followed, the bathroom will remain neat throughout the day.

daily care by the home health aide

Bathrooms are used frequently throughout the day and can easily become dirty. The

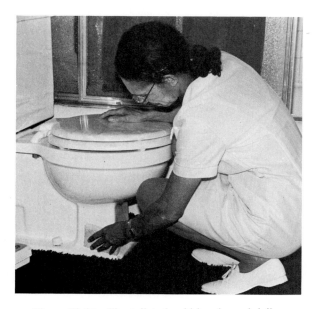

Figure 23-15 The toilet should be cleaned daily.

aide should encourage family members to help in keeping the bathroom neat. In addition, a thorough cleaning reduces the risk of spreading disease. The following duties should be done on a daily basis.

- Wash and rinse all surfaces in the bathroom. The outside of the toilet as well as both sides of the toilet seat should be cleaned daily, figure 23-15. The shower floor and walls, wall tiles, shower curtain, towel racks, windowsills and radiator should also be cleaned daily. Use hot water, detergent and disinfectant.
- Use a damp cloth to remove water spots from the walls around the sink. Clean the bathroom mirror with a glass cleaner, figure 23-16. Also rinse off the soap dish and wipe off the toothbrush holder.
- Damp mop bathroom floor (scrub as needed).
- Using bathroom cleanser and sponge or cloth, clean and rinse sink and tub.
- Using brush and bowl cleaner, clean the inside of the toilet bowl. Be sure to scrub the area under the top rim of the bowl.
- Clorox in water can be used to remove mildew and mold.

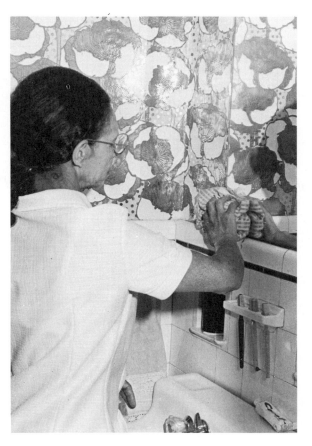

Figure 23-16 The bathroom mirror should be cleaned daily with a glass cleaner.

- Empty wastebasket contents into brown bag or plastic bag. Secure the top of the bag before placing it in the *incinerator* or garbage can. Line the clean wastebasket with a brown bag or plastic liner.
- If needed, place a new roll of toilet paper on the roller. If the existing roll is running low, place a fresh roll nearby for easy replacement.
- A laundry hamper which is kept in the bathroom should be wiped out regularly using hot water and detergent. **Caution:** The client's dirty linens and clothing should be kept separate from the family laundry. It is

best to wash the client's linens daily. When emptying the family laundry hamper, transfer clothing directly to a laundry basket. Never put soiled clothing on the floor. Germs from the clothing can be transferred to the floors or pathogens on the floor can be transferred to the clothing. People walking across the floors can transfer these germs to all areas of the home. Hold dirty laundry away from the body as it is transferred from place to place.

- If possible, open the bathroom window and ventilate the room for a few minutes. Spray around the tub and sink drain with a disinfectant or air freshener.
- Add fresh towels and face cloths to the towel racks. Make a note of any bathroom supplies which need to be purchased such as shaving cream, toothpaste, soap, tissues, toilet paper, etc.
- Do not use the same container for both dirty and clean laundry.

weekly care by the home health aide

Some tasks do not need to be done daily. The duties with each home assignment vary. The aide makes the judgment as to how often duties should be done. The following tasks can be done weekly or whenever necessary.

- Wash the inside and outside of the wastebasket.
- Launder bath mats as needed. **Caution:** Do not put rubber backed mats into the dryer.
- Tidy the linen closet to make it neat, figure 23-17.
- Clean the medicine chest. With permission of the family, throw out old medications. Prescription medicines are normally dated and are marked as to length of time they may be safely used. All medicines should be labeled. It is unsafe to use medicines from unlabeled bottles.

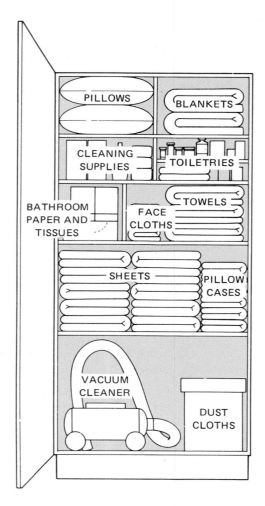

Figure 23-17 A well-organized bathroom closet

summary

- Certain household tasks must be done daily, others once or twice a week, and still others on a weekly or bimonthly basis.
- The home health aide should develop a cleaning schedule that works well. The aide should try to keep to that schedule so the working day is evenly paced and the chores don't become overwhelming.

Unit 24

Marketing and Meal Preparation

key terms

staple items   perishable   produce
convenience foods   fermented   delicatessen
bulk

learning objectives

After studying this unit, you should be able to:
- List four guidelines for planning menus.
- State eight guidelines for buying foods.
- List four guidelines for storing food.
- Name five guidelines for preparing meals.

Marketing and meal preparation requires time and use of special skills. Planning nutritious menus and buying foods the family can afford requires knowledge and use of judgment. Storing foods properly is also important. The aide, like the homemaker, develops these skills with study and practice.

menus and shopping lists

Most meal planning is done for an entire week. Weekly planning saves the aide from making frequent trips to the market. The following steps are helpful planning guides.

- Sit down with the client and/or client's family and ask what foods and menus they want. This could be an important activity for the client as it may foster the client's feelings of being useful and in charge of the care.
- Plan menus for a full week. Make sure that the menu follows any specific guidelines provided by the client's physician.
- Be sure all **staple items,** such as spices and seasonings that are needed for each planned meal are on hand, figure 24-1.
- Make up a shopping list and include all items needed in the household. Shopping time can be reduced by organizing the shopping list so that all items of one type are under one heading, figure 24-2.
- Look in the newspaper and check the prices of products advertised. Cut out any coupons of items on the shopping list.
- Plan to use only the amount of money which is budgeted for food and supplies.

purchasing food

Purchasing food is simplified when planning is well thought out. Planning which

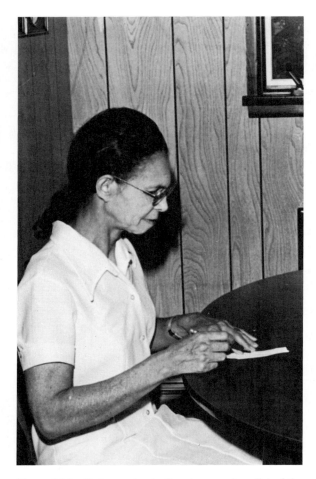

Figure 24-1 Before going to the store, make a list of the items needed.

is done in the home saves the aide time in the store. Marketing should be done at a time when the client can be safely left alone. The aide can sometimes shop while the client has a visitor. Shopping at home is an excellent activity for the housebound client and this is especially true of food shopping. It has several advantages. The client can become involved and interested in choosing foods, planning meals, and, even more importantly, saving money. This activity helps the client remain aware of the "life beyond illness" and can actually make the client feel better and more hopeful

about the future. How do you shop at home for food? By reading newspaper and magazine ads and clipping coupons and company offers. In the appendix are several pages of actual ads found within a four day period in newspapers. One can actually see how prices differ from store to store within a single geographic area. If the client is able to read and has the energy to look through papers and magazines, this might be a challenging and economical way to pass the time.

A smart shopper plans ahead. Sometimes the supermarkets are inconvenient to reach. If it is necessary to expend extra time, bus or taxi fares, or gas and wear and tear on the car to get there, then it is unwise to use that store. If, however, several markets are located within the same general area, then it pays to take advantage of money-saving brand or store coupons and buy items at the store where the price is lowest. When prices are particularly low on staple items such as paper and household cleaning supplies or canned goods, then, if money and storage space are available, extra amounts may be purchased. Practical guidelines for shopping are presented in the following list.

- Avoid going to the grocery store when hungry. Sweets and foods not on the shopping list are more likely to be bought when the shopper is hungry.
- If there is time, walk through the store with the shopping list in hand. Compare prices and decide on the best buys for the budget. If the allowed money won't cover all the items, make substitutions. For example, if beef prices are very high, buy ground beef instead of cube steak. If the quality of fresh **produce** is poor, buy frozen or canned vegetables.
- Select the needed foods by starting at one side of the store and moving from aisle to aisle. Compare the prices of brand names and store brands, figure 24-3. Read labels. Do

	SHOPPING LIST			
Fresh Foods	**Meats**	**Dairy**	**Canned**	**Frozen**
lettuce potatoes tomatoes apples	ground chuck veal roast chicken	skim or low fat milk butter or margarine cheese	peas okra tomato juice	cauliflower corn carrots
Paper Goods	**Dried Foods**	**Desserts**	**Beverages**	**Misc.**
toilet paper paper towels	milk beans	junket vanilla pudding	coffee (inst.) tea soda	detergent scouring pads

Figure 24-2 List needed foods and supplies under headings to help reduce the time spent in the store.

not be swayed by advertising slang such as jumbo, king size, giant, or economy. Buy the size best suited to the needs of the client or family. Large quantities are not practical if they cannot be stored.

- Do not buy sale items unless the client normally uses them and has storage space for them. A bargain the client cannot use is no bargain at all.
- When possible, avoid buying **convenience foods.** These include frozen dinners, foods seasoned in the package or fully prepared.

Convenience foods are usually more costly than other products.

- **Delicatessen** and brand name items usually cost more than store brands.
- Powdered or dried milk is an excellent money saver. Dry milk mixed with water can be added to a quart of skim or whole milk. The flavor may be the same or better and it costs less. The nutritional value is the same as in whole milk.
- Fresh fruits and vegetables are less expensive during their growing season. Compare fresh

	Least Expensive	Most Expensive
Preparation	Dried eggs Dried milk	Fresh eggs Fresh milk
Packaging	Tea in bulk Cheese in pounds	Tea in bags Cheese in prepackaged slices
Distributor	Store brand bread Store brand salami	Brand name or bakery bread Delicatessen cut

Figure 24-3 Price and quality can vary with the brand, preparation or package.

vegetable prices with canned and frozen vegetable prices while vegetables are in season. Out of season produce is quite costly.

- Eggs have the same food value whether they are jumbo, extra large, large or small. Brown or white shelled eggs are equally tasty and nutritious. Large eggs look better when served fried, boiled or poached. However, for cooking or scrambling, small eggs are the best buy.
- When buying meat, consider how the meat will be prepared. Most meat cuts have the same food value. Cheaper cuts can be just as tasty when prepared with imagination and care. When comparing the price per pound, consider the waste due to bones and fat. Figure the number of servings needed and the cost per serving.
- When selecting poultry, buying the whole bird is the best choice. Buying separate parts such as the breast, legs, or thighs is more expensive.
- If there is enough freezer space in the home, meats can be purchased in **bulk;** there is a considerable saving in the cost per pound. At home, meat can be rewrapped for the freezer in smaller meal-size portions. However, do not buy more than can be used. Waste occurs from overstocking the freezer. Most meats can be safely frozen for up to six months. Some meats lose flavor and food value when stored longer. Foods not properly wrapped can be ruined by freezer burn.
- Make sure meats purchased are fresh. If they do not smell, look, or feel right, do not buy them. Fresh meat will regain its shape when poked with a finger. If the meat feels slimy, slick or soft, don't buy it. If the color is off, the meat may be already spoiled.
- Don't buy damaged cans, no matter how low the price. Cans with bulging tops, dents or rust may contain spoiled food.
- Purchase **perishable** foods last. These include foods which spoil easily such as milk, meats and frozen foods.

storing food

After returning from the market, the aide should properly store the purchased foods. Putting foods and supplies away should be done before any other major task is begun.

- Always refrigerate perishable foods immediately. Lettuce can wilt and milk will spoil if they are not refrigerated.
- Frozen fruits and vegetables should be placed in the freezer as soon as possible. Do not overstock on frozen foods.
- Wash and clean poultry before refrigerating. If poultry is not planned for a meal within two days, wrap and freeze it.
- Dried and packaged foods should be stored in airtight containers, figure 24-4. Examples of airtight containers are cannisters, glass jars with lids, or plastic bags. Many containers of food can be refrigerated if there is room. Otherwise they should be stored so that roaches, ants or rodents cannot get to them. If safe storage space is limited, buy only small amounts of these foods.

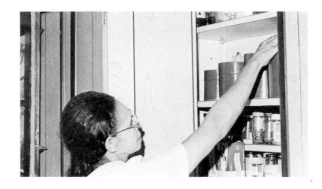

Figure 24-4 Airtight containers are useful for storing dried foods.

- Canned goods store easily and keep very well. They should not be stored near hot water pipes or near any other source of heat.
- Paper goods and other supplies should be stored nearest the place where they will be used. Toilet paper should be stored near the bathroom, and laundry supplies near the washing machine. Cleaning products should always be stored in a closet or cabinet out of the reach of children.

meal preparation

In order to prepare nutritious meals, the aide must use foods from the Basic Four food groups. In addition, the aide should check to see if the client has a special diet ordered or if the client is allergic to any foods. The aide should use the following guidelines when preparing meals:

- Follow the Basic Four food formula when planning meals.

  2–3 servings of milk or milk products
  2 servings of meat or meat substitutes
  4 servings of fruits and vegetables
  4 servings of bread and cereal

- Make any special diet the doctor has ordered for the client.
- Avoid fried foods as much as possible. Fried foods add more fat to the diet than is necessary.
- Most people should limit the number of eggs per week (*not* including eggs used in preparing a dish such as custard).
- Do not overcook frozen or fresh vegetables.
- When opening cans, wash the top of the can before piercing with a can opener, figure 24-5. This will keep dirt and pathogens from entering the food. If the contents spew out or are foamy or appear to have bubbles they

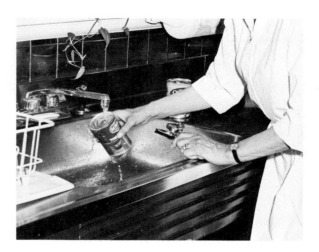

Figure 24-5 The tops of all cans should be washed before they are opened.

may have spoiled and must be discarded. After a can has been opened, unused portions should be transferred to a refrigerator container and covered tightly before refrigerating.

- Check food for spoiling: sour milk, rancid butter, moldy bread, **fermented** fruits, spoiled meats.
- Plan for variety. Throughout the week serve different vegetables, meat, poultry, fish, and meat substitutes. Different spices and herbs may also be used to add variety to meals, figures 24-6 and 24-7.
- Consider how each meal will look on the plate. For example, mashed potatoes, cauliflower, fish and a pear (for dessert) would not look appetizing because each is white or colorless.
- Fresh fruit and vegetables should be served raw if possible because of greater nutritional value. They should be cooked unpeeled to give the most food value. Steaming instead of boiling preserves both flavor and food value. The water from fresh vegetables is high in vitamins. This water may be added to meat stock and used for making tasty soups.

SEASONINGS AND SPICES*	USES
ALLSPICE	Particularly good with pot roast, in puddings and cereals. (Tastes like cinnamon, clove and nutmeg.)
ANISE	In tossed green salad and other vegetable salads. It can be used with pot cheese.
CARAWAY SEEDS	Give flavor to bread, pot cheese, cabbage, cauliflower, cereals and cookies.
CARDAMON SEEDS	Good with curries, soups and meats.
CAYENNE	Few grains will be enough to season vegetables, meats, fish, poultry, soups; vegetable, meat, fish, poultry or egg salads.
CHILI PEPPERS	Seasoning soups, rice, dried peas or beans, meat, fish, pot cheese.
CINNAMON	Flavors cereals, bread, pot cheese, vegetables such as beans, cabbage, cauliflower, carrots, cucumbers, eggplant, lentils, onions and peas.
CLOVES	Can be used in much the same way as cinnamon; particularly nice for flavoring tea.
CORIANDER SEEDS	For seasoning stews, curries, soups and fish.
CURRY POWDER	To season soups, stews, rice, chicken, eggs, meat, fish and vegetables.
GARLIC	Flavors soups, sauces, salads and salad dressings, meats, fish, poultry, pot cheese, dried peas or beans.
GINGER	Used in much the same way as cinnamon.
MACE	Flavors meats, fish, poultry, soup, sauces, stews, potatoes, carrots, snap beans, peas, cabbage and cauliflower.
DRY MUSTARD	Seasons meats, fish, salad dressings, vegetables, eggs, pot cheese, fish, poultry, and all salads.
NUTMEG	Used the same way as mace.
PAPRIKA	Gives a bright garnish to vegetables, meats, eggs, pot cheese, fish, poultry, and all salads.
PEPPER	Adds flavor to meats, fish, poultry, eggs and vegetables.
POPPY SEEDS	Used as toppings for bread, rolls, cookies and cakes. Good with pot cheese and in salad dressings.
SESAME SEEDS	Used on rolls, buns and bread.
TURMERIC	Seasons meats, fish and poultry.

*Spices and many seasonings are highly perishable unless kept in tightly closed containers. They should be bought in small quantities and renewed at least once a year.

Figure 24-6   Seasonings and spices add variety and taste to meals.

HERB AND PART USED	USES IN COOKING
BASIL — leaves	Italian tomato dishes, soups, ragouts, salads, meats, sauces, fruit drinks.
BAY — leaves	For flavoring soups, stews, sauces.
CHERVIL — leaves, and sometimes fleshy roots	In place of parsley, in fine herbs*, salads, sauces, soups. In omelettes.
CHIVES — leaves	In fine herbs*, salads, omelettes, or anything for which a delicate onion flavor is desired.
DILL — seed and young tips	Added to melted sweet butter or salt-free margarine, it makes a fine sauce for fish. In mashed potato, in tossed green, potato, fish or vegetable salads. Sprinkled on broiled chops.
SWEET MARJORAM — leaves	Sprinkled over beef, lamb or pork. Used in veal stew, chopped meat, meat balls. In fine herbs*, salads, and fish dishes. Cooked with zucchini.
MINT — leaves	Flavors sauces, vegetables, jellies, fruit drinks, vegetable and fruit salads, custards, puddings.
OREGANO	Can be rubbed over meat before roasting or broiling or it can be put in the water during the cooking of meat and fish. Used with veal, pork, soups, potatoes, vegetables and fresh salads. (Closely related to marjoram and has a similar flavor.)
PARSLEY — leaves	In fine herbs*, for soups, sauces. Popular with boiled potato and many other vegetables. With meat, fish, eggs and with vegetable, meat, or fish salads.
ROSEMARY — leaves	To flavor roast lamb and veal, meat stews, poultry sauces, stuffings.
SAGE — leaves	In stuffing for meat, poultry, fish. In fish chowder.
SAVORY — leaves	Excellent with snap beans, dried peas, lentils. Also good in chopped beef, gravy, meat stew, and croquettes. Can be sprinkled over fish before baking or broiling.
TARRAGON — leaves	Flavoring for vinegar, sauces, and salad dressings, chicken and other meats. For egg and tomato dishes, sandwiches. In fine herbs*.
THYME — leaves	In fine herbs*, in stews, soups, sauces, salad. With meat, poultry, fish, tomato dishes. Can be combined with melted butter and served over carrots, onions and peas.

*Fine herbs: A finely minced mixture of four or five herbs in different combinations, but always including chives and either parsley or chervil.

Figure 24-7 Herbs may also be used to enhance the taste and appeal of many foods.

- Save whole milk for drinking. Use dry milk in preparing sauces and gravies. The food value and flavor of dry milk is equal to whole milk.
- Use leftover meats in a creative way. Add fresh mushrooms to leftover beef and make a brown sauce. Turkey hash, creamed turkey, chicken salad or sandwiches can all be made with leftovers.
- Foods which are not in season may not be the best buy. However, they do have excellent flavor and they make a pleasant change in the diet. Fresh vegetables should be purchased in the exact amount needed to prevent waste.
- Practice cooking and serving meals. A good cook uses clean, unspoiled raw meats and vegetables and follows recipes. Food should be attractive and served on an attractive table or tray. The home health aide should be pleasant when serving food, figure 24-8.

cooking in a microwave

Microwave ovens have been in general use for a few years, but they are not a standard appliance in all homes. If one has not had oc-

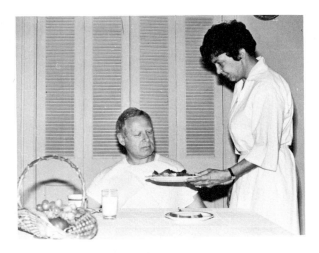

Figure 24-8 Meals should be nourishing, attractive, and served with a smile.

casion to use a microwave oven here are a few simple rules.

NEVER place anything metal in the microwave. It will ruin the oven and probably the metal also. There are special microwave utensils, plates, and dishes which can be used as well as glass, china, and paperware. Most microwave owners will have a simple manual with instructions for proper use. Here are a few examples of ways to make use of a microwave.

- Baked Potato: Wash and dry thoroughly, then prick the skin with a fork so the steam can escape. Place the potato on a paper towel or paper plate and put in the oven following instructions for timing. It can take 3 to 5 minutes to have a perfect baked potato.
- Leftovers: Place in microwave plate or dish, cover with paper towel or wax paper as recommended, and heat at the recommended setting and time. It can take as little as 2 or 3 minutes to heat up leftovers.
- Frozen vegetables: Follow instructions on package. This is an excellent way to prepare frozen vegetables as they remain crisp and taste fresh. Seasoning is done after the food is cooked so that vegetables prepared in the microwave can be appropriately seasoned to fit the needs of any diet.
- Defrost: The microwave may also be used to defrost frozen foods quickly so that they can be chosen and prepared at the last minute. Meats seem to taste better when cooked by traditional methods on top of the stove or in oven or broiler. However, there are recipes in the microwave manual for cooking all sorts of food.
- Reheat: If for some reason, a client's food has become cold (a telephone call interrupting the meal or an emergency of some sort), a microwave proof dinnerplate can be placed directly in the microwave and in just a minute, the meal will be heated thoroughly without loss of flavor or appetite appeal.

summary

- Meal preparation and marketing are an important part of the home health aide's responsibilities.
- The aide must follow any specific guidelines provided by the client's physician when preparing meals.
- The desired food of the client and client's family should be included in menus whenever possible.
- When purchasing food, the aide must keep within budget limits.
- Food should be properly stored.

Unit 25
Laundry Duties

learning objectives

After studying this unit, you should be able to:
- Identify two ways to sort clothes for washing.
- Identify the best time to perform mending.
- Identify several methods for removing stains.

Clothes and household linens are a major expense for most families. The home health aide must be responsible for giving suitable care to these items. Correctly sorting, washing, and ironing clothes requires careful attention.

sorting clothes and linens

Most clothing can be machine washed. However, some articles of clothing must be dry cleaned; others must be hand washed. Most of today's clothes have labels with instructions for proper care. If an item is not labeled, the aide must be able to judge from its appearance. If there is any doubt, the aide should ask a family member which washing method is best.

In general, cotton fabrics can be washed in hot water. Blends of cotton and polyester and cottons of light color should be washed in warm water. Chlorine bleaches are only used for white cottons. There are special bleaches for nylon and **polyester fabrics.** Be careful to follow instructions when using bleaches. Dark fabrics are washed separately from light fabrics. Many homemakers wash dark clothes in cold water with cold water detergent. When sorting clothes for the laundry, use the following tips:

- Sort the clothes on newspapers spread on the floor, figure 25-1. Do not allow clothing to come in contact with the floor. If possible, place clothes in separate laundry baskets for each load.
- Make a separate pile of clothes which must be hand washed or dry cleaned.
- As each item is sorted, check it for spots which might require special care. Collars of shirts and dresses, and spots from food or other stains may need special care, figure 25-2.
- Turn pockets inside out, figure 25-3. Be sure to remove pens, pencils, paper, coins or other items in the pockets.

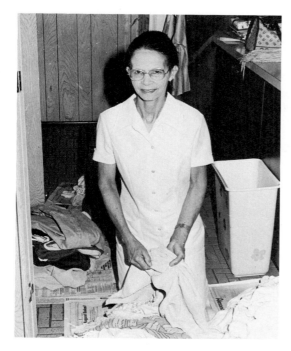

Figure 25-1 Spread newspapers to keep clothes from contacting the floor.

- Shake dirt, sand or grass out of clothing before placing it with the other clothes.
- Remove belt buckles or ornaments which might be ruined in the washer.
- Hand wash separately those fabrics in which the colors run or bleed.
- Make sure dark socks do not get mixed with the light or white loads.

loading the washing machine

Loading differs depending on whether the family has a top or front loading machine, figure 25-4. Before operating the washing machine, the aide should read the directions. If the aide is still in doubt, a family member should be asked to assist. Improper use of a machine could cause personal injury or damage to the clothing or the machine.

- For top loading machines, allow the machine to fill with water before adding the clothes. Pour in the correct amount of detergent. Add the correct type of bleach if it is needed. Make sure the bleach mixes well with the water. Distribute the load evenly around the **agitator** in the center. Close the lid and turn on the machine. (With some top loading machines, the clothes can be added before the machine fills with water. Check directions with each machine.)
- For front loading machines, add the detergent and bleach where indicated. Put in the clothing and close the door tightly. Turn on the machine.
- unload clean clothes into a clean container.

Some clients will not have washing machines and dryers. In that case, you may have to take the dirty linens and clothing to a laundromat. Some apartments do have laundry rooms that are used by the tenants. If it is necessary to use laundromats or laundry rooms, the home health aide should schedule laundry time when it is safe and convenient to be away from the client and, when using an apartment laundry room, at a time when the machines are available. It might be a good idea to talk to the apartment superintendent and arrange for a regular time for you to use the machines.

When using laundromats and laundry rooms the aide will need quarters or other small change and should make certain that there is plenty of change on hand. Usually, it is best to take the soap, bleach, and other necessary supplies from the client's home. If you purchase them from vending machines, the cost is much more. A good idea when using "community" machines (ones that are used by many people), is to wipe them on the inside with a damp cloth before starting to do the wash.

STAIN	HOW TO REMOVE
Blood	Presoak in cold water; if stain is stubborn rub in detergent, then launder using safe bleach.
Butter, oils	Rub cornstarch on spot or use powdered cleaning product or cleaning fluid according to instructions.
Chocolate	Soak in cold water, and rub detergent directly on stain. Launder in water as warm as the fabric allows.
Coffee, tea	Pour hot water directly on spot then wash as usual. Use water as hot as the fabric allows.
Cosmetics	Presoak in detergent and water, then launder.
Crayon and candle wax	Scrape off as much as possible. (Crayons have a wax base.) Place blotting paper under spot and on top of spot. Rub hot iron over blotter. The wax should melt into the blotter. Launder, using safe bleach and detergent.
Deodorants	Presoak area with white vinegar, rinse and launder.
Fruits	Rinse in cold water. If stain is stubborn, put 1 tablespoon of baking soda in a quart of water to neutralize the acid. Rinse and launder.
Grass	Rub detergent into the spot. Launder with safe bleach and detergent.
Ink, magic marker, felt tip pens	Remove washable ink by rubbing cold water and detergent into the spot. Ballpoint pens make a stain that can be removed with dry cleaning fluid. Permanent or nonwashable inks must be removed by a professional dry cleaner.
Lipstick	Remove with cleaning fluid. Make sure the fluid will not ruin fabric by first testing on an inside seam area.
Meat juice, eggs	Scrape off then sponge area with cold water. Rub in detergent and launder.
Rust	Use dry cleaning fluid then wash as usual.
Scorch (mark from hot iron)	Dampen a white cotton cloth in cold water to which a small amount of bleach has been added. Quickly rub over the scorched spot. Turn the iron to a cooler setting—wait until the spot has dried, then proceed with ironing. Deeply scorched items may need to be patched.

Figure 25-2 Guidelines for removing stains

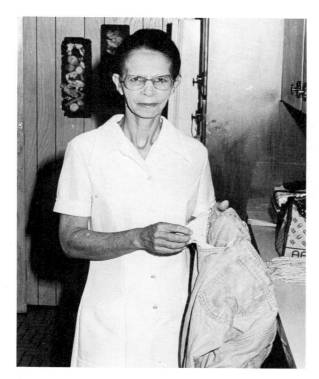

Figure 25-3 Turn pockets inside out to empty them of articles.

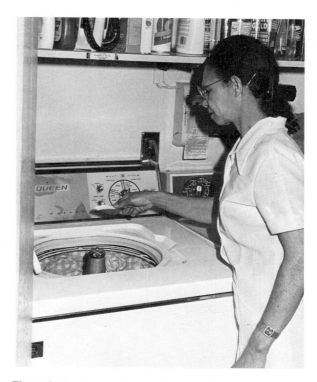

Figure 25-4 Top loading machines are the most common type found in today's homes.

drying, ironing and mending

Not all clothing requires high heat or long drying cycles. Towels, heavy pants and sweat shirts usually take the longest time to dry. Nylon, polyester, or any **permanent press** fabrics can be dried quickly. Permanent press clothing should be removed from the dryer as soon as the tumbler has stopped. If clothes are hung or folded at once, few wrinkles will form in them.

Large items such as sheets and blankets should be placed in the dryer separately or no more than two at a time. Folding sheets and blankets as soon as the drying process is finished helps to prevent wrinkling. Figure 25-5 shows how to properly fold a fitted sheet.

Cotton clothing which needs to be ironed should be folded neatly. Folding cloth-

ing before ironing keeps out unwanted creases and makes ironing easier.

- Set up the ironing board and set heat to correct temperature for steam or dry ironing.
- Gather hangers to be used for those items which will need to be hung.
- Prepare needles and thread of various colors. Stick the needles at the broad end of the ironing board ready to be used to replace buttons or mend small tears or split seams. Just a few extra minutes spent while handling the ironing to make these small repairs will save time and trouble later. The clothes will be ready for use or storage at once.
- While the ironing is being done, other loads can be put through the wash and dry cycles. Clean the lint traps in the washer and dryer after use, figure 25-6. Wipe the inside and

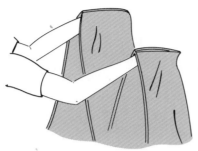

A. Place hands inside fitted ends on each side.

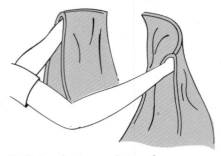

B. Bring the two ends together.

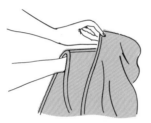

C. Fit the two ends of one side over each other.

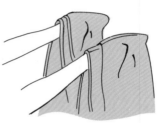

D. Do the same for the other side of the sheet.

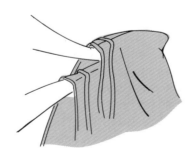

E. Bring all four corners neatly together.

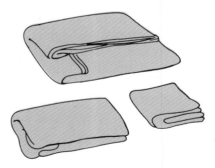

F. Fold compactly avoiding unnecessary wrinkling.

Figure 25-5   How to fold a fitted sheet for storage.

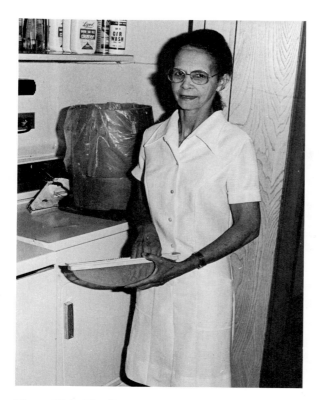

Figure 25-6 The lint traps which are found in washers and dryers collect loose dirt and fabric threads. They must be cleaned after doing the laundry.

outside of machines so they will be ready to use the next time.

- Take the clean and ironed items and store them properly.

summary

- By following instructions on the washing machine, sorting clothing before placing in the machine, using the proper detergent and the correct water temperature, a client's laundry should present no problems.
- When using a commercial machine (in a Laundromat or in an apartment laundry room), take a damp cloth and wipe out the machine before using it. Some people are careless and leave the machines dirty. Wiping the machines before use will help to ensure clean laundry.
- When doing a client's laundry and ironing, the aide should take care to do it properly; this is taking suitable responsibility.
- Unload clean clothes into a clean container.

section 7

Health Care Services

Unit 26

Introduction to Client Care Procedures

learning objectives

After studying this unit, you should be able to:
- List the rules for carrying out client care procedures.
- Describe how to provide privacy for the client during procedures.
- State when the aide's hands should be washed.
- Explain why it is necessary to give an explanation to the client before doing any procedure.
- Recognize those procedures which you, as a home health aide, are not permitted to do because of state mandated guidelines.

There are some procedures that an aide may not perform. For instance, in New York State, an aide may not, under any circumstances, inject medication such as insulin or pain killer. An aide may not irrigate an ostomy. In some states, an aide is not permitted to give decubitus care. These are situations where an aide must follow the instructions of the public health nurse, agency nurse, or agency supervisor. If it is against the state laws for an aide to provide a particular service, then the aide must obey the law.

In some cases, a client may be receiving special and unusual treatments at home which require special machines. These pieces of equipment are known as "durable equip-

ment." Very often rental of such equipment is expensive. Decisions as to the use of such items is made by the doctor and the client or client's family. For the most part, an aide will not be permitted to handle such equipment. For instance there are home dialysis machines (for use by those who have little or no kidney function). It requires several hours on the machine to remove the impurities from the blood. An aide may be expected to check the client's progress and make sure that the machine is functioning. Other durable equipment sometimes used in home care includes respirators, tube feeding, or intravenous feeding equipment, and oxygen tanks, to name a few. Unless an aide is specially trained, qualified, certified, and permitted by law to operate such equipment, she must not attempt to do so. However, an aide will probably be shown by the supervisor what to look for, what to observe, and what to report when such equipment is in use.

You already know that there may be more than one way to perform a procedure. Also, you should be aware that new pieces of equipment and new designs of old equipment are being constantly developed. Thus, some of the procedures included in these pages may seem outmoded. However, there are still areas of the country where the old ways are still practiced or where there is no money to buy new equipment. It is true that the hot water bottle and ice cap are out-of-date, but if they are all that is available, then you should know how to use them properly and safely.

It would be nice to use a digital thermometer or blood pressure cuff so that all you had to do would be read off the numbers and record them. Again, these items of equipment are not in general use throughout the country and it is always good to have the ability to do things the "hard way" just in case the modern equipment fails to work correctly.

As a home health aide goes from case to case, the client care procedures vary. Each client has special needs and will require different procedures. As experience is gained, the home health aide develops a pattern of providing safe and proper care. However, no amount of experience excuses taking shortcuts in giving client care.

Figure 26-1 provides a list of the client care procedures covered in this text. When performing any of these procedures, the aide should always keep in mind the following basic guidelines.

1. Involve the client as an active participant in each procedure. If possible, allow the client to decide when care such as bathing, shaving, etc. is to be done. This allows clients to feel more in control of their lives and is good therapy.
2. The aide's hands should always be washed before carrying out any procedure.
3. The aide should plan ahead and know what equipment and supplies will be needed.
4. Equipment and supplies should be placed as close as possible to save time and energy while giving the client care.
5. Explain to the client what is going to be done and the reason for doing it. The aide should keep in mind that being cared for may make clients feel they do not have control of their lives. Clients may feel they are being forced to do things they do not want to do. It is extremely important for the aide to get the client's cooperation and consent before doing any procedure. If the aide communicates in an easy and natural way, clients feel more important and are usually more cooperative. For example, in the morning ask whether the client needs the bedpan or urinal or needs help getting to the bathroom. Help the client to wash and brush teeth before breakfast. You might say, "Good morning. Did you sleep well? It's about time for breakfast." Let the client talk and LISTEN to what the client is saying. At bathtime and bedchanging time say, "After your bath and back rub I will get your bed ready for the day." Try to get the client interested in what is being done. Participation makes the client more cooperative and understanding of treatments.
6. Provide privacy for the client during a procedure. The client should have privacy when using the bedpan, having a bed bath, or while having the bed linens changed. Talk to the client before these procedures. Plan what to do in case the phone or doorbell rings while in the middle of such procedures. Perhaps a "Do Not Disturb" sign

UNIT 27 PERSONAL CARE AND COMFORT MEASURES

1 Handwashing
2 Giving a Bed Bath
3 Giving a Back Rub
4 Assisting with Oral Hygiene
5 Caring for Dentures
6 Shaving the Male Client
7 Helping the Client to Dress and Undress
8 Giving Nail Care
9 Shampooing the Hair of the Bedridden Client
10 Assisting with the Tub Bath or Shower
11 Helping the Client with Self-Administered Medications
12 Feeding the Incapacitated Client

UNIT 28 VITAL SIGNS

13 Taking an Oral Temperature
14 Taking a Rectal Temperature
15 Taking an Axillary Temperature
16 Determining the Pulse and Respiration Rate
17 Measuring Blood Pressure

UNIT 29 SPECIAL TREATMENTS AND DRESSINGS

18 Giving an Alcohol or Tepid Water Sponge Bath
19 Applying a Clean Dressing
20 Applying Bandages
21 Observing and Caring for Casts
22 Caring for Decubitus Ulcers
23 Caring for the Urinary Catheter
24 Changing the Ostomy Bag
25 Using Oxygen Safely

UNIT 30 ELIMINATION NEEDS AND FLUID INTAKE AND OUTPUT

26 Assisting with the Use of the Bedpan or Urinal
27 Assisting with the Use of the Bedside Commode
28 Measuring Fluid Intake and Output
29 Giving an Enema or Rectal Suppository
30 Bowel Retraining

UNIT 31 COLLECTING AND TESTING SPECIMENS

31 Collecting a Stool Specimen
32 Collecting Urine Specimens
33 Testing Urine for Sugar and Acetone

UNIT 32 BEDMAKING

34 Making an Occupied Bed
35 Making an Unoccupied Bed

UNIT 33 HOT AND COLD APPLICATIONS

36 Applying the Ice Bag, Cap, or Collar
37 Applying the Hot Water Bag
38 Applying the Heating Pad
39 Applying Hot and Cold Moist Dressings

UNIT 34 SUPPORT, EXERCISE, AND LOCOMOTION

40 Applying Binders and Other Supports
41 Moving a Client Up in Bed
42 Assisting the Client to Sit Up in Bed
43 Assisting with Range of Motion Exercises
44 Assisting with the Use of Crutches, Walkers or Canes
45 Following Safety Rules for Transferring Clients
46 Stand-Pivot Transfer
47 Assisting with the Sliding Transfer

UNIT 35 POSTPARTUM CARE

48 Assisting the Mother with Breastfeeding and Breast Care
49 Giving the Infant a Sponge Bath
50 Bathing the Infant Using a Bathinette or Basin
51 Bottle Feeding the Infant

Figure 26-1 Client care procedures

can be put on the door and the phone taken off the hook. (Remember to tell other family members if this is done.) The client will be able to relax without worry of interruptions.

7. Complete client care procedures as quickly and carefully as possible. Procedures cannot be timed. However, if the client is on the bedpan and there are no results, remove the bedpan. Do not wait until the client becomes uncomfortable. Tell the client to call when the bedpan is again needed.

8. Do not embarrass the client in any way. Aides should treat clients as they themselves would wish to be treated.

9. After a client care procedure is completed, remove all equipment and supplies. Clean and store the equipment and supplies at once so that the client's room is neat and orderly.

10. THE AIDE'S HANDS SHOULD BE WASHED BEFORE AND AFTER EACH PROCEDURE IS DONE.

11. The aide should keep a pad and pencil handy in order to make notes of signs and symptoms which need to be reported (temperature, pulse, respiration, enema results, etc.)

summary

- Caring for the physical and medical needs of the client involves both the aide and the client.
- It is vital to gain the cooperation and participation of the client.
- If the client is helpless, the aide must do all the work as efficiently and safely as possible.
- For the client who is able, the aide should let the client actively assist in the procedures.
- The aide must always provide safety, privacy and an explanation of what is being done and the reason for the procedure.
- The aide must recognize the procedures he/she is not permitted to perform because of state mandated guidelines.

Unit 27

Personal Care and Comfort Measures

learning objectives

After studying this unit, you should be able to:
- Demonstrate clear ability to perform all the procedures.
- Explain the purpose of each procedure.
- State when the procedures should and should not be done.
- Identify precautions to be taken for each procedure.

NOTE: All procedures are not allowed in all states. Make sure you are aware of limits as outlined by state guidelines.

client care procedure

1: HANDWASHING

purpose

- To prevent the transfer of disease-producing organisms from person to person or place to place.

NOTE: The hands of the home health aide must be washed before and after each client contact, before preparing food, before and after each meal, after blowing the nose or sneezing, combing hair, after using the bathroom, and after handling soiled items such as linens, clothing or garbage.

procedure

1. Collect the items needed for handwashing and bring them to the bathroom or kitchen sink:
   soap
   soap dish

towel (paper towels preferred)
wastebasket
hand lotion
washbasin (if needed)
orange stick, if available

2. Turn on water using a clean paper towel and adjust to a warm temperature. All homes are not equipped with running water. In these cases, obtain a pitcher of water and heat it in a tea kettle. When the water reaches a warm temperature, pour it into a basin for handwashing.
3. Rinse the bar of soap.
4. Lather the hands well, rinse the bar of soap, and return it to the soap dish.
5. Rub hands together briskly using friction with hand brush if available. Lather between the fingers and around and under fingernails for at least 3 minutes, figure 27-1. Using an orange stick, clean under fingernails. While washing, hold the hands

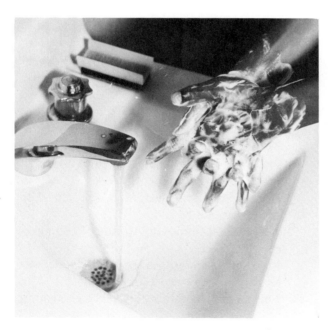

Figure 27-1 Lather between the fingers (courtesy of Louise Simmers, *Diversified Health Occupations*, Delmar Publishers, Albany, NY, 1983).

down to prevent water from dripping toward the arms and elbows, figure 27-2. Wash hands a second time. Discard soapy water.
6. Rinse hands under running water.
7. Dry hands with a paper towel. Use a cloth towel if paper towels are not available.
8. Use the towel to turn off the water faucet. This practice protects the clean hand from touching the contaminated faucet.
9. Discard the paper towel in the wastebasket. Hand towels can be placed in the laundry hamper.
10. Use hand lotion if hands are dry or chapped.

client care procedure

2: GIVING A BED BATH

purpose

- To clean and refresh the client.
- To stimulate circulation.
- To observe the body for signs of irritation or changes in condition of skin.

NOTE: The bed bath is usually given in the morning. This procedure is one of a series of procedures which are performed in the same time period. This will require the home health aide to organize and plan ahead. All materials and supplies needed can be gathered and placed conveniently so that each separate procedure can be completed easily.

- If client needs to use the bedpan, offer it before the bath.
- Gather supplies needed for making the bed and put them near at hand, figure 27-3 (linens, laundry hamper).
- Organize materials needed for oral hygiene and denture care in order to move easily into those procedures if needed.
- Prepare items for nail care and set them nearby.

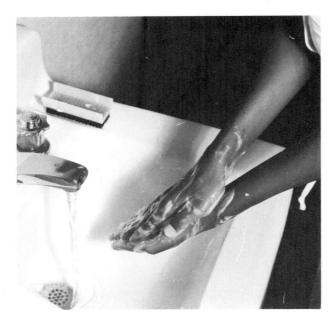

Figure 27-2 Fingertips should be pointed down while washing hands (courtesy of Louise Simmers, *Diversified Health Occupations,* Delmar Publishers, Albany, NY, 1983).

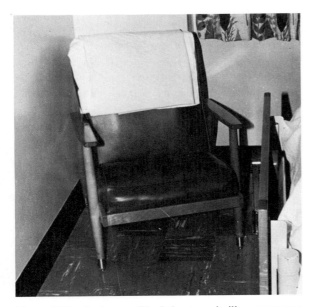

Figure 27-3 A change of bed sheets and pillow cases can be laid across a chair near the bed until needed.

procedure

1. If possible, choose a time for the bed bath which is suitable for the client.
2. Gather supplies needed for the complete series of procedures, including:
   bath basin, ⅔ filled with warm water
   soap and soap dish
   washcloth
   face and bath towels
   fresh gown or pajamas
   orange stick
   body lotion
   bath powder
   change of bed linens
   Chux, if client is incontinent
3. Close windows to prevent a draft from blowing on the client. Place a "Do Not Disturb" sign on the door to avoid interruptions.
4. Wash your hands before beginning the procedure.
5. If needed, give oral hygiene or denture care.
6. Remove blankets, leaving the top sheet covering the client. Place one pillow under the client's head.
7. Pull out bottom part of top sheet (from mattress) so it covers client loosely, figure 27-4. Remove client's gown or pajamas. Place hot water bottle at client's feet to avoid chilling the client.
8. Place a basin of water on the chair or dresser at the bedside.
9. Assist client in moving to side of bed nearest you.
10. Moisten washcloth, squeeze out excess water, and apply soap to the cloth.
11. Form a mitt by folding a washcloth around one hand, figure 27-5.
12. Wash and rinse the client's eyes first. No soap is used for the eyes. Wipe from the inner corner to the outer corner of the eye.

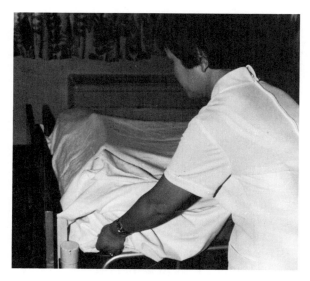

Figure 27-4 Before starting the bath, loosen the bedcovers at the foot of the bed so you will be able to wash the client's feet and legs.

Wash the face, ears, and neck. Pat dry with the face towel.

13. Lift client's arm and lay a bath towel under the area to keep bed dry. Wash, rinse, and pat dry, making sure the arm, underarm, and hand are cleaned and thoroughly dry. Repeat for other arm. Apply underarm deodorant or bath powder if client desires.

14. Give nail care using an orange stick to clean the nails.

15. Place towel over client's chest, then pull sheet down to waist. Working under the towel, wash, rinse, and dry chest. Rinse, dry and powder area under female's breasts carefully to avoid skin irritation. Replace sheet over chest.

16. Have client bend one knee. Fold sheet up from the foot of the bed. Expose the thigh, leg and foot. Place a towel under the area,

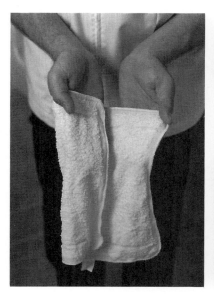

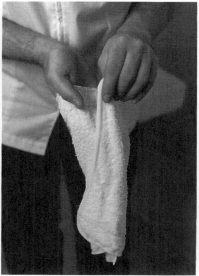

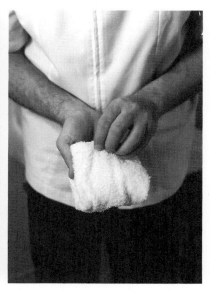

A. Fold one side of the washcloth towards you.

B. Fold over the other side so that the washcloth fits snugly around the hand.

C. Fold up the end of the washcloth and grasp it with the thumb.

Figure 27-5 The washcloth is folded like a mitt to prevent water from dripping.

and put the basin on the towel, placing client's foot in basin. Wash and rinse leg. Move the foot from the basin and wash it well.

17. Remove the basin from the bed, and dry leg and foot.
18. Follow the same procedure for the other leg and foot.
19. Massage lotion into the client's feet.
20. Change the water in the basin before proceeding with the bath. If at any time during the bath, the water becomes dirty or cool, change it.
21. Assist the client to turn onto the side away from you. Assist the client to move toward your side of the bed. Place bath towel lengthwise by the client's back. Wash, rinse and dry neck, back, and buttocks. Use long, firm strokes while washing back.
22. Give the client a back rub.

23. Help client to turn onto the back.
24. Prepare washcloth with soap and have client wash the genital area, if able. Rinse the cloth and have client wipe the genitals. Have the client dry the genitals thoroughly.
25. Spread a towel under client's head and comb or brush hair.
26. Place used towels and washcloth in laundry hamper.
27. Assist the client into a clean gown or pajamas.
28. Move the basin and the other equipment away from the bed.
29. Change the bed linens using the procedure for making an occupied bed.
30. Leave the client in a comfortable position. After all the activities, the client may require a rest period.
31. Wash your hands thoroughly.

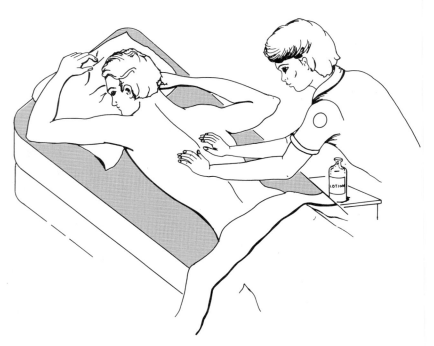

Figure 27-6 Giving the client a back rub increases the blood circulation to the client's back and provides the aide with an opportunity to inspect the back for signs of skin breakdown.

3: GIVING A BACK RUB

purpose

- To increase the blood circulation to the back area.
- To give comfort to the client and provide relaxation.
- To allow the home health aide to observe the skin for signs of decubiti.

NOTE: The back rub may be included as a part of the morning bed bath. However, when the client cannot be bathed daily, the back rub should be given at some time during each day. A back rub increases the blood circulation to the client's back, and also gives the aide an opportunity to inspect the back for signs of skin breakdown, figure 27-6. Daily care is important in preventing decubitus ulcers.

procedure

1. Ask the client when a back rub is preferred.
2. Gather the supplies needed:
   lotion—set in warm water to warm.
   towel
   notebook or daily record sheet and pencil
3. Provide privacy for the client.
4. Wash your hands before beginning the procedure.
5. Turn client to one side or on the stomach. Loosen or remove clothing in order to expose client's back.
6. Place a small amount of lotion on your hand. Rub hands together to warm the lotion.
7. Begin the rub by starting at the base of the spine; rub toward the neck in the center of the back. Use both hands in one long stroke.
8. When reaching the neck, continue back down the sides of the back. When reaching the base of the spine, rub up the center again. Repeat several times.
9. If necessary, add more lotion and use a spiral motion for several minutes, figure 27-7.
10. After 10 to 15 minutes, remove excess lotion and reposition the client comfortably.
11. Wash your hands thoroughly after the procedure.
12. Record and report any signs of skin irritation.

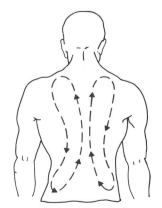

A. Begin with long, smooth strokes to soothe the client.

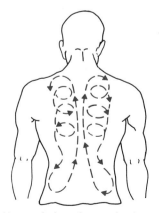

B. Use a spiral motion on the downstroke to stimulate circulation in the skin.

Figure 27-7 Strokes used in a back rub can be varied to produce different effects.

4: ASSISTING WITH ORAL HYGIENE

purpose

- To keep client's teeth and gums healthy.
- To refresh client's mouth and improve appetite.

NOTE: Clients who are helpless cannot give themselves oral care. In these cases the aide must give special mouth care:

- Depress the tongue with a padded tongue blade, figure 27-8.
- Dampen a cotton-tipped applicator with mouthwash. Clean the teeth, tongue and the inside surfaces of the mouth. Hold an emesis basin under the client's chin.
- Rub the lips with a lemon glycerine or vaseline swab in order to keep the lips moist.

procedure

1. Gather the equipment and supplies needed: toothbrush

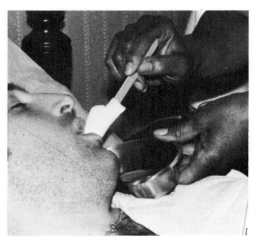

Figure 27-8 The part of the tongue blade used in the mouth must be padded to avoid injury. Be gentle when giving mouth care to the ill and helpless client.

toothpaste, tooth powder, or baking soda
glass of fresh warm water
small bowl or basin
tissues or damp washcloth
towel

2. Wash your hands before beginning the procedure.
3. Help the client prepare to brush teeth. Position the client comfortably (sitting up if allowed).
4. Place a towel over the client's chest and under the chin.
5. Rinse toothbrush and apply toothpaste or tooth powder.
6. Let client brush the teeth, if able. If not, carefully brush the client's teeth.
7. Give the client a glass of water. Be sure client thoroughly rinses the mouth. Hold a basin under the client's chin to catch the water used in rinsing.
8. Give the client a tissue or washcloth to wipe the mouth.
9. Reposition client for comfort.
10. Wash your hands thoroughly after procedure.
11. Clean the supplies used and store them properly.
12. You may need assistance with the unconscious client. Use a tongue depressor with gauze wrapped around it as illustrated in figure 27-8.

5: CARING FOR DENTURES

purpose

- To clean dentures and refresh client's mouth.
- **To provide opportunity to examine client's gums for sore spots or irritation.**
- **To stimulate client's appetite.**

procedure

1. Gather the equipment and supplies needed:
   denture cup or 2 small bowls padded with
      gauze
   denture paste or powder
   toothbrush
   mouthwash
   cup
   towel (if needed)
   damp washcloth
2. Wash your hands before beginning the procedure.
3. Ask client to remove dentures, helping if necessary. Place dentures in a padded bowl or denture cup. Position client comfortably.
4. Place a towel in the sink first. Fill sink half-full of water to prevent breakage if dentures are dropped.
5. Clean dentures under running water, using brush and denture cleaner.
6. Rinse well, place in padded basin and return to client.
7. A client who has a partial denture plate still has some natural, permanent teeth. Assist these clients to brush their teeth as in giving regular oral care.
8. For clients with a complete set of dentures, assist them to rinse their mouth and gums with mouthwash. Hold basin near mouth for waste disposal. Wipe the outside of the mouth with a cloth or tissue.
9. Inspect the gums for irritation, redness, sores or blisters.
10. Assist the client to replace the dentures in the mouth. Some older clients may wish to leave dentures out for a few hours. In such cases, fill a small bowl or denture cup with warm water and let dentures soak. Place them near the client so they can be replaced when desired.
11. Reposition client comfortably.
12. Wash your hands thoroughly after the procedure.
13. Clean all materials used and store them in the bathroom.

client care procedure

6: SHAVING THE MALE CLIENT

purpose

- To make the client comfortable and to maintain client's appearance, figure 27-9.

NOTE: Shaving can be planned for the same time the bed bath is given. For shaving, the electric razor is usually the easiest to use. However, it may be necessary to use a safety razor or a straight edge razor.

procedure

1. Ask the client if he desires a shave. Some clients may decide to grow a beard.
2. Gather the equipment and supplies needed:
   razor with fresh blade
   soap or shaving cream
   basin of hot water
   washcloth and towel
   shaving lotion (if used)
3. Wash your hands before beginning the procedure.
4. Position client comfortably and place a towel under his chin and across his chest.
5. Wash the client's face with soap. Rinse it and leave it wet.
6. Rub a small amount of shaving cream into the beard. If using soap instead of shaving cream, make a good, heavy lather.
7. With one hand, pull the skin tight above area to be shaved.
8. With razor in other hand, gently take short, even strokes. Shave in the direction the hair grows.
9. Rinse the razor frequently.

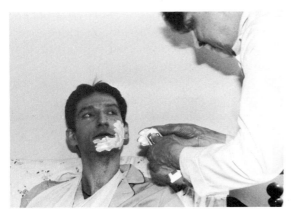

A. Apply shaving cream to the client's face.

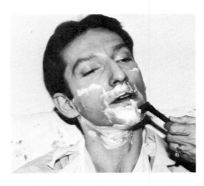

B. Shave the client's face using downward strokes on the cheeks and chin. NOTE: Whenever necessary, the client's skin should be stretched taut in order to avoid nicks and cuts.

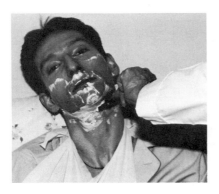

C. Use upward strokes on the client's neck.

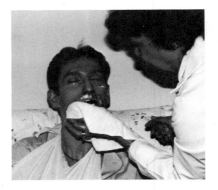

D. Rinse the face with a wet washcloth.

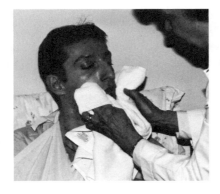

E. Pat the skin dry with a towel.

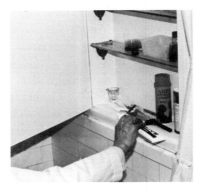

F. Return supplies to the proper location.

Figure 27-9 Shaving the male client.

10. Change water in basin when shave is completed. Rinse the client's face in clear water and pat dry.
11. Apply after-shave lotion if the client is accustomed to using it.
12. Return equipment and supplies, clean and store.
13. Reposition client unless following with a bed bath.
14. Wash hands thoroughly after the procedure.

client care procedure

7: HELPING THE CLIENT TO DRESS AND UNDRESS

purpose

- To keep the client clean and comfortable.
- Client is given help in order to reduce discomfort and reduce risk of strain or injury.

procedure

1. Wash your hands before beginning the procedure.
2. Collect fresh articles of clothing needed:
   clean gown
   pajamas
   daytime clothing as required
3. If client is able, help the client to sit at the edge of the bed and dangle the legs. If the client is too weak to sit up, have client lie flat on the bed. Place a sheet over the body to avoid embarrassing or chilling the client.
4. First assist the client into clean pajama bottoms or underpants. If the client has an injured or a weak leg, place that leg in the pajamas or underpants first, then the other leg. If client can stand, pull the garmet up to the waist. If client must remain on the bed, ask the client to press the heels into the bed and raise the buttocks. While the client is in this position, quickly slide the pants up to the waist. Assist client as necessary. If trousers are to be worn, start with the injured leg first and follow the same procedure. Brush or pull out wrinkles in the garment.

5. To dress the client in a pajama top, shirt, slip, or dress, first help the client place the arms into the armholes, figure 27-10. If client has an injured arm, put that arm into the armhole first. Slip the neck of the garment over the client's head. Pull down smoothly and gently. Fasten buttons or zippers. If client is lying down, ask the client to push down with the heels and raise the buttocks. Straighten the back of the garment. Do not allow the client to lie in wrinkled bed clothes. Wrinkles irritate the skin.
6. To dress the client in socks, turn each sock down to the toe end. Slide client's toe into place and, with one arm on each side of leg, pull the sock up. Make sure socks are smooth over the feet and legs. Wrinkles can cause skin irritations. In most cases, clean, white cotton socks will be used. A woman's stockings should never be fastened with round garters as round garters cut off circulation to the legs. If client is ambulatory, a garter belt may be used to hold up stockings.
7. To undress the client simply reverse the instructions for dressing. If the client has a weak arm or leg, undress the weak limb last. Provide the client with clean nightclothes.
8. Wash hands thoroughly after the procedure.

client care procedure

8: GIVING NAIL CARE

purpose

- To keep the client's nails clean and well groomed.
- To observe for signs of irritation.

NOTE: Nail care is usually given at bath time, or when there is a need because of a broken nail or hangnail. There are times when a mani-

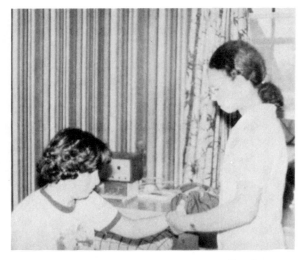

A. Gather the sleeve to slip it over the client's hand.

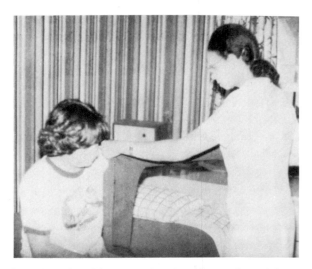

B. Bring the shirt over the shoulder and straighten the sleeve.

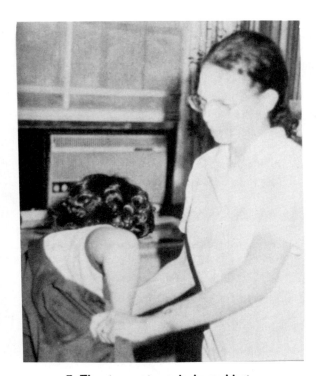

C. The strongest arm is dressed last.

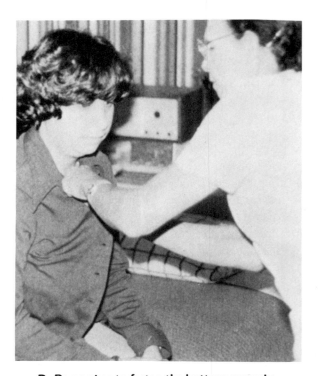

D. Remember to fasten the buttons securely.

Figure 27-10 Helping the client put on a shirt.

cure makes the client feel more attractive. **Caution:** Toenail care is not to be given by the home health aide. If the client needs toenail care, inform supervisor or family member.

procedure

1. Gather the supplies and equipment needed:
   soap and water
   basin
   nail brush
   towel
   small scissors
   emery board or nail file
   orange stick or flat toothpick
   lotion
2. Wash your hands before beginning the procedure.
3. Wash client's hands in soap and water, letting the fingertips soak for a short time.
4. Brush nails with nailbrush. Rinse well. This removes loose skin and dirt.
5. Dry hands and nails, gently pushing back the cuticle with the towel.
6. If nails are too long, make a straight cut off the tip of the nail. Use emery board or file to smooth the edges. **Caution:** Do

this cutting only with the permission of the nursing supervisor.
7. Clean under the nails with an orange stick, figure 27-11. Work gently so as not to injure skin under the nails.
8. Massage hands with lotion, moving from tips of fingers toward the wrist.
9. Wash your hands thoroughly after the procedure.
10. Make a note of any sign of skin irritation. Report unusual conditions to supervisor.
11. Clean the basin, brush and scissors. Return equipment to storage area.
12. **Caution:** If the client is diabetic, check with the supervisor regarding nail care.

client care procedure

9: *SHAMPOOING THE HAIR OF THE BEDRIDDEN CLIENT*

purpose

- To clean the hair and scalp.
- To stimulate circulation in the scalp.
- To make the client comfortable.
- To prevent accumulation of dandruff or formation of crusts.

procedure

1. Ask client if a shampoo is desired.
2. Bring to bedside:
   shampoo (or soap)
   2 large bath towels
   a quart pitcher or plastic bottle
   a large plastic sheet or clear plastic bag
   newspapers
   client's comb and brush
   1 large empty basin
   1 large basin of warm water
3. Provide for privacy during the shampoo.
4. Wash hands before beginning the procedure.
5. Position client so that the head rests over the edge of the bed. The back and shoulders

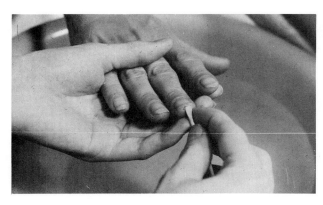

Figure 27-11 Use the blunt edge of an orange stick to remove the dirt under the client's nails (courtesy of Louise Simmers, *Diversified Health Occupations*, Delmar Publishers, Albany, NY, 1983).

should rest on the edge. (The instructor will demonstrate this technique.)

6. Remove clothing from around client's neck. Place a towel around the neck.

7. Spread a newspaper on a chair and set the empty basin on the newspaper. Move the chair with the basin to a position beneath the head of the client.

8. Slide a plastic sheet under the client's shoulders. Let the other end of the plastic fall into the basin. This allows the water to go from the head into the catch basin.

9. Fill the pitcher or bottle from the filled basin of water. Wet the hair.

10. Apply shampoo to the head, lathering well and massaging the scalp.

11. Pour water through the hair, making sure to remove all traces of soap or shampoo.

12. If necessary, reapply shampoo, lather well and rinse thoroughly.

13. Dry client's hair with a large towel. Wrap towel like a turban around the head. Return the client to a comfortable position. A cream rinse or medicinal alcohol may be rubbed into hair to help remove snarls and tangles.

14. Remove basins from the bedside.

15. Completely dry the client's hair. A hair dryer can be used if it is available.

16. Comb and brush hair into a style agreeable to the client, figure 27-12. Leave the client in a comfortable position.

17. Wash hands thoroughly after the procedure.

client care procedure

10: ASSISTING WITH THE TUB BATH OR SHOWER

purpose

- To clean and refresh the client.
- To check client's skin for signs of irritation.
- To stimulate circulation in the skin.

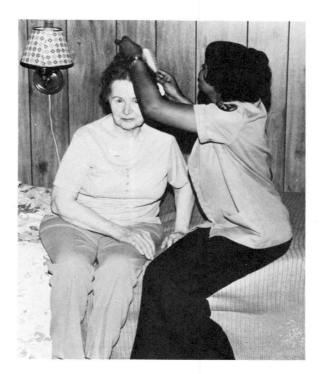

Figure 27-12 When dry, comb and brush the hair, and arrange it in a style preferred by the client.

procedure

1. If possible, plan the tub bath or shower for a time which is convenient for the client. A tub bath or shower should not take more than 10 minutes unless there is a special reason for a longer bath.

2. Get needed supplies and place in bathroom:
   fresh clothing
   bath seat or stool
   2 wash cloths
   towel
   soap and soap dish
   shampoo (if needed)
   metal or plastic pitcher
   hose attachment
   comb and brush
   skidproof bath mat

3. Wash hands before beginning procedure.

4. Fill tub one-third full with warm water. **Caution:** Test the temperature with a thermometer or on inside of wrist to be sure it will not burn the client. Place a skidproof bath mat in the bottom of the tub. If client is taking a shower, regulate the flow and be sure the temperature is correct. The water should be about 115°F (46°C).

5. Assist the client to sit on a chair or on the closed toilet seat. Help the client undress. Place soiled clothing in the hamper. Close the bathroom door so the client will not be chilled.

6. For a tub bath, help client to sit on the edge of the tub. If there is a safety bar, have client hold on to it. When client has gained balance, help the client to turn and lift both legs into the tub. Give assistance by supporting the client under the arms and helping the client to slowly sit down in the tub facing the faucets. If the client cannot sit in the tub, place a bath stool in the water. Help the client to sit on the stool.

7. If the client needs a shampoo, wet the hair and rub in shampoo, lather and massage skull. If possible, have the client tilt head back. Pour rinse water over the head using the pitcher or attach the hose to the faucet and use it to rinse the head. Repeat shampoo, massage and rinse. Client may hold a washcloth over the eyes during the shampoo to prevent suds entering the eyes.

8. Give the client a washcloth and soap. Allow clients to do as much as they can for themselves. If shower is running, make sure the flow is not too heavy; check water temperature often.

9. Remain beside the tub at all times during the bath or shower. **Caution:** Be ready to help the client at any moment. If the client should become faint, empty water from the tub, cover the client with a towel to avoid unnecessary chilling, and lower the client's head between the client's knees.

10. For a tub bath, help the client raise out of the water. Assist the client to sit on the edge of the tub. Bring client's legs over to outside and assist the client to stand. Allow the client to sit on the closed toilet seat or the chair.

11. Make certain that the client's body is thoroughly dry. Help dry difficult areas such as the back and shoulders. Be sure underarms and area under breasts are completely dry. Pay special attention to the feet. Dry soles of feet and between toes.

12. For a shower, make sure the client is completely washed and rinsed and then turn off the shower. Towel dry and assist client out of the shower area.

13. Assist client to dress in clean clothes.

14. Help client back to bed, to a wheelchair, or to a lounge chair.

15. Make a note of any skin or scalp irritations observed on the client.

16. Return to the bathroom and put supplies away. Drain and clean the tub. Place soiled towels in the hamper.

17. Wash hands thoroughly following procedure.

client care procedure

11: HELPING THE CLIENT WITH SELF-ADMINISTERED MEDICATIONS

purpose

- Medications are prescribed by the doctor to relieve pain and other symptoms, to help the body fight infections, and to treat illness.
- Assistance is given in order to encourage the client to take the prescribed medication at the right time, in the right dosage/amount, and in the right manner.
- The following information should be gathered by the supervisor and be made available

to the homemaker/home health aide to assist the aide in ensuring that the client takes the proper medications.

• Name of each medicine
• What each medicine is for
• Description of medicine (physical characteristics)
• How medicine should be taken
• At what time(s) of day medicine should be taken
• How long medicine should be taken
• Possible side effects
• The homemaker/home health aide should be aware of common reactions to medications so the supervisor and/or physician can be called if symptoms appear.

NOTE: The home health aide does not give medications. Aides help clients to take their own medications, figure 27-13. **Caution:** Certain medications, especially strong pain killers, can be dangerous. The home health aide must never let a client take more medication than ordered. If the client is in severe pain, call the doctor and/or the supervisor at once. Never allow the client to take extra medication.

The aide must take special care in assisting blind clients with their medications. Be sure that medications are coded so that the client can find the correct bottles when they are needed. Medications for the blind client must be kept in exactly the same spot so that an error will not be made. Special arrangements should be made by the doctor or public health nurse in setting up the coding.

procedure

1. Have the supervisor or nurse prepare a list of medications prescribed, and write the times at which they should be taken. Some medications are given 3 times a day, usually before or after each meal. Others may be ordered 4 times a day or every 6 hours. A medication taken every 6 hours could be

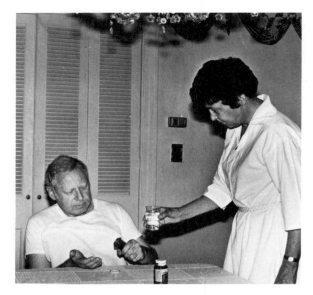

Figure 27-13 Aides help clients to take their own medications. Aides do not give the medications.

given at 6 A.M., 12 noon, 6 P.M., and 12 midnight. The doctor or nurse usually tells the client which times the medications should be taken.

2. Set up a schedule to be followed daily. After each medication has been taken, check it off. This informs the aide and the client that the medicine has been taken. Refer to the schedule and remind the client when medicine is due.

3. Make sure the correct medication is given. Check the prescription label before giving the medicine bottle to the client.

4. Make sure the method of taking the medication is followed. For example, some medicines are taken with juice or milk instead of water. Others are taken before, after, or with a meal.

5. Place certain medications such as nitroglycerine tablets within the client's reach at all times. Nitroglycerine tablets are used by clients who have angina. The client places these tablets under the tongue the moment any chest pain occurs.

FACTS A DOCTOR SHOULD BE TOLD ABOUT THE CLIENT'S MEDICAL HISTORY

- Have you had allergic reactions to drugs or foods in the past?
- Are you taking medicines or vitamins, including over-the-counter drugs or birth control pills or insulin? (These might interact with a new prescription and cause unwanted side effects.)
- Are you now undergoing medical treatment under the supervision of another doctor?
- Are you pregnant or breastfeeding?
- Do you have a kidney or liver disease or any other condition such as diabetes?
- Are you on a special diet?

QUESTIONS THE CLIENT SHOULD ASK THE DOCTOR

- The name and spelling of the medicine prescribed.
- What does the medicine do? Relieve pain? Reduce fever? Lower blood pressure? Cure infection?
- How will you know if the medication is working?
- Are there some medicines you should not take while taking this prescription?
- What are the best times of day to take the medicine? Before, during or after meals? Should you wake up at night to take a dose?
- How long should you continue to take the medicine? Just until you feel better, or for a specific period of time?
- Are there any foods you should not eat while taking the medicine? (Some antibiotics will not work if you drink milk or eat milk products. You should not drink alcoholic beverages when taking some medications.)

HOW TO GET THE MOST FROM PRESCRIPTION DRUGS

- If, after taking medication for 48 hours, you do not feel better, you should call the doctor.
- If you have any bad reactions or side effects to medication, such as dizziness, nausea, or headache, call the doctor at once.
- Read labels for storing instructions. Some drugs should be kept cool and dry, others protected from light. Some are dated and are not good or safe to use beyond a certain date.
- Do not transfer medicines from the original containers. Containers are designed to keep the drug properly protected. Also, if the medicine is placed in another container, it may be mistakenly taken by you or someone else.
- Discard any remaining medication when you have no further need to take it.
- Never give medications prescribed for yourself to another person.

Figure 27-14 The client should be knowledgeable about the medication that is being taken.

6. Put away sleep and pain medications after each use. Sleeping pills and other addicting drugs are to be used only as ordered by the doctor. There is always the danger of an accidental overdose of sleeping pills.

7. Review the evening medication schedule with the client. Be sure the client knows the method and time to take medications when no assistance can be given. Leave the medications within easy reach of the client.

Encourage the client to take nighttime doses in a well-lit room.

8. If the client has questions about the medications, encourage the client to ask the doctor. The client should be knowledgeable about medications that are being taken, figure 27-14 on page 295.

figure 27-14 on page 295.

client care procedure

12: FEEDING THE INCAPACITATED CLIENT

purpose

- To provide proper nutrition for the client.
- To provide suitable food, based on client's condition, meeting standards of the Basic Four food groups.
- To provide a pleasurable experience for the client.
- To observe the quantity of food ingested and report any problems that may arise.

NOTE: Feeding can and should be a pleasant experience for the client. The food should be served with hot foods hot, and cold foods cold. Food should be attractively presented to the client.

While the food is cooking, ask the client if the urinal or bedpan is required. If client uses either, make certain that you wash your hands both before and after presentation.

procedure

1. Wash the client's hands and face and situate the client comfortably in bed or at the table.
2. Wash your hands thoroughly.
3. Bring the food to the client.
4. How you feed an incapacitated client depends on the handicap or physical problems. If your client has only one arm, for example, you should pre-cut items requiring cutting. If the client has no teeth, the food should be soft so that there will be no discomfort to the client. **Caution:** The client should

never be embarrassed because of any physical incapacity.

5. Ask the client which food is desired first. (Getting the client's cooperation and participation is very important.)
6. If the client must be totally fed by you remember:
   - Feed slowly; let the client set the pace, figure 27-15.
   - Feed small amounts.
   - Make sure the consistency of food is appropriate. (A person with dentures, for example, may not be able to have corn on the cob.)
   - Do not rush the client. However, do not let the client dawdle until food is cold and unpalatable.
7. Wash your hands following the procedure.

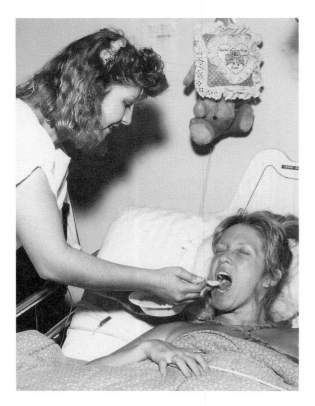

Figure 27-15 Feeding the helpless client in bed

Unit 28
Vital Signs

learning objectives

After studying this unit, you should be able to:
- Demonstrate clear ability to perform all the procedures.
- Explain the purpose of each procedure.
- State when the procedures should and should not be done.
- Identify precautions to be taken for each procedure.
- Recognize abnormal readings.
- Record vital signs properly.

NOTE: All procedures are not allowed in all states. Make sure you are aware of limits as outlined by state guidelines.

client care procedure
13: TAKING AN ORAL TEMPERATURE

purpose

- To measure the client's body temperature in the most appropriate way.
- To routinely check the temperature in order to note any significant change.

NOTE: Using an oral thermometer is the most convenient way to obtain a person's temperature. However, it is not the most accurate method. If the client has taken a cold or hot drink, the temperature of the mouth changes. Smoking also affects the accuracy of the reading. In addition to accuracy, the aide must consider safety as it is possible that the thermometer might break in the client's mouth. **Caution:** The oral thermometer can only be used when the client is able to hold it in the mouth properly. If for any reason the client cannot keep the thermometer in the mouth, call the supervisor for instructions. In some of these cases, a rectal temperature may need to be taken with a rectal thermometer. Sudden changes in temperature or temperatures above 101°F (38.3°C) should be reported to the supervisor at once.

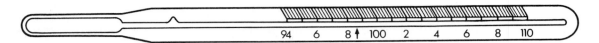

A. The bulb end of the oral thermometer is long and slender.

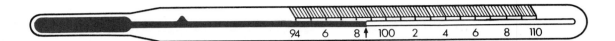

B. The mercury rises from the bulb end to the temperature mark.

Figure 28-1 Normal oral temperature is 98.6° Fahrenheit.

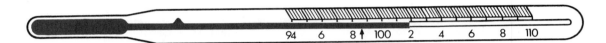

Figure 28-2 An elevated oral temperature such as 101.8°F should be reported to the supervisor at once.

procedure

1. Ask the client not to drink any liquids or smoke 15 minutes before the temperature is taken. Otherwise an inaccurate reading could result.
2. Gather the equipment needed:
   oral thermometer with cover
   tissues
   pad and pencil
   watch with second hand
   alcohol
3. Wash your hands thoroughly.
4. Ask the client to find a comfortable position, either in a chair or in a bed.
5. If necessary, clean the thermometer with soap and cold water or alcohol. Rinse well.
6. Hold thermometer by stem end and read mercury column. It should register 96°F (35.5°C). If it does not, shake down the thermometer with a snap of the wrist. Shake the thermometer down until it reads 94°F (35.5°C).

7. Insert bulb end of thermometer under client's tongue. Slant it toward the side of the mouth. Ask the client to close the mouth and keep the thermometer under the tongue.
8. Be sure the client holds the thermometer under the tongue for a minimum of 3 minutes and then remove the thermometer.
9. Gently wipe the thermometer with a tissue from the stem to the bulb end. Discard the contaminated tissue. If using a cover, discard it.
10. Read the thermometer at eye level and record the measurement. Normal oral temperature is 98.6°F (37°C), figure 28-1. Mark down the time the reading was made. Report any temperature which reads above 101°F (38°C), figure 28-2.
11. Clean the thermometer by washing it with a small amount of soap and cold water, figure 28-3. Rinse all soap from the thermometer. A tissue wet in alcohol may also be used to clean the thermometer. Wipe

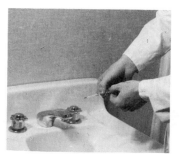

Figure 28-3 Clean the thermometer by washing it with a small amount of soap and cold water.

from stem end to the front, bulb end (clean to dirty).

12. The client may have an electric thermometer with a digital readout.
13. Return thermometer to the proper storage place, figure 28-4.
14. Wash your hands after the procedure.

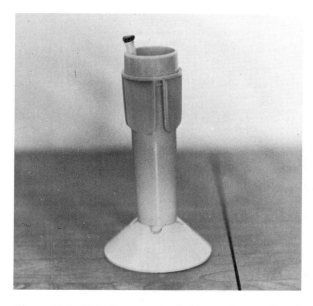

Figure 28-4 This thermometer holder makes a safe and clean storage container. A clean cotton ball should be placed inside on the bottom to avoid breaking the bulb end.

14: TAKING A RECTAL TEMPERATURE

purpose

- To obtain the most accurate measure of the client's temperature.
- To obtain the temperature of a person who cannot hold an oral thermometer in the mouth.
- To routinely check the temperature in order to note any significant change.

NOTE: A rectal temperature is sometimes taken instead of an oral temperature. At times this is done because the rectal temperature is more accurate. If a person breathes through the mouth or used oxygen an oral temperature would not give an accurate reading. Drinking fluids or smoking before a reading also alters it. In these situations clients must have rectal temperatures taken. A rectal temperature is necessary for those who cannot hold a thermometer in the mouth. Infants, small children, and adults who are seriously ill or mentally confused cannot hold a thermometer properly. In addition, rectal temperatures are taken for any person with a history of convulsions.

The rectal thermometer is shaped differently than the oral thermometer. The bulb end of the rectal thermometer is thicker and more rounded. This shape adds to the safety and comfort of the client, figure 28-5. The normal rectal temperature (99.6°F) is one degree more than the normal oral temperature (98.6°F).

procedure

1. Gather the equipment needed:
   rectal thermometer with cover, if available
   lubricant
   tissues
   pad and pencil
   watch with second hand
   alcohol
2. Wash your hands thoroughly.

3. Tell the client that you plan to take a rectal temperature. Provide for privacy. Do not expose the client unnecessarily.
4. Shake down the thermometer to 96°F (35.5°C).
5. Position client on left side, Sims position. Cover the client with a sheet or blanket and remove the client's clothing from the lower part of the body.
6. Lubricate the bulb tip of the thermometer with a water-soluble jelly and a tissue. This makes insertion easier and more comfortable.
7. Fold back the sheet or blanket to expose the client's buttocks. Raise top buttock with your hand and, with the other hand, gently insert bulb end of thermometer into the client's rectum about 1½ inches.
8. Redrape the client and hold the thermometer in place for 3 to 5 minutes. **Caution:** Do not let go of the rectal thermometer.
9. Remove the thermometer; wipe it from stem to bulb end (clean to dirty).
10. Discard contaminated tissue.
11. Read the thermometer and record the temperature. Record the time and place the letter *R* (rectal) beside the temperature reading.
12. Return the client to a comfortable position.

13. Clean the thermometer using soap and cold water or alcohol. Rinse it thoroughly. Store properly.
14. Wash your hands thoroughly after the procedure.

client care procedure

15: TAKING AN AXILLARY TEMPERATURE

purpose

- To obtain the client's temperature reading when a rectal or oral reading is not possible.

NOTE: The axillary temperature is not the most accurate method of taking a temperature. However, it may be ordered by the doctor or supervisor when an oral reading is not possible. Taking an axillary temperature is more convenient than taking a rectal temperature and is less embarrassing for the client. An axillary temperature is usually 0.5° to 1.0°F (0.28° to 0.56°C) lower than an oral temperature.

procedure

1. Wash your hands before beginning the procedure.
2. Rinse the thermometer in cool water and wipe it dry with a tissue.

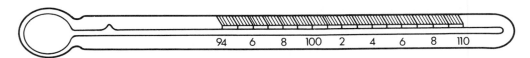

A. The bulb end of the rectal thermometer is thick and rounded.

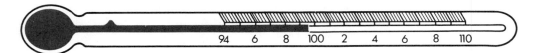

B. Normal rectal temperature is 99.6°F, one degree higher than the oral temperature.

Figure 28-5   The round bulb of a rectal thermometer makes insertion easier and safer.

3. Shake down the thermometer so the mercury is below 96°F (35.6°C).
4. Dry the client's armpit with a tissue.
5. Place the thermometer in the center of the client's axilla (armpit) with the bulb end toward the client's head. This position rests the bulb end against the blood vessel and a more accurate reading can be obtained.
6. Position the client's arm close to the body and place the client's forearm over the client's chest. This position enables the arm to hold the thermometer in place.
7. Leave the thermometer in place for ten minutes.
8. Remove the thermometer and wipe it clean of any perspiration.
9. Read the temperature indicated on the thermometer. (A normal axillary temperature is 97.6°F.)
10. Record the temperature. An axillary temperature is recorded with an *Ax* beside the number, e.g., 97.6°F Ax.
11. Shake down the thermometer, clean it, and return it to its proper place.
12. Wash your hands following the procedure.

client care procedure

16: DETERMINING THE PULSE AND RESPIRATION RATE

purpose

- To measure, record, and observe the character of the client's pulse rate with confidence and accuracy.
- To count the rate and observe the character of respirations.
- To report changes or abnormal rates to the supervisor, nurse or doctor.

NOTE: A pulse is taken to determine its regularity, strength, and rate. Regularity is described as either regular or irregular. An irregular pulse may indicate skipped heartbeats or changing rhythm patterns. An irregular pulse should always be recorded.

Strength is described as bounding, strong, weak, or thready. If the strength has changed, the aide should call the supervisor.

Pulse rate is described as the number of beats per minute. The age, size, and sex of the client may influence the rate. Normal ranges in pulse rates are:

60–90 adults
70–90 children over 6 years of age
80–100 children under 6 years of age
100–130 infants

procedure for determining pulse rate

1. Gather the equipment needed:
   wrist watch with a second hand
   note pad and pen or pencil
2. Wash your hands before beginning the procedure.
3. Tell the client that you are going to check the pulse rate. Ask the client to help by remaining quiet and still while you are counting.
4. Have the client sit in a comfortable chair or lie in bed with arms resting gently on the chest.
5. Place the tips of your first three fingers on the pulse site. The radial pulse on the inner wrist is most often used. **Caution:** Do not use your thumb to feel the client's artery. Using the thumb can result in an inaccurate reading.
6. Count the pulse beats for one full minute.
7. Record the pulse rate, regularity, and strength. Also record the time the pulse was taken. If irregular, take apical for 1 minute and record apical pulse.

procedure for determining respiration rate

NOTE: Character of respirations is described as regular or irregular; labored, difficult, shallow or deep; and noisy or quiet.

Normal respiration rate for adults is 16 to 20 breaths per minute.

1. Gather equipment needed:
   wrist watch with a second hand
   note pad and pen or pencil
2. After client's pulse has been taken, leave the fingers in position on the wrist. By doing this, the client is not aware that you are counting respirations, figure 28-6.
3. One rise and fall of the chest counts as one respiration. Count the number of respirations during a full one-minute period.
4. Note how deeply the client breathes. Also check the regularity of the rhythm pattern. Note the sound of the breathing.
5. Record the number of respirations occurring in one minute. Record the character of the client's breathing.
6. Report changes from the client's usual way of breathing. Report any difficulty in breathing to the supervisor at once.
7. Wash your hands following the procedure.

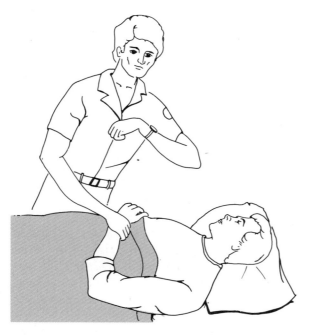

Figure 28-6 The aide rests the client's lower arm across the chest to take the pulse and respirations. Note that the aide's fingers are over the inner part of the wrist where the radial artery is located. Also, the aide can see and feel the breaths being taken by the client.

17: MEASURING BLOOD PRESSURE

purpose

- To take blood pressure correctly.
- To accurately report blood pressure readings to the supervisor, nurse, or doctor.

NOTE: Blood pressure is taken by the use of a sphygmomanometer (an instrument with a cuff, rubber bulb, and dial gauge for recording pressure) and a stethoscope (a listening device that magnifies sound), figure 28-7.

Two readings are recorded: the systolic pressure is recorded first. This is the pressure that is felt in the artery when the heart con-

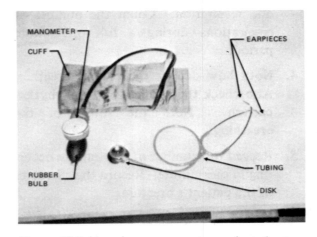

Figure 28-7 A sphygmomanometer and stethoscope used for taking blood pressure

tracts. The diastolic pressure is recorded second. This is the pressure that is felt in the artery when the heart is in the relaxation stage. The systolic rate is always higher than the diastolic rate. Normal blood pressure for an adult is about 120/80, although it may vary depending on age, sex, emotional state, exercise and weight.

The cuff should be the right size for the client's arm otherwise an incorrect reading may be obtained. Cuffs come in various sizes: child, normal adult, and extra large. It is important to read the mercury at eye level; therefore, it is best to take the readings while you are sitting down, next to the client.

procedure

1. Gather equipment needed:
   sphygmomanometer
   stethoscope
   alcohol sponges or cotton balls
2. Wash your hands before beginning the procedure.
3. Explain to the client what you are going to do. Have the client sit or lie in a comfortable position with one arm extended at the same level as the heart. The palm should be upward. (Either arm may be used, unless otherwise indicated by the doctor. What is important is that the blood pressure be taken on the same arm each time.) Arm should be in resting position.
4. Pick up the stethoscope. Wipe the earpieces, figure 28-8. Place the stethoscope around your neck.
5. Pick up the cuff and wrap it securely around the client's arm, about one inch above the elbow. Fasten. (Some cuffs have a Velcro fastener; others have hooks at the end of the cuff.)
6. Attach the manometer (the dial gauge) to the top of the cuff so you can read it, figure 28-9.
7. Tighten the small round valve that is lo-

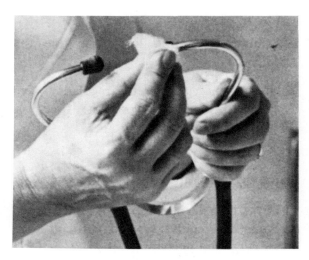

Figure 28-8 Clean the earpieces of the stethoscope with an alcohol sponge or cotton ball.

cated along the side of the rubber bulb. (This valve controls the pumping you will do later.)

8. With the tips of your fingers, locate the artery on the inside of the client's elbow. When you feel a throbbing beat, you have located the artery. Keep your fingers on the spot. Never use your thumb since it, too, has a pulse beat.

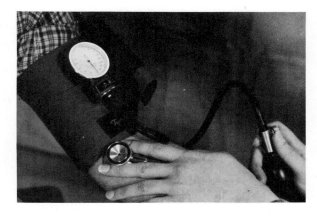

Figure 28-9 The gauge on the manometer should be positioned for easy visibility (courtesy of Louise Simmers, *Diversified Health Occupations*, Delmar Publishers, Albany, NY, 1983).

9. Place the round disk of the stethoscope over the artery you located on the client (slipping your fingers to hold it in place), figure 28-10. With your other hand, insert the earpieces in your ear.

10. Take the rubber bulb in your hand. Look at the dial gauge while you pump air into the cuff by squeezing the bulb. Pump until the reading on the dial gauge is about 180–200.

11. Listen with the stethoscope placed in your ears and the disk over the artery. You should not hear any sound.

12. While listening, slowly release the air by opening the valve located beside the bulb, using the thumb and forefinger. (This will cause air to escape from the cuff and the reading on the manometer will drop.) You may have to tighten the bulb valve if the air escapes too fast.

13. Listen carefully. When the first thumping sound is heard, remember the number seen on the dial gauge. This is the systolic pressure.

14. Watch the dial continue to fall as the air escapes. When the thumping sound becomes a muffled sound, remember the number. This is the diastolic pressure.

15. Release the remainder of the air from the cuff and remove it, leaving the valve open.

16. Record the two readings. Blood pressure reading is written as a fraction with the systolic (top) listed first and the diastolic (bottom) written under the line; for example, BP $\frac{120 \text{ (systolic pressure)}}{80 \text{ (diastolic pressure)}}$

17. **Caution:** Be careful not to pump the pressure too high. Remember that the pressure of the cuff can cause the client discomfort so it is important to release the air and work quickly when taking the blood pressure. If it is necessary to repeat the procedure, wait a few minutes before inflating the cuff; this allows the circulation to return to normal.

18. If you are unsuccessful in obtaining a blood pressure reading after three attempts, move to the client's other arm and try again, repeating the same procedure. (A reading taken after three attempts would probably

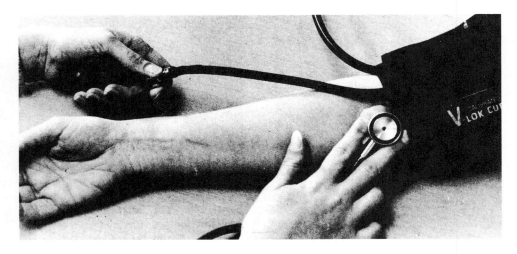

Figure 28-10 Place your fingers over the disk as you pump air into the cuff. Adjust the valve on the bulb to control the flow of air (courtesy of Louise Simmers, *Diversified Health Occupations*, Delmar Publishers, Albany, NY, 1983).

be inaccurate and the client would become uncomfortable.) Never guess. If a blood pressure is hard to take or you are not sure, tell the supervisor or nurse.

19. May use other side of stethoscope for hard to hear blood pressures.
20. Wash your hands following the procedure.

Precautions
- If you are taking the blood pressure of a stroke client use the unaffected arm only.
- If your client is having home dialysis (as part of a kidney treatment), or is receiving intravenous (I.V.) fluids, take the blood pressure on the unaffected arm.

Unit 29

Special Treatments and Dressings

client care procedures

18. Giving an Alcohol or Tepid Water Sponge Bath
19. Applying a Clean Dressing
20. Applying Bandages
21. Observing and Caring for Casts
22. Caring for Decubitus Ulcers
23. Caring for the Urinary Catheter
24. Changing the Ostomy Bag
25. Using Oxygen Safely

learning objectives

After studying this unit, you should be able to:
— Demonstrate clear ability to perform all the procedures.
— Explain the purpose of each procedure.
— State when the procedures should and should not be done.
— Identify precautions to be taken for each procedure.

NOTE: All procedures are not allowed in all states. Make sure you are aware of limits as outlined by state guidelines.

client care procedure

18: GIVING AN ALCOHOL OR TEPID WATER SPONGE BATH

purpose

- To reduce client's temperature if it reaches 104°F (40°C) or higher.
- To give relief and comfort.

NOTE: An alcohol or tepid water sponge bath should only be given on the direction of the supervisor or doctor. When a temperature is elevated to 104°F or more, the client may display mental confusion or be irritable. The home

health aide should try to soothe the client. The aide should explain that the sponge bath will bring down the temperature. The client must be told that the sudden cold may be startling. **Caution:** The home health aide should stop the sponge bath at once if the client's lips turn cyanotic (blue), or if the client shivers. Also, the aide should watch for changes in the pulse rate. If any of these changes occur, cover the client and call the supervisor or doctor at once.

procedure

1. Gather the supplies and equipment needed: basin containing tap water

3 washcloths
3 towels
ice bag with cover or plastic bag of ice
    chips
bath blanket or cotton blanket
fresh gown or pajamas
rubbing alcohol, if ordered
watch with second hand
pen and note pad

2. Wash your hands before beginning the procedure.
3. Prepare a basin with cool water. If an alcohol sponge bath is indicated, add alcohol 70% to the water. **Caution:** Never apply alcohol to the client's face.
4. Take and record the client's temperature, pulse and respiration. Note the time at which these signs were taken.
5. Fold bed sheets and blankets to the foot of the bed.
6. Cover the client with a bath blanket. Remove the client's gown or pajamas.
7. Place a warm hot water bottle at the client's feet to avoid unusual chilling. The feet are furthest from the heart and circulation may be poorest in the foot area, especially among older people.
8. Moisten a washcloth in the water (or alcohol mixture), figure 29-1. Squeeze out the excess liquid. Sponge the face and dry it with a towel. **Caution:** Do not sponge the eye area. Place an ice bag on the forehead.
9. Lift one arm from under the bath blanket. Place a towel under the arm. Sponge and dry one arm and then the other.
10. If the client is displaying no bad effects, continue with the sponge bath. Sponge the arms for 5 minutes, the chest for 5 minutes, the legs for 5 minutes and the back for 5 minutes. The entire procedure should take about 30 minutes. **Caution:** Do not sponge the eyes, the abdomen, or the genital area.
11. Dress the client in a clean gown or pajamas. Pull the covers over the client.

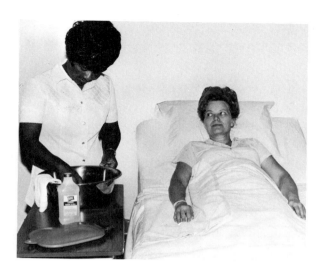

Figure 29-1 Preparing to give a sponge bath.

12. Take and record the client's temperature, pulse, and respiration (TPR) as soon as the procedure has been completed. Notify the supervisor of the results.
13. Wash your hands thoroughly after the procedure.
14. Clean the supplies and store them. After 30 minutes, take and record the TPR again.

client care procedure

19: APPLYING A CLEAN DRESSING

purpose

- To absorb drainage from wound or incision area.
- To protect area from contamination.
- To reduce odor and keep client comfortable.

NOTE: Most dressings will be changed as ordered by the doctor or supervisor, q.d. (once a day), or p.r.n. (whenever necessary). When changing dressings, the home health aide should observe and record the amount of drainage, the progress of healing, and the surrounding skin condition. **Caution:** Before changing dressings, the home health aide must have the approval of the supervisor. Dressing changes can only be made as ordered by the supervisor.

procedure

1. Gather supplies and bring to bedside:
   hydrogen peroxide or cleansing agent
   six to eight 4 × 4 gauze pads
   antibiotic ointment (if prescribed)
   nonallergenic tape
   waste bag
   note pad and pen
2. Wash your hands thoroughly.
3. Position the client comfortably, exposing only the area to be dressed.
4. Open the package of gauze pads without touching the pads, figure 29-2. Place supplies within easy reach. Open the bottle

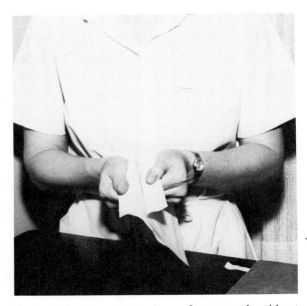

Figure 29-2 Open the package of gauze pads without touching the pads (courtesy of Caldwell and Hegner, *Health Care Assistant,* Delmar Publishers, Albany, NY, 1985).

of cleaning solution and the tube of ointment if used.

5. Remove the used dressing. If the dressing does not lift off easily, pour hydrogen peroxide over it to help loosen it. Tape may be loosened by using a special adhesive solution. Handle area gently to avoid further irritation. Nonstick pads are available in most drugstores. If possible, they should be used. Discard used dressing in open waste bag.
6. Dampen a clean gauze with hydrogen peroxide. Do not allow the bottle to touch the gauze.
7. With one straight stroke, wipe from the center of the wound outward. Drop contaminated pad into open waste bag. Do not put hand inside of waste bag. Be sure to use a clean, moistened pad for each stroke. Clean the entire area. Never move back and forth across the wound. The wound is considered cleaner than the surrounding skin. For this reason, cleaning away from the wound is moving from clean to dirty.
8. If an ointment has been prescribed, place proper amount on the center of an opened gauze pad. Only the outer edges of the pad should be held. Place pad over the wound and tape in place. Leave the edges of the gauze free to allow for air circulation.
9. Discard waste bag. Return supplies to storage. Follow aseptic techniques.
10. Record observations of the wound and skin condition. Report signs of redness, swelling, heat, or foul odor. In addition, report to the supervisor if the client complains of pain around the wound.
11. Return client to a comfortable position.
12. Wash your hands thoroughly.

Specific orders for this procedure are given by the supervising nurse.

20: APPLYING BANDAGES

Bandages are long continuous strips of material that are applied to different parts of the body. They serve many purposes such as a covering for a wound to prevent infection while healing takes place or to give support to an injured joint, muscle, or bone. There are many different types of material used for bandages. Ace bandages are very common. Gauze bandages are frequently used also. Kling and Kerlix are other common types of bandages.

purpose

- Provide a covering for a wounded area.
- Secure traction or a splint in place.
- Apply pressure to a body part.

procedure

1. Wash hands before beginning procedure.
2. Place the part to be bandaged in good body alignment and normal positioning. Client will usually be lying down—in bed. Support the body in the appropriate places, head and arms if necessary.

SHOULDER DRESSING

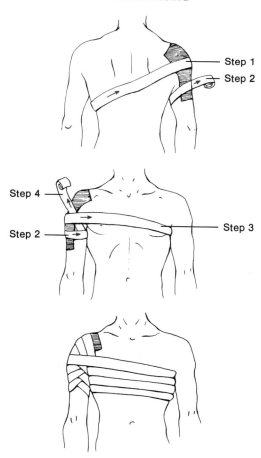

Figure 29-3   Shoulder dressing.

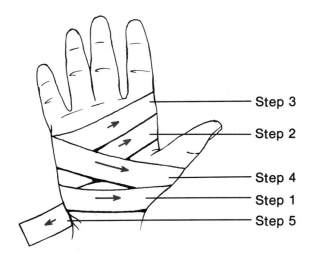

Figure 29-4 Hand dressing.

3. Apply the bandages from the farthest part of the body to the nearest part of the body. Refer to figures 29-3 to 29-7.

4. Be sure to make secure your first turns of the bandage (one to two turns in place). Always make certain all areas of the bandage are of the same pressure. The bandage should not be so tight as to cause edema at either end. Check the skin color and temperature after bandaging a part of the body. Secure the bandage with clips or adhesive tape. Wrinkling of the bandage may cause trauma and edema to the part bandaged.

5. If possible, leave the toes or fingers exposed for viewing after bandaging is completed.

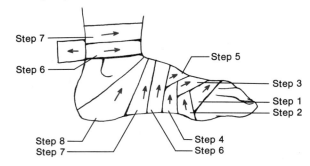

Figure 29-5 Foot bandage.

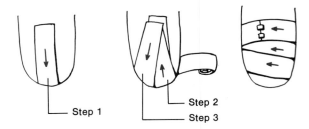

Figure 29-6 Stump bandage.

6. Types of Bandages:

a. Circular	Each turn of the bandage overlaps the previous turn.
b. Spiral	Each turn of the bandage slightly overlaps the previous turn, so that the bandage moves upward.
c. Spiral Reverse	The beginning turns are circular in nature, then with the following layers the top of the bandage is turned under.

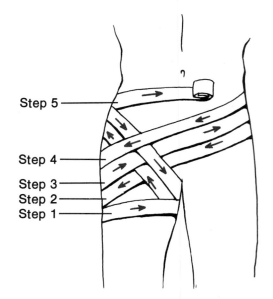

Figure 29-7 Upper thigh and trunk.

d. Spica — This is the same as for the spiral reverse, but covers a much larger area.

7. Be sure to record your observations of the part bandaged. Report any unusual observations to the supervising nurse.
8. Ace bandages may be washed and reused when dry. Gauze bandages must be discarded and not reused at any time.
9. Return client to a comfortable position.
10. Wash hands thoroughly when procedure is completed.

NOTE: Bandaging takes practice. Be sure to review this procedure with your supervising nurse.

21: OBSERVING AND CARING FOR CASTS

Casts are used to provide immobilization of an extremity or/and joint following trauma, fractures, or to correct a body bone/joint defect, figure 29-8. Casts may be applied to an extremity or to the entire body. Casts may be made of plaster of Paris, fiberglass, polyester, or cotton.

purpose

- Promote healing of injured area that is casted.
- Provide comfort to the client.
- Prevent skin irritations and possible skin breakdown.

procedure

1. Observe the new cast every 2–3 hours for the first two days and then daily.
   a. note the color of the skin at the farthest end of cast (normal pink, warm to touch, and movable toes or fingers by the client).
   b. note for edema at both ends of the cast (report and record this information).
   c. note for response to touch (that is the response of the nerves to stimulation) report and record this information.
2. Observe the cast daily for roughness around the edges. This may cause skin irritation and may be filed or covered with a soft padding. Request a visit by the supervising nurse and ask for the appropriate material to prevent skin breakdown.
3. Observe the cast itself, noting any redness that may indicate bleeding or drainage from under the cast. Circle the area with a magic marker noting the date and time that you first noticed the marking. Record and report immediately.
4. Observe the cast constantly for any cracks. Cracks are unsafe and the doctor should be notified of this crack. You must state the exact location and length of the crack as well as the depth of it.
5. When the cast is near the perineal area protect it from moisture. Ask the supervisor for permission to use a waterproof substance or plastic around the casted area. Protect the cast and skin by preventing any dirt, sand, or small articles from getting inside the cast. This may cause an infection under the cast. Note that plaster of Paris casts tend to crumble and become soft when moist; therefore this type of cast must always be kept dry.
6. Ask the client if he/she has pain in any particular area under the cast. This may indicate a pressure point and skin breakdown under the cast. Note the diagram. Report and record immediately.

general information

1. Check the house for throw rugs or objects on the floor. Remove any hazard that may cause the client to fall.

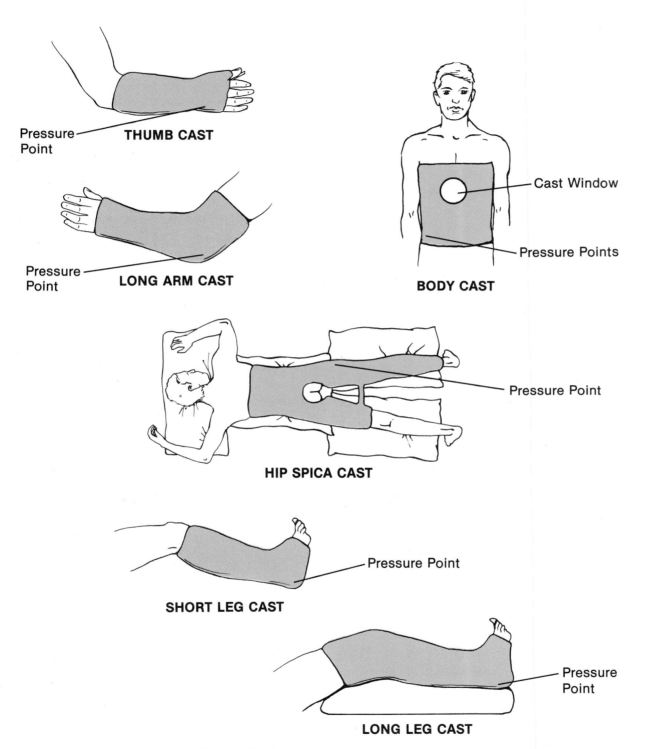

Figure 29-8 Casts that are frequently applied.

2. Remember that at first the client may not have a good sense of balance and may be unsteady in walking. Arrange the furniture so that the client may hold on to furniture or handrails while walking.

3. Assist the client in making changes in eating, dressing, writing, toileting, and walking. Note whether the dominant hand/arm is casted so that the client is helped in activities of daily living.

4. Ask the supervising nurse for specific orders for passive range of motion exercises. A physical therapist may come to assist the client with specific exercises. A home health aide may not perform these exercises without orders.

5. Check for the composition of the cast by asking the supervising nurse. Plaster of Paris casts take at least 24 hours to dry, while polyester, fiberglass, and plastic casting tape take 5–15 minutes to dry. Additional information needed: time that the client may ambulate, that is, to bear weight. This time may vary also: plaster of Paris casts take 48 hours until a sling or crutches may be used while the others vary from 15–30 minutes. Good body alignment is necessary while the client is at rest.

6. Check for specific orders for the client in a body cast. You will need instruction for toileting this client.

client care procedure
22: CARING FOR DECUBITUS ULCERS

purpose

- To promote healing of ulcer.
- To increase circulation and prevent further breakdown of skin.
- To keep skin around ulcer area clean.
- To provide a chance to observe the progress of treatment.

procedure

1. Gather supplies needed.
   waste bag
   six 4 × 4 gauze pads
   nonallergenic tape
   hydrogen peroxide or solution prescribed by doctor
   ointment (prescribed by doctor)
   heat lamp (if ordered by doctor)

2. Wash your hands thoroughly.

3. Position and drape the client comfortably. Expose only the ulcerated area.

4. Open a package of sterile gauze pads. Separate the package at one end. Avoid touching the pads.

5. Open the bottle of hydrogen peroxide or whatever solution the doctor orders.

6. Remove soiled dressing. Check the drainage on the dressing for the amount, color, and odor. Observe whether the ulcer has become wider or deeper.

7. Drop soiled dressing into an open waste bag. **Caution:** Do not touch the sides of the bag as touching it would contaminate the hands.

8. Dampen a gauze pad with hydrogen peroxide. Do not contaminate pad by touching it with the peroxide bottle.

9. Wipe from the center of the ulcer outward. Use only one pad for each stroke. Use one stroke from the center to the outer edge. Discard each pad in waste bag as soon as it has been used.

10. Repeat each time, using a fresh pad and fresh peroxide. Use four strokes in all. Clean from the center to each side, from center to top, and then center to bottom. Do not rub back and forth across area. If the ulcer is infected, this motion could cause the infection to spread. Use a fresh pad for each stroke. Drop each pad into waste bag after use.

11. If heat lamp has been prescribed, use as ordered. **Caution:** Never place the heat

lamp closer than 18 inches to the client. Time the treatment and follow the doctor's orders exactly.

12. If an ointment has been prescribed, drop the prescribed amount in the center of a fresh pad. Do not touch the pad with the ointment tube. Place the pad over the ulcer.

13. Apply tape by placing two strips through the center. Allow for proper air circulation; do not close off the edges of the gauze, figure 29-9.

14. Return client to a comfortable position.

15. Replace supplies and discard waste bag following aseptic techniques.

16. Wash your hands thoroughly following the procedure.

17. Remember to turn and reposition the client every two hours to relieve pressure points.

23: CARING FOR THE URINARY CATHETER

purpose

- To clean the skin where the catheter enters the body.
- To prevent infection of the urinary tract.
- To remove odors and make the client comfortable.
- To protect aide (client with AIDS)

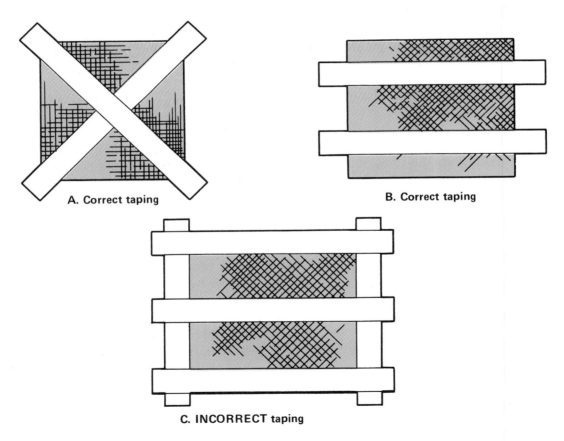

A. Correct taping

B. Correct taping

C. INCORRECT taping

Figure 29-9 Correct taping allows for proper air circulation. Ends of gauze should never be taped down.

NOTE: A urinary catheter is a tube inserted into the bladder to drain urine. Germs can easily enter the bladder while the catheter is in place. Therefore, cleaning around the urinary opening is important.

Because of the danger of contamination and infection, in many areas caring for the urinary catheter is no longer a standard procedure. Rather, the nursing supervisor replaces the catheter when given orders from the physician. The catheter may be replaced weekly or once a month.

The urinary collection leg bag is smaller than the bedside urinary collection bag. The leg bag is attached to the client's thigh (upper leg). The leg bag allows for greater mobility for the client *but* must be emptied more frequently. It must be checked every 2–3 hours. A client may use the leg bag while up in the wheel chair or ambulating and then can be connected to the bedside drainage urinary collection bag when in bed for the night. The leg bag must be rinsed thoroughly with warm water and hung in the bathroom to drain (over bath tub water handle or bath assistance bar). A clean stopper must be used for the tubing while the bedside urinary collection bag is not in use. Some collection bags have a particular place to insert the tubing. Be certain to check with the supervising nurse for the appropriate care and procedure regarding leg bags and bedside urinary collection bags.

suggested schedule of bag change

1. Leg bag—sterile, new one used weekly.
2. Bedside collection bag—sterile, new one used weekly.
3. Catheter—sterile, new one inserted per physician's instructions by the supervising nurse, weekly or monthly.

procedure

1. Bring to bedside:
   disposable gloves

commercial ointment/cleansing agent
antiseptic swabs (if ordered by doctor)
mild soap
basin of warm water
washcloth or gauze pads
waste bag
antiseptic or antibiotic ointment (if prescribed)
cotton-tipped applicator
2. Wash your hands thoroughly.
3. Position the client on the back. Expose only a small area where the catheter enters the body.
4. Put on the gloves to reduce spread of germs from your hands to the client.
5. Using soap and warm water, take a cloth or gauze pad and wash skin area surrounding catheter.
6. Using antiseptic swabs or gauze pads dipped in warm water, wipe the catheter tube. Make only one stroke with each swab or pad. Throw away the pad after one stroke. Start at the urinary opening and wipe away from it. Be careful not to dislodge the catheter. Clean the catheter up to the connection of the drainage bag hose.
7. An antiseptic or antibiotic ointment may be prescribed to prevent infection. Drop ointment onto a cotton-tipped applicator. Do not let ointment container touch the applicator tip as this would contaminate the tip.
8. Apply ointment where the catheter is inserted into the body.
9. The client may be using a drainage bag which attaches to the leg. If a leg bag is used, make sure the bag is kept lower than the bladder. If urine flows from the container back to the bladder there is danger of infection. The client should sit or lie so that the leg with the bag is lower than the bladder. The container may be attached to the frame of wheelchair.
10. If the client is using another type of drain-

age bag, follow instructions as given by supervisor or doctor.

11. Drainage bags should be emptied as they become filled, or at least every 8 hours. To empty, hold a measuring pitcher or basin at the lower end of the drainage bag, figure 29-10. Open the tube and release the collected urine. If the client's fluids are being measured, be sure to record the amount collected. Close the tube tightly.

12. If the tube from the catheter to the drainage bag appears clogged or dirty, report this to the supervisor. Urinary drainage equipment can only be replaced by a qualified person. This is a sterile procedure.

13. Return the client to a comfortable position.

14. Return unused supplies to storage. Clean equipment and store. Dispose of waste bag.

15. Wash your hands thoroughly.

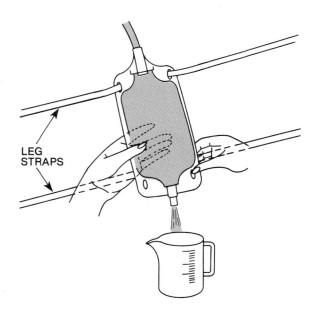

Figure 29-10 Leg drainage bags should be emptied every 2–3 hours.

client care procedure
24: CHANGING THE OSTOMY BAG

purpose

- To keep the client clean.
- To prevent skin breakdown around the stoma.
- To regulate and establish a daily routine for removing wastes.

NOTE: An ostomy bag is sometimes called a stoma bag. It is used for clients who have had a surgical operation called a colostomy, jejeunostomy, or an ileostomy. In these operations, the intestine is cut and brought to the outside of the body. Body wastes are expelled through an opening in the abdomen instead of the rectum. The ostomy bag is placed over the opening to collect the wastes.

Until a client has adjusted to using the ostomy bag there may be strong feelings of embarrassment. The home health aide can help the client accept the inconvenience by being understanding. The aide should not show displeasure in assisting the client. An ostomy bag should be changed daily. It is best to change it at about the same time each day. In some cases, the client wears a gauze pad instead of a bag.

In addition to changing the bag, the client must wash out the intestine. Most clients have been taught at the hospital how to irrigate (wash out) the intestine. An aide may help the client. However, the aide may not do the procedure unless advanced training in the procedure has been learned and state requirements for certification have been met. The bag is changed frequently in the beginning. For colostomies of longer duration, colostomy bag may remain on for as long as 10 days. A gum powder prevents skin breakdown. Older colostomy openings may need irrigation due to constipation that resulted from a lack of fluids and/or bulky foods in the diet.

procedure

1. Gather supplies:
   basin half filled with warm water (may use sink in bathroom)
   clean ostomy bag
   waste bag
   washcloth and towel
   mild soap
   skin ointment (if prescribed)
   4 × 4 gauze pads
2. Wash your hands thoroughly.
3. Gently remove used ostomy bag from the stoma (intestinal opening). Flush contents down toilet. Drop the bag into waste bag.
4. Wash area around stoma using a mild soap, warm water and a soft cloth. Rinse all soap from area and pat it dry with gauze pads. Wipe stoma clean with water and washcloth or wet gauze pad, and pat the area dry.
5. Apply ointment if prescribed. Remove self-stick backing from new ostomy bag.
6. Fit stoma through bag opening, press firmly in place working from the stoma outward. Ostomy bags are sized to fit different size stomas. The nurse or doctor can determine the correct size for the client.
7. Make sure the plastic clip at the bottom of the bag is securely closed. This prevents leakage of fluid.
8. Help client as needed. Dress and transfer the client to a chair or back to bed. Leave the client in a comfortable position.
9. Store unused supplies. Following aseptic procedure, discard waste bag.
10. Wash your hands thoroughly following the procedure.

25: USING OXYGEN SAFELY

purpose

- To check equipment in order to ensure that the client receives oxygen correctly and breathes easier.
- To avoid misuse of oxygen equipment and careless practices which risk causing fires, explosions, or injury.

procedure

1. Check the meter to be sure that there is enough oxygen in the tank being used. If the supply is low, call the supervisor. Bring out the reserve tank if one is stored in the house. Call to order a replacement tank.
2. Wash your hands before beginning the procedure.
3. Fit the oxygen mask or nasal cannula securely for the client, figure 29-11.
4. Check to see that the client has set the flow meter correctly.
5. Check that all safety precautions are being observed.
   - Do not smoke in or near rooms where oxygen is used or stored.
   - Do not use matches, candles, or open flames where oxygen is used or stored.
   - Do not use electrical appliances during oxygen therapy. This includes heating pads, electric razors, televisions or radios.
   - Do not use silk, wool or man-made fabrics as clothes or blankets around a client using oxygen. Only cotton is allowed. The other fabrics could cause static electricity sparks which can cause fires.
   - Do not give alcohol baths while oxygen is in use.
   - Do not allow oil or grease to come in contact with any part of the oxygen equipment.

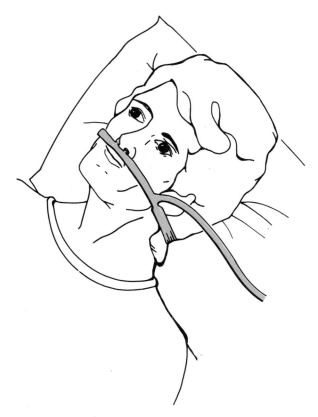

- Check for leakage from valves or connections to tank.
- Do not touch safety valves or devices on oxygen cylinder.
- Instruct client to turn off flow meter before opening the main cylinder valve.
- Instruct the client to open the cylinder valve slowly.

6. Check to be sure there is an adequate water supply for nebulizer or humidification. Humidification means adding moisture to oxygen. Oxygen is dry and can be irritating if used alone. Nebulizer is the name of the mechanism used for adding moisture and medications to the oxygen flow.

7. Wash your hands following the procedure.

Figure 29-11 The home health aide may help the client to properly place the oxygen cannula.

Unit 30

Elimination Needs and Fluid Intake and Output

learning objectives

After studying this unit, you should be able to:
- Demonstrate clear ability to perform all the procedures.
- Explain the purpose of each procedure.
- State when the procedures should and should not be done.
- Identify precautions to be taken for each procedure.
- Record and report results of all procedures.

NOTE: All procedures are not allowed in all states. Make sure you are aware of limits as outlined by state guidelines.

client care procedure

26: ASSISTING WITH THE USE OF THE BEDPAN OR URINAL

purpose

- To provide for routine elimination of bladder and bowel.
- To observe or measure urine or feces output.

NOTE: The bedpan and urinal are used for clients who are confined to bed, figure 30-1.

The bedpan or urinal should be given whenever the client requests it. The client may be undergoing retraining for bowel and bladder habits. The aide should follow a regular schedule of offering the bedpan or urinal. If the client does not remember to ask, the home health aide should offer to bring the bedpan or urinal. The aide can politely remind the client by asking, "Do you need to use the bedpan or urinal?"

A woman client will use the bedpan for both urinating and defecating. A male will need a urinal if he needs to urinate, figure 30-2. Be-

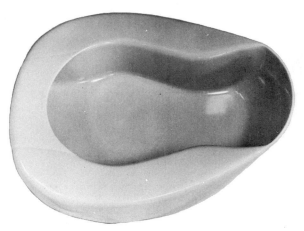

A. A regular bedpan supports the client in a sitting position.

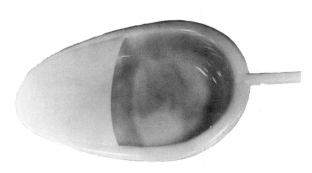

B. A fracture bedpan is most useful for a client who cannot move around in bed easily.

Figure 30-1 The bedpan is used for clients who are confined to bed (courtesy of Durr-Fillauer Medical Inc.).

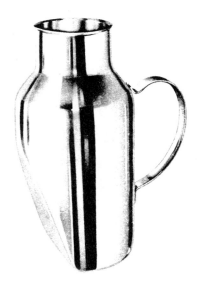

Figure 30-2 A male urinal (courtesy of Caldwell and Hegner, *Health Assistant,* Delmar Publishers, Albany, NY, 1980).

cause it is smaller and of a better shape for urinating, the urinal is preferable to the bedpan for male clients when they need only to urinate. It is also less bother for the aide.

The urinal should be presented with a small amount of water in the bottom, unless output is to be measured or if a urine test is required. As in the case of bedpan presentation, the privacy of the client is of great importance.

procedure

1. Gather equipment and supplies needed:
   bedpan
   toilet tissue
   talcum powder or cornstarch
   newspaper or paper towel (cover)
   basin of warm water
   soap, washcloth, towel
2. Wash hands before beginning the procedure.
3. Provide privacy by closing bedroom door.
4. If a metal bedpan is used, first warm it by running hot water over the rim. Dry the rim and sprinkle it with talcum powder or cornstarch. The powder prevents the

client's buttocks from sticking to the bedpan.

5. Place prepared bedpan near the bed. Put toilet tissue near the client's hand.
6. Fold top blanket and sheet at an angle. Raise the client's gown or lower pajama bottoms.
7. To raise the buttocks, have the client bend knees and push on the heels. As the client lifts, place your hand under the small of the client's back, or you may need to turn the client on the side, then return to the back. The aide holds the bedpan in place when the client is lying on his/her side and then turns the client.
8. Lift gently and slowly with one hand. Slide the bedpan under the hips with the other hand. The client's buttocks should rest on the rounded shelf of the bedpan. The narrow end should face the foot of the bed. If the client cannot assist, turn the client to one side and position the bedpan over the buttocks, figure 30-3. Roll the client onto the bedpan. Make sure the client's head is elevated.
9. Pull sheet over client for added privacy. Make sure the client is as comfortable as possible. An extra pillow under the head may be used.
10. While client is using the bedpan, the aide should prepare a basin of warm water and bring it to the bedside along with soap, a washcloth and towel. These items will be used for handwashing.
11. Remove the bedpan when the client is finished using it. Do not leave the client sitting on the bedpan longer than 5 minutes. Remove the bedpan by having the client bend the knees and push on the heels. Place one hand under small of client's back and lift. Remove the bedpan with the other hand.
12. If possible, have clients wipe themselves. If they are not able to do this, the aide

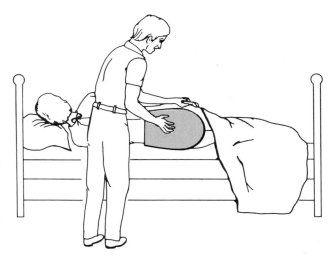

Figure 30-3 The client is rolled away from the aide. The aide's hand is placed on the client's hip and arm for support. With the other hand, the aide places the bedpan over the client's buttocks. The client is then rolled toward the aide onto the bedpan.

must wipe the clients. Discard tissues in the bedpan (unless a specimen is to be taken).
13. Replace the bedclothes. Have clients wash their hands after using the bedpan. Give the client a warm, wet cloth and soap.
14. Take the bedpan to the bathroom and collect specimen (if required). Observe the contents and note if the color or odor seems abnormal.
15. Empty bedpan into toilet. Flush. Fill bedpan with cold water from the tub and empty into the toilet. Clean the bedpan by using warm, soapy water and the toilet bowl brush. Empty water into toilet and flush.
16. Rinse bedpan with warm water and dry with paper towels. Cover and store.
17. Discard paper towels in waste basket or garbage can.
18. Wash your hands well.

27: ASSISTING WITH USE OF THE BEDSIDE COMMODE

purpose

- To provide the client with an opportunity to eliminate body wastes.
- To make the client more comfortable.
- To provide the aide with the opportunity to observe quantity and quality of elimination.

procedure

1. Wash hands before beginning the procedure.
2. Bring the commode to the bedside. Provide toilet paper and other supplies needed.
3. Put a small amount of water in the commode's collection container, unless a specimen is to be collected.
4. Provide privacy.
5. Using proper body mechanics, transfer client from chair or bed to chair commode, figure 30-4.
6. When client has completed elimination, transfer client back to chair or bed.
7. Wash client's hands and make client comfortable.

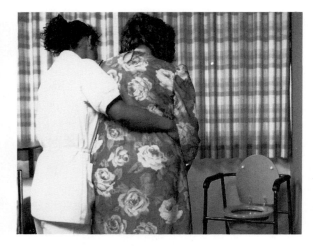

Figure 30-4 Assisting the client to the commode.

8. Take the collection container to bathroom and clean.
9. Wash your hands thoroughly after the procedure.

28: MEASURING FLUID INTAKE AND OUTPUT

purpose

- To keep an accurate record of the amount of fluid the client drinks and excretes.

NOTE: Intake is a measure of all the fluids or semifluids that a person drinks. Output is all the fluid that passes out of the body. The abbreviation for measuring fluid intake and output is I & O. Figure 30-5 shows the fluids that should be included in the measurement of both intake and output.

Measure for Intake	
ice	gelatin
ice chips	any other clear
bouillon	liquids
juices	
water	
coffee	
tea	
milk	
broth	
gruel	

Measure for Output
emesis (vomit)
urine
blood from wound
drainage from wounds
liquid stools

Figure 30-5 Various fluids and substances are measured and recorded as intake and output.

procedure

1. Gather the needed supplies and equipment: record sheet and pen
   1 glass measuring cup or container for intake
   1 large glass measuring container or cup for output
2. Wash hands before beginning procedure.
3. Measure and record all liquids taken by the client. This includes all fluids taken with meals and between meals: coffee, milk, fruit juice, tea, water, soup, etc.
4. Ask the client to use a urinal or bedpan for all voiding. All urine must be collected so that it can be measured.
5. Pour urine from bedpan or urinal into a

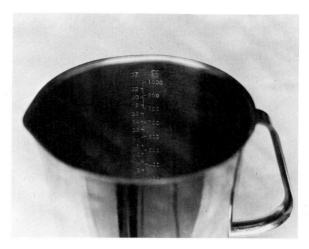

Figure 30-6 This measuring container shows ounces and cubic centimeters on the inside.

COMMON WEIGHTS AND MEASUREMENTS			
1 drop	= .01 ml.	2 Tbsp.	= 30 ml.
15 drops	= 1 ml.	375 ml.	= 1.5 cups
1 tsp.	= 60 drops	500 ml.	= 2 cups
1 tsp.	= 4 ml.	1 liter	= 1000 ml.
1 kg	= 1 liter	1 liter	= 4 cups
1 kg	= 1000 ml	4 liters	= 4000 ml.
1 kg	= 4 cups	4 kg	= 16 cups

ml = millimeter   kg = kilogram

COMMON HOUSEHOLD MEASUREMENTS		
1 tsp.	= ⅛ fl oz or 1 dram	fl = fluid
4 tsp.	= 1 Tbsp	oz = ounce
1 Tbsp	= ½ oz or 4 drams	Tbsp = tablespoon
16 Tbsp	= 1 cup (liquid)	tsp = teaspoon
12 Tbsp	= 1 cup (dry)	lb = pound
1 cup	= 8 fl oz	
1 glass	= 8 fl oz or ½ pint	
16 fl oz	= 1 lb	
1 pint	= 1 lb or 2 cups	
1 quart	= 4 cups	
1 gallon	= 16 cups	

Figure 30-7

measuring cup, figure 30-6 on page 323. Record the amount. (4 cups are equal to 1 quart or 1 liter; 1 liter = 1000 cc or mL; 1 oz = 30 cc or mL), figure 30-7 on page 323.

6. Be sure to explain to the client how to keep exact records, figure 30-8. The client will need to record the fluids at times when the aide is off duty.
7. Clean equipment after each use.
8. Wash hands thoroughly after the procedure.

29: GIVING AN ENEMA OR RECTAL SUPPOSITORY

Many states do not allow home health aides to perform this procedure.

purpose

- To relieve the client of constipation.
- To make the client more comfortable.

DAILY INTAKE AND OUTPUT RECORD   DATE *Apr. 5, 1988*

TIME	INTAKE			OUTPUT	
	LIQUIDS INGESTED	AMOUNT		BODY EXCRETIONS	AMOUNT
7- 8 A.M.	Water	180 cc			
8- 9				Urine	200 cc
9-10	Fruit Juice	90 cc			
10-11					
11-12					
12- 1 P.M.	Coffee	120 cc			
1- 2	Milk	180 cc		Emesis	40 cc
2- 3					
3- 4					
4- 5				Urine	140 cc
5- 6					
6- 7					
7- 8					
8- 9					
9-10					
10-11					
11-12					
12- 1 A.M.					
1- 2					
2- 3					
3- 4					
4- 5					
5- 6					
6- 7					
24 HOUR TOTAL	INTAKE			OUTPUT	
COMMENTS: OBSERVATIONS:	Urine Cloudy				

Figure 30-8 Sample of an Intake and Output record

NOTE: Enemas and suppositories provide temporary relief from constipation. Regular use is not advisable because a dependency or habit can form. In most cases, proper diet and exercise will prevent constipation. Both are needed to stimulate normal bowel activity. However, after abdominal surgery, clients may be constipated. They are afraid to have a bowel movement because of the pain. At these times, the doctor may order an enema, suppository, or laxative. Only a prepackaged enema kit may be used if an enema is given by the home health aide. **Caution:** An enema or rectal suppository may be given only on orders from the doctor.

A rectal suppository softens the stool so that it can be expelled. A suppository is cone-shaped for easy insertion. A rectal suppository can only be inserted by a person who has had special training. A home health aide is seldom authorized to give an enema or rectal suppository to a client in the home. **Caution:** The aide may give an enema or rectal suppository, if authorized, only if instruction on how to do so has been received.

procedure

1. Supplies needed:
   commercial prepackaged enema
   lubricating jelly
   basin of warm water
   protective pad
   bedpan
   toilet paper
   washcloth and towel
   note pad or record and pen
2. Wash hands before beginning the procedure.
3. Provide for the client's comfort and privacy.
4. Have client turn onto the left side. Turn covers back to expose only the buttocks.
5. Slide protective pad under the client.
6. Warm enema in basin of water. Lubricate tip of enema tube, if needed (most commer-

cial prepackaged enema tips are already lubricated).
7. Separate buttocks and insert tip in rectum about 3 inches. Be gentle so as to avoid injuring tender rectal tissues.
8. Slowly squeeze the flexible plastic bottle. This forces the solution to flow evenly into the rectum.
9. Remove enema tip while holding the client's buttocks together. Ask client to retain fluid as long as possible.
10. Position client on bedpan. Remove bedpan after client has expelled feces and enema solution. Clean area around anus and buttocks.
11. Return client to a comfortable position. Remind the client to call if the bedpan is needed again. It may be necessary to leave the protective pad in place until the effects of the enema are complete.
12. Empty contents of bedpan into the toilet and flush the toilet. Make a note of the contents including amount, color, and consistency.
13. Clean bedpan and replace supplies in storage.
14. Wash hands thoroughly following the procedure.

inserting a rectal suppository

1. Before beginning the procedure read the instructions printed on the label of the suppository.
2. Wash your hands and put on disposable gloves before beginning the procedure.
3. Turn the client to one side.
4. Ask the client to place the upper leg over the lower leg so as to expose the rectum. Provide privacy for the client.
5. Remove wrapper from the suppository, lubricate first, then insert the suppository into the client's rectum, figure 30-9.
6. Present bedpan to client (following instruc-

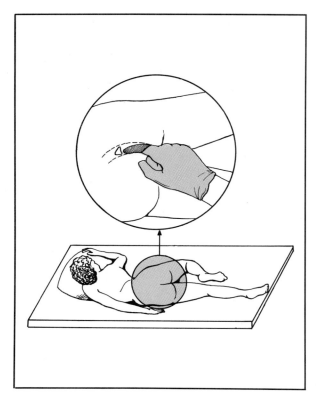

Figure 30-9 Carefully place the rectal suppository into the rectum about 3 inches for adult clients.

tions recommended by product used) or when client requests the bedpan.

7. If client is mobile, assist the client to the bathroom.
8. Observe results of elimination.
9. Record and report results.
10. Wash hands thoroughly after the procedure.

client care procedure

30: BOWEL RETRAINING

purpose

1. To relieve the client of constipation.
2. To make the client more comfortable.

Constipation can result from illness, poor eating habits and/or unhealthy eating habits. Con-

stipation causes the client added discomfort when it occurs in addition to all other physical ailments. Under the instructions of a doctor, nurse, or supervisor, a home health aide can assist the client in a program of bowel retraining.

Older people can become overly "bowel conscious" and have a misconception of what normal elimination should be. The frequency of bowel movements may range from three times a day for one person to only once every two or three days in another. Therefore, the term constipation should not be used to describe a missed movement or two, but only to unusual retention of fecal matter along with infrequent and/or difficult passage of stony, hard stools.

Among the elderly, constipation is very often encountered. If a client is unable to exercise and move about regularly, bowel action becomes sluggish. Sometimes medications used for treating an illness cause constipation. If a client has hemorrhoids, there may be a fear of pain and so the client avoids trying to have a bowel movement.

Untreated constipation can lead to the following symptoms:

- fullness or pressure in the stomach
- gas
- belching
- bad taste in the mouth
- coated tongue
- dizziness
- dull headache
- loss of appetite
- impaction
- development of hemorrhoids, fissures and ulcers.

procedure

1. To provide immediate relief (ONLY IF SO INSTRUCTED) administer a Fleet Enema.
2. Commence a planned diet (AS RECOM-

MENDED BY THE PHYSICIAN OR NUTRITIONAL THERAPIST). Among the foods that can help prevent or overcome constipation are: bran, whole grain cereals, wild rice; broccoli and leafy vegetables such as cabbage, brussels sprouts, spinach, lettuce, turnip greens; fresh, dried or stewed fruits, plums, prunes and figs; olive, corn or safflower oil. In addition to adding the above foods to the daily diet, a client should be encouraged to drink water (unless, for medical reasons, water intake should be limited), perhaps eight or more glasses per day.

3. Set up a regular schedule to have client go to bathroom, or use bedpan or commode. (Of course, this also means that a regular time schedule for eating also be established.) Half an hour after eating is probably the most effective time as bowel activity (gastro-colic reflex) is very slight during the night, but increases dramatically about one-half hour after food is ingested.

   a. Have client go to bathroom at approximately the same time each day (after breakfast, lunch and/or dinner).

   b. Use the same bathroom (this reinforces the habit pattern) and have client remain seated for about 15 minutes to one-half hour. Remind the client to avoid straining. (Follow doctor's instructions as to length of time client should remain on toilet)

   c. If possible have client in a squatting position with thighs pressed against the stomach and the back curved. (Adults with short legs may sit on the toilet seat with both feet resting on a footstool to assist in positioning most effectively).

NOTE: It will take from one to four weeks to retrain and develop regular bowel habits. Most clients will prefer to be alone while using toilet, bedpan or commode. Make sure the client is as comfortable as possible, then give your client privacy. An aide's encouragement is an important part of this daily routine. When the client is relaxed and reassured about the importance of this procedure, he or she will be more cooperative.

Unit 31

Collecting and Testing Specimens

learning objectives

After studying this unit, you should be able to:

- Demonstrate clear ability to perform all the procedures.
- Explain the purpose of each procedure.
- State when the procedures should and should not be done.
- Identify precautions to be taken for each procedure.
- Recognize abnormal conditions.
- Record and report observations.

NOTE: All procedures are not allowed in all states. Make sure you are aware of limits as outlined by state guidelines.

client care procedure

31: COLLECTING A STOOL SPECIMEN

purpose

- To provide stool sample for a diagnostic test of the client's condition.
- To monitor the client's ongoing condition.

NOTE: Some stool specimens must be examined immediately. In other cases, the specimen must be kept cold or frozen. The supervisor or doctor will give specific instructions depending upon the tests which must be made.

procedure

1. In bathroom set out:
   specimen container or clean, small jar tight-fitting lid
   tongue blades or plastic spoon
2. Wash hands before beginning the procedure.
3. If possible, offer the bedpan at a time when the client usually has a bowel movement.
4. Give the client the bedpan following regular bedpan procedure. However, ask the client not to urinate after moving the bowels. Do not contaminate the specimen with toilet paper.

5. Cover bedpan and take it to the bathroom, figure 31-1.
6. Using tongue blades or spoon, place small amount of stool into a clean jar or specimen container, figure 31-2. Cover tightly. Discard the spoon or tongue blade.
7. Wash your hands well.
8. Follow the nurse's instructions regarding storing and labeling the specimen.
9. Clean all equipment and supplies. Return them to the proper storage place.
10. Make sure the client is clean and comfortable.

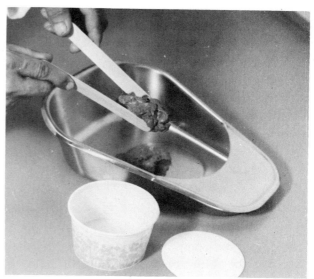

Figure 31-2 Use tongue blades to transfer the stool specimen from the bedpan to the specimen container (courtesy of Louise Simmers, *Diversified Health Occupations,* Delmar Publishers, Albany, NY; 1983).

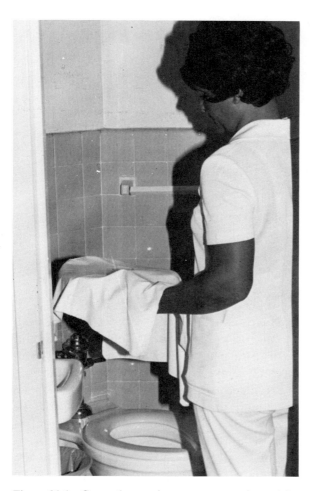

Figure 31-1 Cover the specimen to prevent air particles from settling on it and contaminating it.

client care procedure

32: COLLECTING URINE SPECIMENS

purpose

- To provide a urine sample for a diagnostic test.
- To monitor the client's ongoing condition.

NOTE: A clean catch specimen is sometimes requested in order to obtain a urine sample that is relatively free of contamination. It is very important that the specimen not become contaminated.

procedure

1. Gather the needed supplies and bring them into the bathroom:
   measuring container or graduate
   specimen container or clean, small jar with tight-fitting cap
   bedpan or urinal

2. Obtain a clean bedpan or urinal. If it is not clean, use soap and water to wash it out. Rinse and dry it well.

3. Wash hands before beginning the procedure.

4. Offer the client the bedpan or urinal. If possible, choose a time which is convenient for the client.

5. Instruct the female client not to deposit any toilet paper in the bedpan after use. The paper would contaminate the specimen.

6. Give the client privacy.

7. After the client voids, assist the client back into a comfortable position.

8. Take the urinal or bedpan into the bathroom. If the client's intake and output are being measured, pour urine from the bedpan into a measuring container, figure 31-3. Measure the amount of urine and record the amount on the chart.

9. Pour a small amount, about 2 ounces (60 cc) into a clean jar or specimen container. Tightly cover the container.

10. Make sure the specimen is properly labeled with the name of the client, the date, the time, and the doctor's name. Also note if the specimen was voided or is a catheter specimen.

11. Clean and replace supplies and equipment.

12. Wash your hands well.

13. Follow instructions of the supervisor or doctor in taking the specimens to be examined. Most urine specimens should be kept cool after they are collected.

clean catch specimen

1. Wash hands before beginning the procedure.

2. Wash the client's genital area, or have the client do so, if able. It is especially important for the urinary opening to be cleansed.

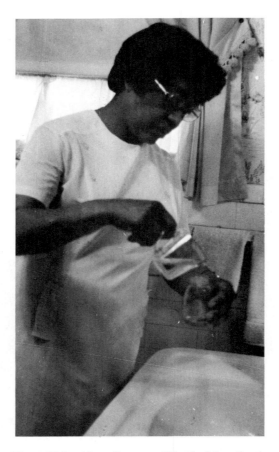

Figure 31-3 About 2 ounces (60 cc) of the client's urine should be poured into a clean jar or specimen container.

3. Give the client a labeled specimen container.

4. Explain the procedure to the client.

5. Have the client begin to void into the bedpan, urinal, or toilet. After a small amount of urine has been voided, have the client catch some of the urine in midstream in a sterilized specimen container. When enough urine has been obtained for the specimen, the client can resume voiding into the bedpan, urinal, or toilet.

6. Immediately place the sterile cap on the container so the specimen will not become contaminated.

7. Both the client's hands and the aide's hands should be thoroughly washed following the procedure.

client care procedure

33: TESTING URINE FOR SUGAR AND ACETONE

purpose

- To measure the sugar and acetone content of the client's urine.
- To routinely check the diabetic client's use of carbohydrates and prevent emergencies such as diabetic coma and insulin shock.
- To check the health status of expectant mothers.

NOTE: All diabetics must remain on a strict diabetic diet. In addition, many take prescribed medication. A daily record of urine tests shows whether the diet and medication are controlling the disease. **Caution:** A sudden change in the sugar and acetone test results should be reported to the supervisor or doctor at once.

There are several commercial testing kits in use. The instructions are clearly written on the label. Usually a diabetic client does the urine testing. However, a home health aide should check the results. Provide the client with specimen jars or containers and testing kits. If the client is blind, or otherwise disabled, the home health aide will be fully responsible for carrying out the tests.

procedure

1. Set up a schedule for testing the urine. The doctor decides how often testing is necessary. Discuss the schedule with the client. These tests are usually made four times a day (q.i.d.).
2. When a client needs assistance, obtain testing kits, and a bedpan or urinal. Begin by using the same procedure described for collecting a routine urine specimen.
3. Wash hands before beginning the procedures and after completing the procedures.
4. Record results of tests on a chart such as the one shown in figure 31-4.

testing for sugar

1. To test the urine for sugar, obtain a bottle of labeled Clinitest tablets. Check the expiration date. Do not use if it is past the date. Read the label carefully for instructions. **Caution:** Do not touch the tablets with the fingers as burns can occur.
2. Carefully follow the directions on the package. Wait for the tablet to dissolve in the urine-water solution. Compare the color of the solution with the color chart. Sugar is recorded as negative, trace, 1+, 2+, 3+, or 4+. The color on the chart begins with blue, meaning negative. The highest sugar level, 4+, is bright orange. This may also be recorded as a percentage.
3. If Tes-tape is used to test for sugar, the color

Date: 10/24/88				
Time	7:30	11:30	4:30	8:30
Sugar	neg.	1+	trace	
Acetone	neg.	neg.	neg.	

Figure 31-4 Sample chart used to record results of urine testing for acetone and sugar.

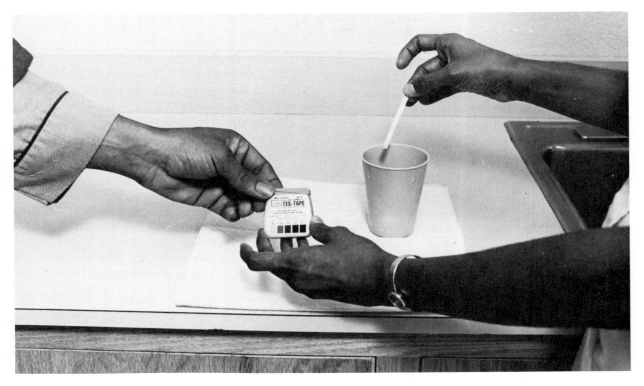

Figure 31-5 To check the presence of sugar in the urine with Tes-tape, compare the color of the urine-soaked tape against the color guide.

of the urine-soaked tape is compared against the color guide, figure 31-5.

4. Record the results of the test.

testing for acetone

1. To test the urine for acetone, obtain a bottle of labeled Acetest tablets. Read the instructions on the label carefully. **Caution:** Do not touch the tablets with the hand as burns can easily occur, figure 31-6. Check the expiration date. If it has expired, do not use.

2. Carefully follow the directions for testing on the package. Compare the color of the Acetest tablet with the color chart, figure 31-7. Acetone is recorded as negative (no change), small (pink), moderate (light purple) or large (dark purple).

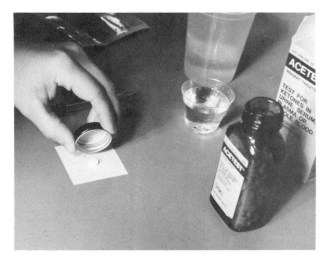

Figure 31-6 Shake one tablet into the bottle cap to avoid possible burn. Do not touch the Acetest tablets (courtesy of Louise Simmers, *Diversified Health Occupations,* Delmar Publishers, Albany, NY, 1983).

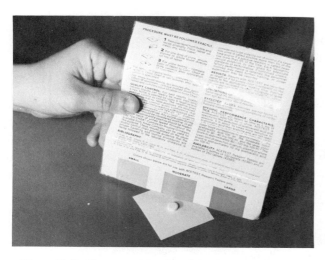

Figure 31-7 Compare the color of the Acetest tablet with the color chart (courtesy of Louise Simmers, *Diversified Health Occupations,* Delmar Publishers, Albany, NY, 1983).

3. Record test results as soon as test is completed.

4. If Tes-tape is used to test for acetone, the color of the urine-soaked tape is compared against the color guide.

5. Make sure the testing materials are properly stored in an air-tight container. Tablets are ruined when exposed to the air for even a moderate length of time.

6. Check the expiration date on the testing materials. If materials bear a date that is before the date on which the test is done, the results may be invalid (incorrect).

7. Report to the supervisor or doctor at once if there is a sudden change in the test results.

8. Report to supervisor or family member if the supply of testing materials is low.

Unit 32
Bedmaking

learning objectives

After studying this unit, you should be able to:
- Make an occupied bed with reasonable speed causing the client as little discomfort and inconvenience as possible.
- Follow safety rules for the client.
- Follow rules of proper body mechanics.
- Properly make an unoccupied bed.

NOTE: All procedures are not allowed in all states. Make sure you are aware of limits as outlined by state guidelines.

client care procedure

34: *MAKING AN OCCUPIED BED*

purpose

- To change the bed linens while the client lies in the bed.
- To add to the client's comfort by removing wrinkled or soiled sheets.

NOTE: When handling the bedclothes, the home health aide should avoid quick and rough movements. The soiled linens may contain pathogens which could be spread by such movements. **Caution:** Soiled linens must always be held away from the aide's body. Never place soiled linens on the floor. Insert them in a pillow case and place them on a chair.

The home health aide should also be constantly alert to the client's safety. A fall from bed could injure the client. The aide should be as gentle as possible with the client during the bedmaking procedure.

procedure

1. Bring to bedside:
   2 clean sheets
   1 clean pillow case for each pillow
   2 straight chairs
   laundry hamper
   Chux, if the client is incontinent

2. Wash hands before beginning the procedure.
3. Provide the client's privacy by closing the bedroom door.
4. Place fresh linens conveniently in order of use.
5. Loosen bedding from under mattress by lifting the mattress with one hand as you pull out bedding with the other hand.
6. Remove covers one at a time, folding each to the foot of the bed.
7. Leave top sheet covering the client to prevent a chill and embarrassment.
8. Place the two straight chairs against one side of the bed. This helps protect the client from falling out of bed. If the bed has siderails this is not necessary. Simply raise the siderail on the opposite side of the bed.

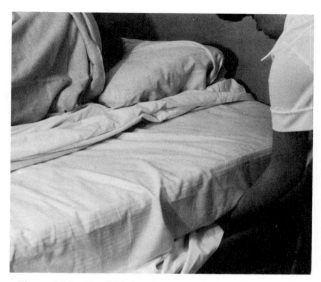

Figure 32-2 Fanfold the clean top sheet at the center of the bed. Make a mitered corner and tuck the sheet in place from the head to the foot of the bed (courtesy of Louise Simmers, *Diversified Health Occupations,* Delmar Publishers, Albany, NY, 1983).

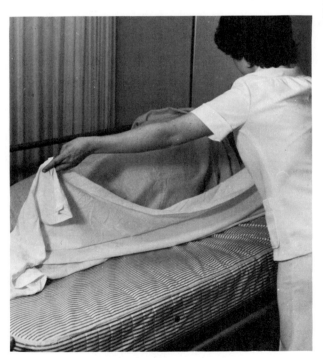

Figure 32-1 The soiled bottom sheet is rolled or fanfolded to the center of the bed close to the client (courtesy of Louise Simmers, *Diversified Health Occupations,* Delmar Publishers, Albany, NY, 1983).

9. Assist the client to turn on the side facing the chairs or siderail. Assist the client to move near the edge of the bed by the chairs. Stand at the other side of the bed.
10. Roll or fanfold (fold in pleats) the soiled bottom sheet to the center of the bed beside the client's back, figure 32-1.
11. Fold the clean bottom sheet lengthwise and place the fold at the center of the bed. Fanfold half of the clean sheet next to the soiled sheet. Tuck the other half under the mattress. Make a mitered corner at the top. Tuck from the top or head of bed and move toward the foot of the bed, figure 32-2.
12. Help client turn toward you onto the clean sheet. Bring the chairs to the other side of the bed for the client's protection (or raise the siderail).
13. Go to the other side of the bed and remove soiled sheet. Drop it into clothes hamper.
14. Pull clean sheet across bed and tuck under mattress. Miter corner at top and tuck

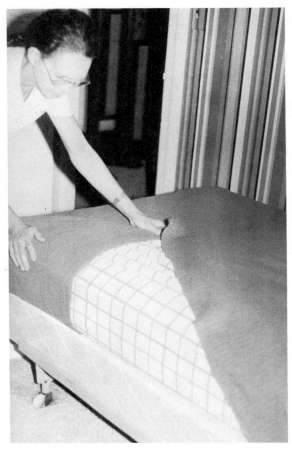

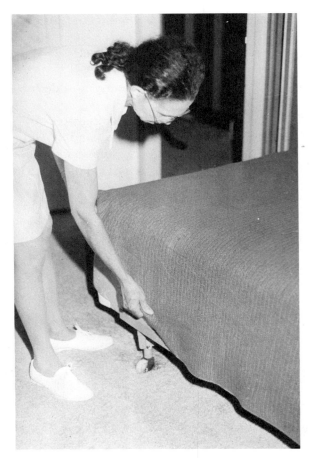

A. Fold up the corner to form a right angle.   **B. A pleasing slant forms at the corner of the bed.**

Figure 32-3   Mitering a corner.

along side from head to foot of bed. Make certain the sheet is tight and wrinkle free.

15. Turn client onto the back in center of the bed. Place clean top sheet over soiled top sheet. Slide the soiled sheet out from under the clean sheet. Have client hold fresh top sheet in place.
16. Drop soiled sheet into hamper.
17. Unfold blankets and replace over top sheet.
18. Tuck in the bottoms of the sheet and blankets (or spread) at the foot of the bed. Miter the two corners, figure 32-3. Leave plenty of room for foot and toe movement.
19. Change the pillow cases and replace pil-

lows under client's head. Put soiled cases in hamper.
20. Return supplies to storage area.
21. Be sure client is comfortable and that the room is neat.
22. Wash your hands following the procedure.

client care procedure

35: MAKING AN UNOCCUPIED BED

purpose

- To air the bed and bedding.
- To add to the client's comfort by removing wrinkled or soiled sheets.

NOTE: If fitted sheets are used, the aide should follow the same general procedure for making the bed, completing one side of the bed entirely before moving to the opposite side. The bottom fitted sheet will have four fitted corners which conform to the shape of the mattress. A top fitted sheet is fitted only on one end; the fitted portion should always be placed at the bottom of the bed. As with regular sheets, the bed linen should be free of all wrinkles.

procedure

1. Bring to the bedside:
   clean top and bottom sheets
   clean pillowcases
   protective pad (if needed)
   laundry hamper
2. Wash hands before beginning procedure.
3. Place linen in order of use near the bed.
4. Strip the bed completely and let it air. Fold blankets and put them nearby. Remove sheets gently so as to avoid spreading pathogens. Hold them at arm's length while gathering them and place them in the hamper provided. Remove pillowcases and place in hamper.
5. Put clean bottom sheet on bed. Unfold the sheet lengthwise with the long fold at the center of the bed. Place lower hemline even with the bottom of the mattress.
6. Open sheet gently; do not shake it. Starting at the head of the bed, miter the corner and tuck in that side of the sheet. A great deal of time is saved by working on only one side of the bed at a time.
7. Place the top sheet over the clean bottom sheet wrong side up. Place the wide hem even with the top edge of the mattress, figure 32-4. Place the center fold at the center of the bed.

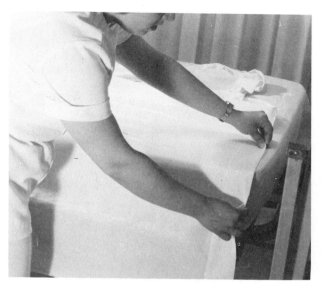

Figure 32-4 Place the top sheet over the clean bottom sheet, wrong side up. Place the wide hem even with the top edge of the mattress (courtesy of Louise Simmers, *Diversified Health Occupations*, Delmar Publishers, Albany, NY, 1983).

8. Place the blankets back on the bed. Put the top edge 12 inches from the top of the mattress.
9. Tuck the blankets and top sheet under the bottom of the mattress. Miter the corners. Fold top sheet over top edge of blankets.
10. Walk to opposite side of bed and repeat steps 6–9.
11. Holding top of sheet and blanket, pull them back toward the foot of the bed. Fanfold as you go.
12. Put fresh cases on pillows. (Replace pillows on bed if needed.)
13. Take soiled linens to bathroom or laundry. Tidy client's room.
14. Wash your hands following the procedure.

Unit 33
Hot and Cold Applications

learning objectives

After studying this unit, you should be able to:
— Demonstrate clear ability to perform all procedures.
— Explain the purpose of each procedure.
— State when the procedures should and should not be done.
— Identify precautions to be taken for each procedure.
— Recognize signs of client discomfort.
— Follow all rules of client safety when doing the procedures.

NOTE: All procedures are not allowed in all states. Make sure you are aware of limits as outlined by state guidelines.

client care procedure

36: APPLYING THE ICE BAG, CAP, OR COLLAR

purpose

~se pain and decrease swelling of local-

is such as an ice bag,
NOT be applied with-
The supervisor will tell
ly ice and how to do it.
ations must be covered

with a cloth. Never apply ice or the cap, bag or collar directly to the skin. A towel, face cloth or fitted cover should be used against the skin. **Caution:** Elderly persons may sustain tissue injury if hot and cold applications are improperly used.

procedure

1. Wash your hands before beginning the procedure.
2. Fill an icebag, cap or collar with ice cubes or crushed ice. Use a spoon to transfer the ice. Fill the container half full so that its

Care Services

weight will not be uncomfortable for the client, figure 33-1.

3. Place the bag on a flat surface with the top in place but not tightened. Hold the neck of the bag upright. Gently press the bag from the bottom to the opening in order to expel the air.

4. Secure lid firmly and wipe dry with paper towels. Periodically test for leakage.

5. Wrap ice bag in towel or soft cloth. Covering it protects the client's skin from direct contact.

6. Apply to affected body area. Make sure that any metal parts face away from the skin. Place an extra towel around the bag if the skin appears sensitive to the cold.

7. Check the client's skin every 5 minutes. Look for signs of redness, whiteness or cyanosis (blue color). If these signs appear, call the supervisor for instructions.

8. If ice melts, replace with fresh ice and continue treatment.

9. Remove ice bag after 20 minutes unless the doctor or supervisor orders differently.

10. Empty bag, allow it to dry. Store it properly.

11. Return client to a comfortable position.
12. Wash your hands following the procedure.

37: APPLYING THE HOT WATER BAG

purpose

- To increase circulation to a body area.
- To relax tension and relieve pain in a small area.

procedure

1. Wash your hands before beginning the procedure.

2. Run water from the faucet and test the temperature, figure 33-2. Test with a bath thermometer or place a few drops on the inside of the wrist. It should be about 120°–130°F (49°–55°C). On the wrist this feels warm but not scalding hot.

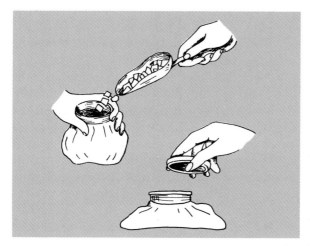

Figure 33-1 An ice bag should be half filled so it can lie flat against the client's body and not cause discomfort due to its weight.

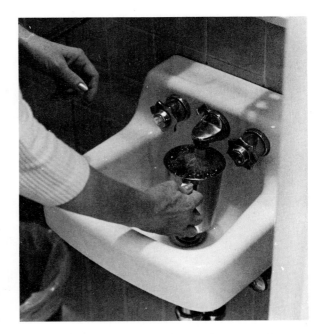

Figure 33-2 Some aides prefer to collect water in a graduate pitcher before testing it for temperature.

3. Fill the hot water bag ⅓ or ½ full.
4. Lay the hot water bag on a flat surface, holding the neck of the bag upright. Cap should be in place but not tight. Press the bag gently from the bottom to the opening to expel the air.
5. Secure cap firmly and wipe outside of bag with paper towels. Check for leaks.
6. Wrap bag with a towel or small pillowcase to keep client's skin from direct contact with the hot water bag. **Caution:** Direct contact can cause burns.
7. Take the client's temperature, pulse and respiration before applying the hot water bag to the affected area. Record the signs on the client's chart.
8. Continue to check the client's skin for redness every 15 minutes. Redness indicates that the skin may be irritated from the heat. Record any observations and note the time.
9. Refill the bag with warm water as often as needed. Remove bag after the prescribed time. Follow the instructions of the supervisor.
10. Remove water from the bag and hang it up until moisture evaporates.
11. Reposition client comfortably.
12. Wash your hands following the procedure.
13. Store the bag, making sure to leave some air inside so the sides won't stick together and ruin the bag. Store other supplies.

client care procedure

38: APPLYING THE HEATING PAD

purpose

- To reduce pain in a small area.
- To stimulate circulation to an area.

NOTE: The electric heating pad produces dry heat. The temperature is controlled by a thermostat so the temperature remains even or constant. **Caution:** A heating pad is never used together with a moist dressing. Water and electricity are a dangerous combination.

A heating pad should be used only if ordered by the supervising nurse. Never use it on an unconscious client. The client must be able to tell the aide if the pad is too hot. A client should be warned not to lie on the pad directly. The heating pad should be removed while the client sleeps because of the possible danger of burns. Rarely used by diabetic clients.

procedure

1. Gather supplies:
heating pad
heating pad cover
2. Wash your hands before beginning the procedure.
3. Connect heating pad to electrical outlet near the bed. Turn switch to high and test for proper operation.
4. Turn thermostat to the heat level ordered by the doctor (usually medium or low).
5. Place a cover over the pad. A towel or light blanket can be used.
6. Place the pad on the area which needs the heat treatment.
7. Note the time, and be sure to observe the client's skin often. Check the order for time of use, usually 20–30 minutes, three times a day. If client is uncomfortable or if the skin becomes reddened, lower heat at once. Avoid burning the skin.
8. Remove the pad when the therapy time is completed. Return pad and cover to storage area.
9. Record any changes in the skin condition. Note the client's reaction to the treatment.
10. Wash your hands following the procedure.

39: APPLYING HOT AND COLD MOIST DRESSINGS

purpose

HOT
- To stimulate circulation
- To reduce pain
- To loosen crust around area

COLD
- To reduce circulation
- To reduce pain
- To reduce swelling

NOTE: There are moist heat electric pads now on the market which can be used instead of the moist dressings described here. Instructions must be followed carefully to avoid burns.

Hot or cold moist dressings must be ordered by the doctor. Dressings are not applied by the aide when there is an open or draining wound. Open wounds that are draining require a sterile dressing. This is applied by a nurse or doctor. A home health aide will be instructed by the doctor or supervisor as to the type of moist dressing needed. Instructions are given as to the length of time the dressing should be kept in place.

Heat dilates the blood vessels. This enlarging increases the blood supply to the treated area. Body metabolism is increased and pus forms more quickly. The tissues of the skin relax, and pain is relieved. Each client reacts differently to heat. Some clients are extremely sensitive to heat and must be watched carefully to avoid burning the skin. Cold constricts or tightens the blood vessels. Cold can relieve pain by lowering the temperature of the surrounding skin. Cold also reduces swelling.

procedure

1. Bring to bedside:
   basin of water at correct temperature
   dressing or small towel
   covering cloth or bandage
   towel or bed protector
   prescribed medication (if ordered)
   bag for waste
   If dressings are to be kept wet, also include:
   four-ounce measuring cup
   hot water bottle or ice bag
2. Wash your hands before beginning the procedure.
3. Prepare a basin of water at the correct temperature. Water for hot dressings should be about 115°F (46°C). Water for cold dressings is cooled by adding ice cubes, figure 33-3. If ordered, add medication to the water.
4. Expose area to be dressed. Place a towel or plastic sheet under the area to protect the bed from becoming wet.
5. Moisten the dressing and squeeze out excess water. Place it on the client's body.
6. Fasten dressing in place with bandage or cloth and pins. Position the client comfortably.

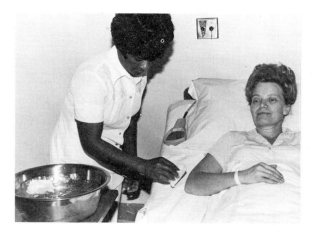

Figure 33-3 Ice cubes in water keep it cold for the application of cold moist dressings.

7. If dressings are to be kept hot, a filled hot water bag may be placed over the dressing, or small amounts of warm water may be poured on dressing. For cold dressings, an ice bag may be placed over the moist dressing.

8. Remove dressing at the prescribed time. Drop used dressing into waste bag. Return supplies to storage area.
9. Return client to comfortable position.
10. Wash your hands thoroughly following the procedure.

Unit 34
Support, Exercise, and Locomotion

learning objectives

After studying this unit, you should be able to:
- Demonstrate clear ability to perform all procedures.
- Explain the purpose of each procedure.
- State when the procedures should and should not be done.
- Identify precautions to be taken for each procedure.
- Use proper body mechanics for both client and aide during each procedure.
- Follow all rules of client safety when doing the procedures.

NOTE: All procedures are not allowed in all states. Make sure you are aware of limits as outlined by state guidelines.

client care procedure

40: APPLYING BINDERS AND OTHER SUPPORTS

purpose

- To provide support and comfort after surgery, accident, or childbirth.
- To hold dressings in place.

NOTE: A binder is a wide piece of heavy cotton or flannelette. It is used to give support and relief from pain. Ace bandages and elastic stockings are also used for this purpose. Binders in common use are the straight binder; the scultetus (many-tailed) binder; the single T-binder; the double T-binder, and the breast binder, figure 34-1.

applying a scultetus binder

procedure

1. Gather materials needed:
   scultetus binder
   2 safety pins, if needed

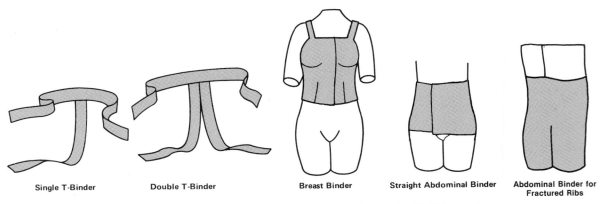

Single T-Binder   Double T-Binder   Breast Binder   Straight Abdominal Binder   Abdominal Binder for Fractured Ribs

Figure 34-1 Types of binders; most binders are fastened with Velcro tabs.

2. Wash your hands before beginning the procedure.
3. The binder should be put on just before the client gets out of bed in the morning.
4. Fold top sheet to pubic area; lift gown to chest area.
5. Have client bend knees and push on heels to lift hips off bed.
6. Slide binder in place, making sure that the lower end of the binder is at the base of the spine.

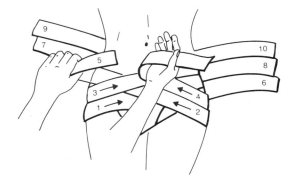

Figure 34-2 Tails of the scultetus binder are alternately crossed over the abdomen beginning at the bottom and working toward the top. The aide must make sure the completed binder is smooth and wrinkle free.

7. Straighten all the straps on each side of the client. Starting at the bottom, bring straps over abdomen one at a time, figure 34-2. First from one side and then the other—right strap, left strap, right strap, etc.
8. Cross each of the last two straps diagonally from top to bottom. If the binder does not have Velcro tabs, secure with safety pins. Check to be sure bandage is not too tight.
9. Return client to a comfortable position in bed or help client out of bed.
10. Wash your hands following the procedure.

applying elastic stockings

purpose

- To help prevent blood clots in immobilized clients.
- To help prevent pooling of blood in the lower extremities.
- To provide support and comfort for the client.

NOTE: There must be a doctor's order for elastic stockings. The client must be measured by a nurse or doctor for proper size of stockings. Stockings should be removed only for a bath and according to the doctor's orders.

procedure

1. Wash your hands before beginning the procedure.
2. Have the client lie down while stockings are being put on.
3. Turn stocking inside out to heel by placing your hand inside stocking and grasping heel.
4. Position stocking over foot and heel of client, making sure the heel is properly placed.
5. Pull stocking up smoothly over calf and ankle. Avoid wrinkles which will constrict the area.
6. Pull stocking over knee and thigh. If stocking has gusset (double thick area) this should be on the inside of the thigh (over the femoral artery).
7. Pull toe of stocking forward for comfort. Smooth hands over stockings to ensure that there are no wrinkles, figure 34-3.
8. Wash your hands following the procedure.

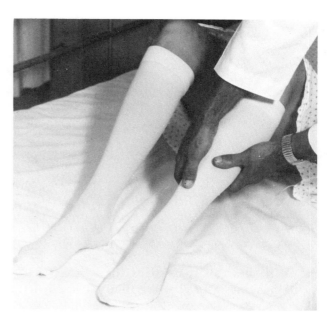

Figure 34-3 Use both hands to smooth the elastic stockings into place (courtesy of Louise Simmers, *Diversified Health Occupations*, Delmar Publishers, Albany, NY, 1983).

client care procedure

41: MOVING A CLIENT UP IN BED

purpose

- To provide for client comfort.
- To relieve pressure on body parts.
- To avoid promoting poor posture.

NOTE: Very often a client will slide down into the bed away from the headboard. This is uncomfortable for the client. The sheets become wrinkled and undue pressure may be placed on the bony prominences allowing the formation of decubitus ulcers.

procedure

1. Wash your hands before beginning the procedure.
2. Tell the client what you are going to do before you do it.
3. Stand with one foot ahead of the other foot. Bend your knees and place one knee securely against the bed.
4. Slide one arm under the client's shoulders and the other arm under the client's back. The client's head should be in the bend of your arm at the elbow.
5. If client is able, have the client bend the knees and place the feet firmly on the bed.
6. Have the client push against the bed with both feet as you slide the client toward the head of the bed. Use good body mechanics and shift your weight from the rear leg to the forward leg as you move the client.
7. Wash your hands following the procedure.

assisting the client to move up in bed

1. If the client is able, have the client grasp the headboard by reaching up and behind. This allows the client to pull the body up

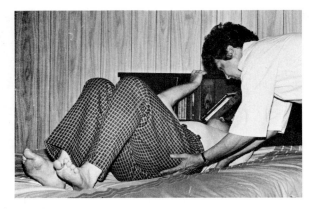

Figure 34-4 The client can assist in moving up in bed by pushing heels into the bed and pulling with the arms.

to the head of the bed as the aide assists by pushing, lifting, and pulling. The client can also push upwards by placing the heels on the bed and pulling with the arms, figure 34-4.

2. When assisting the client, straighten out the bottom sheet. If the client is using pillows, fluff them up and reposition the client comfortably.
3. Wash your hands following the procedure.

client care procedure

42: ASSISTING THE CLIENT TO SIT UP IN BED

purpose

- To make the client more comfortable.
- To change the client's position to improve circulation.
- To change the position so the client can engage in activities such as eating, reading, watching television, etc.

NOTE: If the client is weak or very elderly, the sitting position may be hard for the client to maintain. Supporting the client with pillows may help the client maintain the sitting position.

procedure

1. Wash your hands before beginning the procedure.
2. Tell the client what you are going to do.
3. Face the head of the bed while standing at the side of the bed.
4. Position the leg farthest from the bed ahead of the leg nearest the bed.
5. Place you right hand under the client's right arm at the shoulder and grasp the back of the client's upper arm.
6. Place your left arm under the client's shoulders.
7. Tell the client to hold on to the back of your right upper arm.
8. With your knees bent, move the client to a sitting position.
9. Support the client with pillows to help maintain the sitting position. **Caution:** If the client is weak, stay with the client to be sure the client does not slump or fall.
10. Wash your hands following the procedure.

client care procedure

43: ASSISTING WITH RANGE OF MOTION EXERCISES

purpose

- To increase muscle tone in the client's body.
- To restore function to injured parts of body.
- To avoid permanent disability of client's body.

NOTE: Clients who are ill or disabled may need help in order to maintain or develop muscle tone. After a mastectomy, for example, range of motion (ROM) arm exercises are usually prescribed by the doctor. Many times accident victims must relearn the art of walking. Unconscious clients are unable to exercise their bodies. These clients can be helped by ROM exercises. Each client will be evaluated by the physical therapist before leaving the hospital.

The recommended exercises must be approved by the doctor. These exercises should be carried out on a regular basis. Range of motion exercises not only restore muscle tone, but also maintain good blood circulation. Good circulation to the skin helps stop the formation of decubitus ulcers.

Active range of motion (ROM) exercises are those in which the client exerts effort. Passive ROM exercises may only be done by a registered physical therapist, a nurse or a doctor. If these exercises are not done properly, the client can be harmed. Passive ROM exercises are those in which the client exerts little or no effort, and motions are made largely by the assistant. Active ROM may be carried out by the home health aide following instructions of the supervisor. **Caution:** Joints are always supported during any ROM exercise.

procedure

1. Wash your hands before beginning the procedure.
2. Assist the client into a back-lying position (supine).

3. Exercise the shoulder.
   - Raise the arm above the head keeping the elbow straight, figure 34-5A.
   - Bring the arm out to the side. Turn the palm up and bend the elbow, figure 34-5B. Raise the bended arm above the head.
   - Bring the arm out to the side. Bend the elbow and rest it on the mattress. Raise and lower the forearm.
4. Exercise the elbow.
   - Bend the elbow, keeping the arm close to the body. Bring the fingers to touch the shoulder. Lower the fingers to touch the bed.
5. Exercise the forearm.
   - Bring the arm out to the side. Rest it on the bed. Take the client's hand and rotate the arm, palm up and palm down.
6. Exercise the wrist and fingers.
   - Take the client's hand and move the hand forward and back. Move the hand side to side.
   - Curl the client's fingers and straighten them. Spread the fingers apart and rotate the thumb.

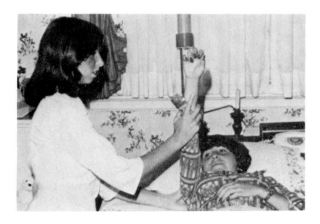

A. Keeping the client's arm straight, raise the arm above the client's head.

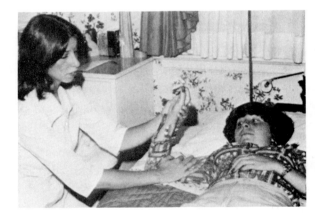

B. With the elbow bent at a right angle, move the forearm toward the client's head and back down toward the client's leg.

Figure 34-5 Range of motion exercises of the arm benefit the shoulder.

7. Exercise the knee and hip while the client is lying on the back.
    - Bend the knee and raise it to the chest.
    - Bring the leg out to the side and back, figure 34-6A.
    - Cross one leg over the other leg.
    - Allow the leg to rest on the bed with the knee straight and the heel resting on the bed. Rotate the leg inward and outward.
    - Raise and lower the leg, keeping the knee straight, figure 34-6B.
8. Exercise the feet.
    - Curl the toes and straighten them.
    - Move the foot back and forward.
    - Rotate the foot inward and outward.
9. Turn the client over to a face down position (prone).

10. Raise the arm, keeping the elbow straight.
11. Raise the leg, keeping the knee straight.
12. Bend the knee, bringing the heel toward the buttocks.
13. Return the client to a comfortable position.
14. Wash your hands following the procedure.

client care procedure

44: ASSISTING WITH THE USE OF CRUTCHES, WALKERS, OR CANES

purpose

- To provide support and maintain balance as client walks.

NOTE: There are three basic walking patterns. With a nonweight-bearing pattern, all the

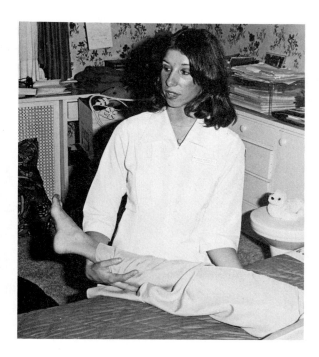

A. Swing the leg out to the side to exercise the hip as well as the leg.

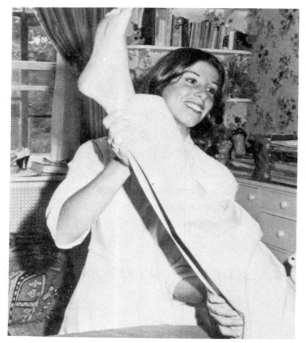

B. Support and raise the leg slowly to prevent straining the client's leg muscles.

Figure 34-6 Range of motion exercises for the hip and leg muscles

weight is placed on the arms and uninvolved leg. Partial weight-bearing means that minimal weight is placed on the toes or forefoot. However, most weight is still on the arms and the uninvolved leg. With a full weight-bearing pattern, full weight is placed on both legs, but a cane is used for balance.

To walk in a nonweight-bearing pattern, the client uses crutches. The doctor or therapist measures the client to select the correct length of crutches. Usually a therapist teaches the client how to walk with them.

To walk in a partial weight-bearing pattern, the client can use crutches but often uses a walker, figure 34-7. The walker is a curved metal frame with four legs. It is a walking aid which gives maximum stability as the client moves. The client steps or hops forward while holding the walker.

A cane is used when the client is strong enough to bear full weight on both legs, figure 34-8. A standard cane should not be used as a weight-bearing aid. A special cane with four

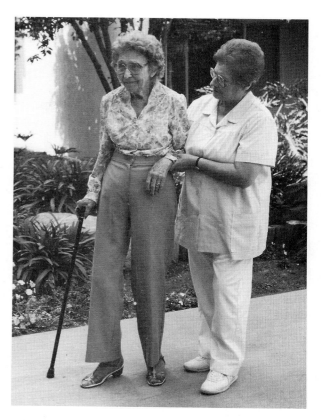

Figure 34-8   Assisting the client using a cane. Mild exercise out of doors is good therapy.

short legs is designed to bear a small amount of weight only. A cane is primarily used for balance. Check rubber tips on all canes, walkers, and crutches to ensure that the tip is firmly attached and that it is not worn down.

procedure

1. Always wash your hands before any client contact.
2. Always walk on the client's weak side. If the client's left leg is fractured, the aide should walk on the client's left side.
3. Walk slightly behind the client. This is a safety measure in case the client should start to fall.
4. For the client using crutches, hold onto the client's belt if the client feels uncomfortable

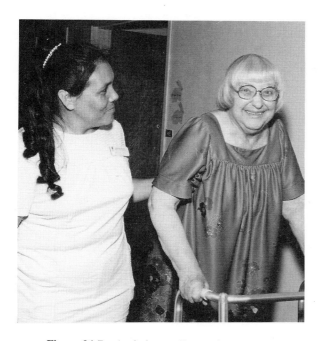

Figure 34-7   Assisting a client using a walker

using the crutches. This often gives the client more confidence. Move forward with the client. Never pull the client backward.

5. For the client using a walker, instruct the client to place the walker firmly before walking. If the client is strong enough, the walker and the weaker leg can be moved forward at the same time.

6. For the client using a cane, instruct the client to hold the cane in the hand opposite the weaker leg, figure 34-9A. If the right ankle has been injured, the client should hold the cane in the left hand.

7. Balance is a judgmental situation. If the client has poor balance, the aide should support the weak side. If the client has good

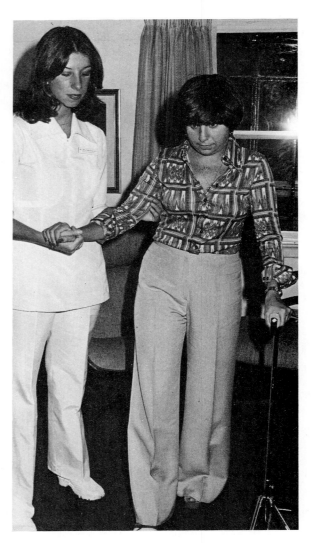

A. The quad cane is held in the hand opposite the weak side.

B. Remaining on the client's weak side, the aide walks along with the client.

Figure 34-9 A cane with four legs provides balance and a limited amount of weight support.

balance and uses no assistive device, the aide should walk on the strong side, and be ready to give support to the client. If the client has good balance and uses an assistive device, the aide should walk on the weak side and be ready to give support to the client, figure 34-9B.

8. Wash your hands following the procedure.

45: FOLLOWING SAFETY RULES FOR TRANSFERRING CLIENTS

purpose

• To move a client from one location to another safely, and without discomfort.

NOTE: Transfer is the term used to describe moving the client from one place to another. Transfers may be needed from bed to wheelchair; bed to toilet; from one chair to another; from chair to bed; or from wheelchair to bathtub. The kind of transfer will vary with the seriousness and type of disability. Figure 34-10 illustrates the steps for transferring the client from the bed to a chair. In all transfers the following rules apply.

procedure

1. Wash your hands before beginning the procedure.
2. Always lock the wheelchair brakes before a transfer, or anchor a chair firmly. The wheelchair should be positioned so that the transfer is done towards the client's stronger side.
3. Encourage the client to push off from a surface in getting up. The client should be discouraged from pulling on the armrest, bed, walker or the aide's arm.
4. Preferably, the client should be wearing shoes during a transfer. If this is not possible

or is not indicated for some reason, the client may be barefoot. Socks or stockings should not be worn as they may cause the client to slip on the floor.

5. Use proper body mechanics during all transfers to prevent muscle strain. Most transfers should be done by guiding, not lifting, the client. When moving the client, the home health aide's knees should be bent and the back kept as straight as possible. The aide should keep equal weight on both legs. This gives the home health aide a broad base of support.
6. Care is needed in helping a client get in and out of the bathtub. The best way to do this will depend on the client's disability, the size of the bathroom, and the equipment available.
   • Place a bath mat on the tub floor.
   • Place a bath seat in the tub for elderly clients.
   • Encourage the client to use grab bars or railings if they have been installed.
   • Discourage the client from holding onto the soap dish or shower handle for support.
   • Help a client with a weak side to get in the tub toward the weak side. Help the client to get out of the tub toward the strong side.
7. Wash your hands following the procedure.

46: STAND-PIVOT TRANSFER

purpose

• To help move a client who can bear at least partial weight on one leg.

NOTE: The stand-pivot transfer is used when a client can put at least partial weight on one

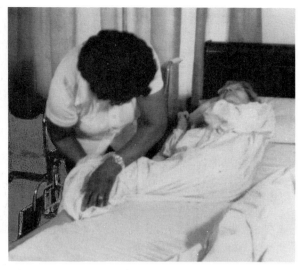

A. Turn the client toward you to reduce the risk of falls. Swing the client's feet off the bed to make sitting up easier. The wheelchair should be at the head of the bed, facing the foot of the bed, with the wheels locked.

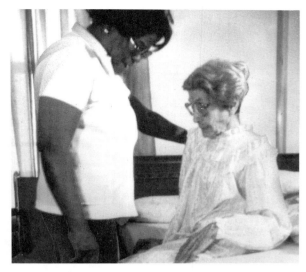

B. Once you have assisted the client to a sitting position, let her rest for a few moments. The change in position may cause dizziness. Once you are sure the client is stable, you can place slippers or shoes on the feet. Remember to squat rather than bend at the waist to prevent back strain. You can then assist the client to stand.

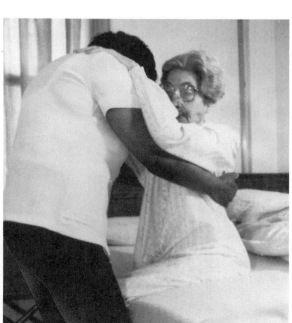

C. The client places her hands on your shoulders. You place your hands on either side of her chest under the arms. Remember good body mechanics-bend your knees and place one foot ahead of the other to stabilize your position and prevent back strain.

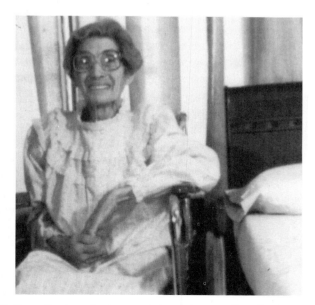

D. Once the transfer is complete, make sure the client is seated securely and comfortably in the wheelchair with feet placed on the foot rests.

Figure 34-10 The principles of body mechanics are applied when transferring the client from the bed to a wheelchair or chair.

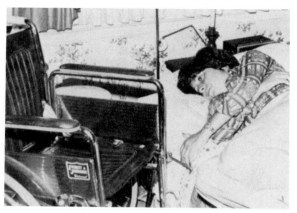

A. With the wheels locked, place the wheelchair near the bed at a 45° angle. Have the client lie close to the edge of the bed with the knees bent.

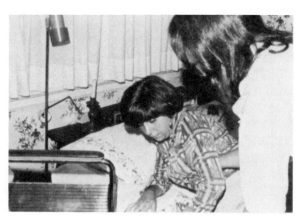

B. Help the client to a sitting position.

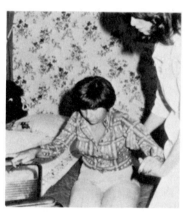

C. Tell the client to use the armrest for support.

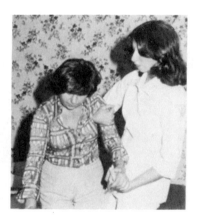

D. Place your forearm under the client's armpit for support.

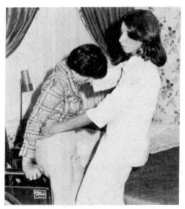

E. Brace the client by pressing your knee against the client's knees.

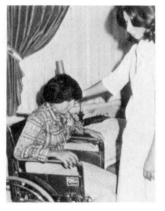

F. Position the client to rest comfortably in the wheelchair.

Figure 34-11 The stand-pivot transfer may be used to move the client from the bed to the wheelchair. Be sure the brakes are locked on the wheelchair.

foot. The transfer is easier if the client can bear weight on both legs or full weight on one leg. Clients who have arthritis or have had a stroke or hip fracture often need this type of transfer. The most common transfer is from the bed to the wheelchair, figure 34-11 on page 353. The transfer can be used for any similar situation. It is used for moves from the wheelchair to an easy chair, from the wheelchair to the toilet or from the wheelchair to a car, figure 34-12.

procedure

1. Wash your hands before beginning the procedure.

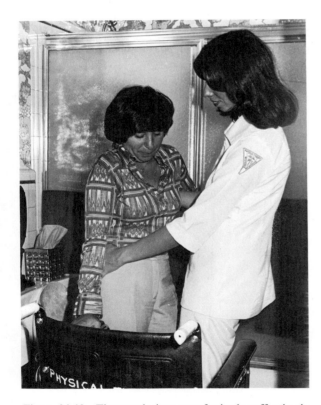

Figure 34-12 The stand-pivot transfer is also effective in moving the client from the wheelchair to the toilet.

2. Position wheelchair toward the client's strongest side at a 45° angle. Lock the brakes and push footrests up out of the way. Some wheelchairs have footrests which can be removed completely during transfer. This makes the transfer easier and safer.
3. Assist the client to sit on the edge of the bed. Be sure both of the client's feet are firmly placed on the floor, slightly apart.
4. Stand in front of the client. Place your foot against the client's weaker foot. Brace your knee against the client's knee. This helps control the weak leg and prevents it from buckling. Move your other foot slightly back for balance. If the client cannot bear weight on the weak foot, place your foot under the client's foot.
5. To rise, the client should bend at the hips and push with the strongest arm and leg. The client can rock back and forth to gain momentum. Place your arms under the client's arms and around the back. Guide the client forward.
6. When standing, have the client pivot (turn) on the good leg. If the right side is stronger, the client should turn counterclockwise (towards the left); if the left is stronger, the client should turn toward the right. As the client pivots, have the client reach with the good arm for the wheelchair armrest. As the client sits, the client can hold on to the armrest for support.
7. Help the client keep the upper body slightly forward when attempting to sit. Leaning forward prevents the client from flopping back into the wheelchair.
8. Use pillows or blankets to make the client comfortable in the wheelchair.
9. Lower the footrests and position the client's feet.
10. Wash your hands following the procedure.

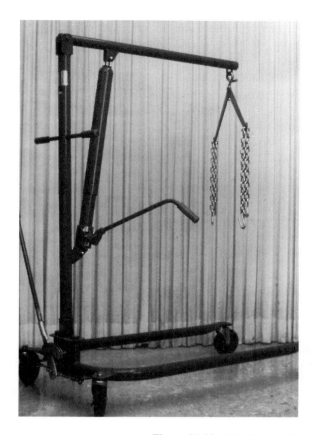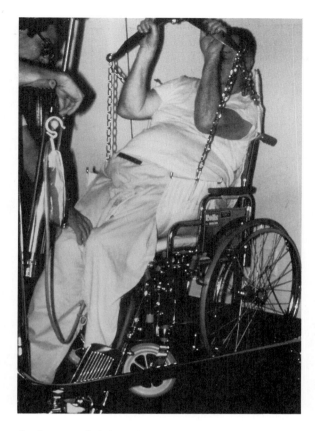

Figure 34-13 The Hoyer lift for moving heavy or helpless clients.

47: ASSISTING WITH THE SLIDING TRANSFER

purpose

• To move the client who has strong arms but cannot bear weight on either leg.

NOTE: Sliding transfers are used when the client cannot put weight on the legs. A person with a double amputation or with both legs paralyzed can usually use this transfer. The sliding transfer can only be done if the client has strong arms. In addition, the client must use a wheelchair with removable armrests. A smooth sliding board is used to form a bridge between the wheelchair and bed. Apply powder to the board to assist in sliding.

procedure

1. Wash your hands before beginning the procedure.
2. Place the wheelchair alongside the bed, as close as possible.
3. Remove the armrest which is nearest the bed.
4. Lock the brakes on the wheelchair.
5. Slide one end of the board under the client's buttocks. The other end of the board rests on the seat of the wheelchair.

6. Instruct the client to use both arms to push up and over toward the wheelchair. The arms must be strong to support the client's entire body weight.
7. Help the client by guiding the client's buttocks along the board. Hold the wheelchair steady as the client slides into it.
8. Wash your hands following the procedure.

In some cases, a mechanical device called a Hoyer lift is used to move very heavy or completely helpless clients into and out of bed, wheelchairs, and bathing facilities. If a Hoyer lift is used, you must be instructed in its use and be checked on your performance before you can operate the equipment. The Hoyer lift is shown in Figure 13 on page 355.

Unit 35
Postpartum Care

learning objectives

After studying this unit, you should be able to:
- Demonstrate clear ability to perform all procedures.
- Explain the purpose of each procedure.
- State when the procedures should and should not be done.
- Identify precautions to be taken for each procedure.

NOTE: All procedures are not allowed in all states. Make sure you are aware of limits as outlined by state guidelines.

client care procedure

48: ASSISTING THE MOTHER WITH BREASTFEEDING AND BREAST CARE

purpose

- To provide for cleanliness and prevention of infection to the breasts.
- To prevent breasts from sagging and losing muscle tone.
- To protect the nipples and observe for cracking or signs of soreness.
- To protect the infant from bacterial infection.
- To provide for the mother's comfort before, during and after nursing the child.

procedure*

1. Provide:
   mild soap
   warm water in basin
   clean washcloth and towel
   clean nursing bra (or well-fitting support bra)
   nursing pads
   cotton balls
   rinse water in basin (at feeding time)
   clock or watch to time nursing period

* La Leche League suggests that washing the nipple before each feeding can lead to drying and cracking and should be avoided. Consult your physician.

2. Wash your hands thoroughly before beginning the procedure.

3. Help the mother to wash her hands before handling the breasts.

4. Help the mother open the front of her dress or shirt top. Have mother wash nipples in warm water and mild soap using a circular motion, washing from the nipple outward, figure 35-1. Rinse and dry the breasts thoroughly.

5. Have mother sit in comfortable position in a rocking chair with footstool to support the feet. If mother is still on bedrest, help her lie on one side.

6. Change infant's diaper; wash your hands thoroughly after the diaper change.

7. Bring child to mother. Make sure infant's nose is not pressed against the mother's breast. The nostrils must be free so the infant can breathe as it nurses.

8. The nursing period is gradually built up from just a few minutes to a maximum of 20 minutes. Some mothers prefer to let baby nurse at both breasts (one at a time) during one feeding period. Others will feed the infant only at one breast for each 20 minute feeding period. They alternate breasts at different feedings.

9. To remove the baby's mouth from the breast, have mother press on two sides of nipple to release the suction.

10. At the end of the feeding period, return baby to crib. Make sure baby has been burped before it is laid down. Change diaper if necessary.

11. Wash your hands before continuing with the procedure.

12. Help the mother with her bra, putting fresh nursing pads over the nipples to absorb any leakage. If nipples are sore or cracked, have the mother contact the doctor. An ointment or medication may be prescribed. Report these problems to the supervisor.

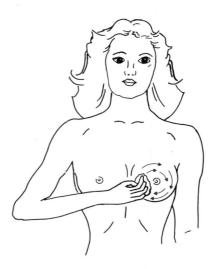

Figure 35-1 Nipples should be washed in a circular motion moving away from the center.

13. Return supplies to storage.

14. Wash your hands following the procedure.

client care procedure

49: GIVING THE INFANT A SPONGE BATH

purpose

- To clean and refresh infant.
- To observe skin tone, activity and signs of abnormality or unusual changes in behavior.

procedure

1. Bring needed supplies to kitchen table or baby's bath table:
   warm water in basin or Bathinette (test temperature)
   towel and washcloth
   bath sheets
   diapers (cloth or disposable paper)
   bath oil
   baby lotion
   diaper pail

change of clothing (undershirt, gown, etc.) mild soap

2. Wash your hands thoroughly before beginning the procedure.

3. Lower siderail of crib. Keep the rail raised to its highest position whenever infant is in crib. Bring infant to bathing area.

4. Place infant on bath sheet and undress. Drop soiled diaper into diaper pail. Close diaper pins and keep out of baby's reach. **Caution:** NEVER leave the baby unattended while it is on the bath table.

5. Cover infant with bath towel. Wash the infant's face with warm water only. Do not use soap on the face. Pat face dry. Make sure ears are carefully dried. Wash neck and pat dry. Rub in small amount of lotion around creases in baby's neck.

6. Apply soap over baby's head and lather well to remove crust. Rinse soap away by holding head over basin as you repeatedly wipe head with wet washcloth. If soap is left on scalp, it will cause scales to crust and collect. Dry scalp carefully. Rub on baby oil.

7. Lather your hands and apply soap to the infant's hands, arms and chest. Rinse completely with washcloth and dry with towel.

8. Apply soap to abdomen and legs and lather well. Rinse with washcloth and dry.

9. Turn infant on the stomach and lather the infant's back; rinse and dry.

10. Wash, rinse and dry genital (perineal) area last. Uncircumcised males should have the foreskin pushed back gently and the area washed with water only. Wash the penis and folds of the scrotum. Apply lotion to folds and creases. Wash the labial area of females with water only.

11. Dress infant and return to crib or playpen.

12. Return supplies to storage. Clean up area where bath was given.

13. Wash your hands following the procedure.

50: BATHING THE INFANT USING A BATHINETTE OR BASIN

purpose

- To clean and refresh infant.
- To exercise infant's body.
- To observe body responses and skin condition.

NOTE: Make certain the infant is not in a draft during bath. Always support the infant's head and hold securely to prevent injury to the child. **Caution:** Always have all needed supplies near at hand so the infant is NEVER left unattended during the bath period.

Bring all supplies to the Bathinette, kitchen sink or bath basin. Test the water temperature by thermometer or skin test at your wrist. Put water to a depth of 3–4 inches.

A full bath is not given until the umbilical cord has dropped off. The cord usually dries up and falls off 5 to 8 days after birth. **Caution:** The cord will detach by itself; do not try to help it along. Circumcised male infants may be bathed in the tub only after circumcision has healed completely.

procedure

1. Collect the needed supplies:
   towel or bath blanket
   mild soap
   change of diaper (cloth or disposable paper)
   gown, undershirt or clothing desired
   receiving blanket
   baby lotion and baby oil
   cotton balls

2. Wash your hands thoroughly before beginning the procedure.

3. Undress infant in crib; wrap in receiving blanket and bring to bath area.

4. Support head and body with one arm and

hand, leaving other arm free to bathe infant. Remove receiving blanket.

5. Wash the part of the eyes near the nose, washing from nose outward using cloth and clear water. Wash rest of face with freshly dampened cloth.

6. To wash the infant's head, use the football hold. Support the baby upright by placing its body firmly under your one arm and resting its body against your hip. Hold the infant's head with your hand spreading your fingers. Hold the infant's head over the tub or basin. Soap and rinse the scalp, then dry thoroughly.

7. While holding the infant securely, immerse the infant's body in water, figure 35-2. Keep the head well above the water level. Bathe starting with neck, arms, front and legs. Wash and rinse carefully in folds of skin. Turn the infant onto the stomach. Support the body holding the infant's head out of the bath water. Wash back, buttocks, legs, feet and between the toes.

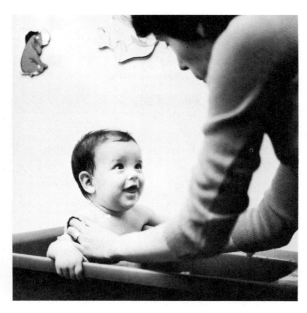

Figure 35-2 Take a firm hold of the infant before lowering the infant into the bath water.

8. Wash genitals, using only water and washcloth. Push back foreskin of uncircumcised male and wash carefully. Replace foreskin over end of penis. For female infants, separate folds of labia. Use a downward stroke only, from front to back.

9. Remove infant from bath water and dry thoroughly. Use baby lotion or powder in folds of skin around neck, arms and legs. Gently dry the ears.

10. Dress infant and return to crib or playpen.

11. Clean up the bath area and return supplies to storage. Place used diapers in diaper pail and dirty clothing and towels in clothes hamper.

12. Wash your hands following the procedure.

<table><tr><td>client care procedure</td></tr></table>

51: BOTTLE FEEDING THE INFANT

purpose

- To provide nutrition.
- To give infant the security of being held, cuddled, and bonded.
- To provide opportunity to observe infant's responses, color, skin condition, etc.

procedure

1. Wash your hands before beginning the procedure.

2. Warm the bottle to temperature so that when tested on the wrist, it is warm, not hot.

3. Change infant's diaper, if necessary, so infant will be comfortable, clean, and dry while eating. Wrap infant loosely in a clean receiving blanket. Leave infant in crib with side rails up.

4. Wash your hands.

5. Bring bottle to table next to a comfortable rocker or arm chair.

6. Support infant's head and back when pick-

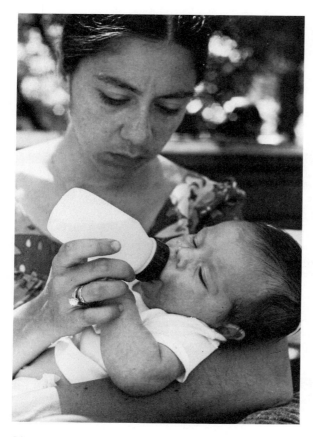

Figure 35-3 Be sure the nipple is full of milk in order to prevent the infant from sucking air.

ing it up from the crib. Sit comfortably in chair, holding child securely in a comfortable position for taking nipple; start to feed the infant. Do not prop bottle, figure 35-3.

7. When infant has had 2–3 ounces, either sit the infant upright on your lap and gently pat back, or hold the infant over your shoulder and pat its back until the infant burps.

8. Continue feeding and burping until infant is finished or shows no interest in eating. Do not force infant to take more than it wants.

9. When the baby is finished, burp it once more then place it in the crib lying it on its side or stomach. **DO NOT PLACE THE INFANT ON BACK.** If infant should regurgitate, there would be a possibility of causing serious health hazard.

10. Wash your hands following the procedure.

Unit 36
Job-Seeking Skills

key terms
diagnosis related groups   infraction
registry service   misconduct
personal reference   pilferage

learning objectives

After studying this unit, you should be able to:
- Accurately fill out an employment application.
- Prepare a resume and/or personal information sheet.
- Present yourself in a professional manner to a prospective employer.
- Make appointments to discuss job opportunities.

One of the hardest tasks faced by anyone is entering a new situation. As a student, you were probably afraid you would not be able to pass the tests, recite in class or demonstrate a skill to the teacher in front of the other students. However, if you have passed your course for home health aide, you have already met these challenges. Now as a graduate, you are facing a new challenge—putting your new found skills to work.

Until now, you have been guided by your instructor(s) and for the most part have worked in a team situation with your fellow students. Now you are on your own. You must "sell" yourself and your skills to an employer.

You must make your own decisions as to what kind of clients you would rather work with. Do you want part-time or full-time work? Do you want a sleep-in job? Would you rather work with elderly clients who mainly need companionship and minimal care, or do you want to use all your skills and deal with complex medical problems? Do you prefer working with children or are you willing to take whatever jobs are open?

trends affecting employment

A new government reimbursement system for medical care according to diagnosis-related groups (DRGs) is expected to bring about an even greater need for home health care. The most recent Medicare data shows that the average annual cost per Medicare beneficiary receiving inpatient hospital care was $3675; for nursing home care, $1710; and for home health care only $819. That same report under Medicaid costs showed that while nursing home care averaged $7854 per patient, home care was only $1281 per client. What this means to you is that more and more people are going to choose home care for economic reasons. Health care services rank in the top five in the nation as far as job opportunities are concerned.

contacting prospective employers

Your first step toward finding a job is to know where to look. There are local and national agencies in most areas that are listed in the telephone book. Your instructor may also be able to give you a list of addresses and phone numbers. You can look in the employment section of your local newspaper; you can contact your local department of social services, and you can see if your hospitals have a *registry service* where you may apply. Some medical groups also have lists of clients who need home health aides.

Make a list of those places you plan to contact; then keep a record of the date you called and any appointments you may set up. Remember, you may register at several agencies and you may work for more than one agency on a part-time basis. When you phone for an appointment, know what you want to say. "I am a graduate of the ABC home health program, and I am looking for work. May I have an appointment?"

the job interview and application form

When you go to your appointment remember that personal appearance is very important. Dress neatly and look your very best.

the application form

Have an information sheet with you listing some facts that usually appear on an application form. This will save you time and you won't make foolish errors when you fill out the application. Some of the facts that you should have on your information sheet are listed in figure 36-1.

If you do not have a telephone, you should leave the number of a neighbor or friend who has agreed to take messages for you. *Personal references* may not be relatives, but may include your minister, doctor, or instructor(s). Be sure that you have permission from those people you list as references to use their names. If possible, obtain letters of recommendation from these people before you go for a job interview. This will save time for the agency, and the person who is giving the recommendation only has to write one letter of reference. The agency can then make a copy of your letters of reference and confirm them by phone.

Each agency will have its own application form, but if you are prepared with the information requested in figure 36-1, you should not have any difficulty completing the form. It is always a good idea to read the application form carefully before completing it. It may include special instructions, such as asking the applicant to type or print all information. Fill out each item neatly and completely. Do not leave any items blank; if the item does not apply to you, write "N.A." (not applicable).

NAME First	Middle	Last	PHONE

ADDRESS (number, street, city, state, zip)	SOCIAL SECURITY NO./ALIEN I.D. No.

HIGH SCHOOL OR OTHER SCHOOL ATTENDED	SCHOOL ADDRESS

HIGHEST GRADE/DEGREE COMPLETED

SCHOOL GRANTING CERTIFICATION AS HOME HEALTH AIDE	SCHOOL ADDRESS

PREFERRED SCHEDULE (days of week/hours per day)

DATE AVAILABLE FOR EMPLOYMENT

PAST EMPLOYMENT (Complete the following section, starting with your most recent position.)

Employer/Supervisor	Address	Phone	Job Title	Salary	Dates of Employment	Reason for Leaving
1.						
2.						
3.						

PERSONAL REFERENCES (other than relatives)

Name	Address	Phone Number
1.		
2.		
3.		

Figure 36-1   Sample application form

Take care to spell words and to punctuate sentences carefully. Do not write in spaces marked "office use only." Review your application before submitting it to the employer.

You should have with you your Social Security card, your alien green card, a driver's license, your certificate, and, if at all possible, a copy of your most recent physical examination showing your immunizations, the results of a TB test, and other facts about your personal physical condition. Some agencies will have their own form to be given to the examining physician, figure 36-2. Remember to take your own pen.

the interview

After the application has been filled out, you will probably be interviewed by a nurse or personnel manager. Make sure that you know the correct date and exact time of your interview as well as the name of the person who will be interviewing you. Check to make sure that you know how to get to the appropriate location, or ask for specific directions.

Dress neatly and conservatively. Make sure that your clothes are clean and well pressed. Avoid excessive jewelry or makeup. Observe the personal hygiene rules discussed in Unit 2 of this text.

Arrive a little early for your interview. This will tell your prospective employer that you are prepared to arrive on time for your assignments if you are hired.

Introduce yourself to the person who will be interviewing you, and shake hands firmly. Always be polite, speak clearly, sit or stand straight, and use correct grammar. Do not chew gum or smoke during any part of the interview. Answer all questions truthfully and directly. Be ready to talk about the training and/or experience you have had. Be honest about the kind of cases you prefer. Listen carefully to your interviewer. Do not immediately ask about salary, benefits, and the like. This information is usually supplied by the interviewer toward the end of the interview. If you are unclear about any information, ask questions.

You should not anticipate receiving a definite indication of a job offer or rejection at the end of the interview. The interviewer will usually let you know when you will be contacted. Be sure to thank the interviewer as you leave.

If you are then offered the job, you have the choice of accepting the agency's terms or looking elsewhere for a position. Once you have accepted a position with an agency, be realistic in your goals. As in any kind of employment, there is a system of progression where the new employees must prove themselves. It is possible that an agency may test you by calling you for weekend or holiday part-time work. Many employers think it is a sign of dedication if you accept the assignments offered. After you have worked for a while, the agency will have a better idea of your abilities and strengths and will work you into a regular schedule.

When you are employed by an agency, you may be asked to sign a document similar to the one presented in figure 36-3. This document will indicate the policies and rules of your agency. You should read it carefully and be willing to accept and abide by the conditions included in it.

New York State has recently implemented a new and very restrictive code for agencies providing home health care. In order to be qualified to operate, agencies must meet exacting standards set by both the Department of Health and the Department of Social Services. Included in the standards required by New York State are:

- A grievance procedure for an agency's employees
- A patient's bill of rights which MUST be ex-

TO THE PHYSICIAN: Please fill out the following medical form as completely as possible. State law requires that our employees have a completed physical on file with a yearly update. Please forward this form immediately upon completion of examination. Pending test results will be followed up by our office. Information required is indicated by a check mark.

NAME OF PATIENT: _____ AGE: _____

ADDRESS: _____
            Street No.   Town (City)   State   Zip Code

PHYSICAL FINDINGS:

BP: _____ Pulse: _____ Resp: _____ Height: _____ Weight: _____

____ Cardiovascular   ____ Gastrointestinal   ____ Musculoskeletal
____ Respiratory   ____ Genitourinary   ____ Nervous

____ Above physical findings essentially normal.
____ Abnormal findings/limitations: _____

_____

HISTORY

Habituation/Addiction
____ Alcohol   ____ Depressants   ____ Stimulants   ____ Narcotics   ____ Other: _____

If any, please explain: _____

Illness/Injury – please indicate any past or present condition that would result in physical, mental or behavioral limitations in normal functioning: _____

MANDATORY IMMUNIZATIONS/TESTS:

DIPHTHERIA/TETANUS – should have booster every ten years.

Date of Last Immunization: _____

RUBELLA – MUST show proof of immunity through direct immunization or *positive* antibody titer test.

Date of immunization: _____ Date of Antibody Titer Test: _____
                                       Results: _____

TUBERCULOSIS — MUST have Mantoux (ppd) skin test every year and follow-up chest X ray if test
   results positive.   Follow-up Chest

Date of Mantoux: _____ Results: _____ X ray date: _____
                                             Pos.   Neg.

ENTERIC PATHOGENS – stool examination and/or culture (only if indicated by check mark)

Date of Examination/Culture: _____ Results: _____

This person (is   is not) physically and mentally capable of performing the functions of an aide in the home setting, and is free from any condition which would endanger his/her safety or the safety and well-being of the clients to be cared for.

DATE: _____ PHYSICIAN'S SIGNATURE: _____

                ADDRESS: _____
                             Street No.   City   State   Zip Code

                PHONE NO.: _____

Figure 36-2 Some agencies have their own forms for physical examinations.

TO THE EMPLOYEE

Because you are important to us, we want to help you develop a good work record. If we feel that you are violating any of our rules and policies, or that you have misunderstood the terms of employment, we will hold a conference with you. Continued *infractions* will cause your immediate dismissal. PLEASE READ THE FOLLOWING CAREFULLY.

1. *Attendance and tardiness record:* Recurring cancellations of promised scheduled workdays may result in dismissal. Absence without call in may result in immediate termination. No pay raises will be granted if attendance and tardiness records are unsatisfactory. We must be able to depend on you. You must call in if you are unable to meet your assignment.

2. *Unbecoming conduct:* Any of the following are considered to be gross *misconduct:* carelessness and inattention to client care; failure to perform duties; violation of safe practices; inefficiency and wasting of materials; refusal to obey direct orders; insubordination; rude, discourteous or uncivil behavior; intoxication, drinking or possession of intoxicating beverages while on duty; gambling on duty; sleeping on duty; unauthorized absence from assignment or leaving early without permission; failure to report an injury or accident concerning an employee or client; soliciting tips from clients or families; sale of services to clients or families; divulging confidential information about client and family; theft and/or dishonesty; *pilferage* of drugs or violation of any law on drug use including use or sale of same; damaging, defacing or mishandling equipment or property; interfering with work performance of another employee; falsifying client or personnel records or any form of misrepresentation.

Employee's statement:

I have read the above rules and regulations and understand my responsibilities to the agency and client. I agree to abide by these terms of employment.

_____   _____
Employee Signature   Date

_____   _____
Supervisor's Signature   Date

Figure 36-3   Once you have decided to accept a position with an agency, you may be asked to sign a document which states that you have read and understand the rules of the agency.

plained to the client (or client's family) in the presence of a witness
- Documentation of certification of all employees
- Proof of an annual physical examination by employees
- Proof of employee's attendance at a minimum number of in-service programs each year
- Proof of citizenship and/or verified alien registration
- Satisfactory completion of an approved Home Health Aide course of study

summary

If you have successfully completed the home health aide program and have a certificate, you should have no trouble finding employment. When you go to an agency or prospective employer, be on time, dress neatly, and be prepared to talk about your training and experience. Do not chew gum or smoke during the interview. Fill out the application form neatly and completely.

appendix

appendix a   temperature conversion chart

NOTE: The following table is provided as an aid for study and comparison of temperatures. Some homemaking duties and client care procedures refer to temperatures in Fahrenheit or Celsius.

DEGREES FAHRENHEIT TO DEGREES CELSIUS AND VICE VERSA											
°F	°C	°F	°C	°F	°C	°F	°C	°F	°C	°F	°C
96	35.6	118	47.8	140	60	162	72.2	184	84.4	206.6	97
96.8	36	118.4	48	141	60.6	163	72.8	185	85	207	97.2
97	36.1	119	48.3	141.8	61	163.4	73	186	85.6	208	97.8
98	36.7	120	48.9	142	61.1	164	73.3	186.8	86	208.4	98
98.6	37	120.2	49	143	61.7	165	73.9	187	86.1	209	98.3
99	37.2	121	49.4	143.6	62	165.2	74	188	86.7	210	98.9
100	37.8	122	50	144	62.2	166	74.4	188.6	87	210.2	99
100.4	38	123	50.6	145	62.8	167	75	189	87.2	211	99.4
101	38.3	123.8	51	145.4	63	168	75.6	190	87.8	212	100
102	38.9	124	51.1	146	63.3	168.8	76	190.4	88	213	100.6
102.2	39	125	51.7	147	63.9	169	76.1	191	88.3	213.8	101
103	39.4	125.6	52	147.2	64	170	76.7	192	88.9	214	101.1
104	40	126	52.2	148	64.4	170.6	77	192.2	89	215	101.7
105	40.6	127	52.8	149	65	171	77.2	193	89.4	215.6	102
105.8	41	127.4	53	150	65.6	172	77.8	194	90	216	102.2
106	41.1	128	53.3	150.8	66	172.4	78	195	90.6	217	102.8
107	41.7	129	53.9	151	66.1	173	78.3	195.8	91	217.4	103
107.6	42	129.2	54	152	66.7	174	78.9	196	91.1	218	103.3
108	42.2	130	54.4	152.6	67	174.2	79	197	91.7	219	103.9
109	42.8	131	55	153	67.2	175	79.4	197.6	92	219.2	104
109.4	43	132	55.6	154	67.8	176	80	198	92.2	220	104.4
110	43.3	132.8	56	154.4	68	177	80.6	199	92.8	221	105
111	43.9	133	56.1	155	68.3	177.8	81	199.4	93	225	107.2
111.2	44	134	56.7	156	68.9	178	81.1	200	93.3	230	110
112	44.4	134.6	57	156.2	69	179	81.7	201	93.9	235	112.8
113	45	135	57.2	157	69.4	179.6	82	201.2	94	239	115
114	45.6	136	57.8	158	70	180	82.2	202	94.4	240	115.6
114.8	46	136.4	58	159	70.6	181	82.8	203	95	245	118.3
115	46.1	137	58.3	159.8	71	181.4	83	204	95.6	248	120
116	46.7	138	58.9	160	71.1	182	83.3	204.8	96	250	121.1
116.6	47	138.2	59	161	71.7	183	83.9	205	96.1	255	123.9
117	47.2	139	59.4	161.6	72	183.2	84	206	96.7	257	125

appendix b sample of weekly time sheet

064-40-0878 SS #

Name: Judy Goldstein

W/E 9 11 89 Month · Day · Year

PRINT THIS TIME SHEET   USE A SEPARATE LINE FOR EACH CASE   SKIP A LINE BETWEEN DAYS

Agency	Case #	CLIENT Last Name–First initial	DATE Mo.	DATE Day	Travel to 1st Case Hr.	Min.	Mi.	Fare	Arrived Hr.	Min.	Left Hr.	Min.	Svce. Hrs.	Miles on Case	Travel to next case Hr.	Min.	Mi.	Fare	Travel to Home Hr.	Min.	Mi.	Fare	Other Exp.	Signature
VNA	2303	Brown, J.	9	6		25	6		9	00	12	00	3							25	6		.10	J. Brown
		Holiday	9	7																				
ERDS-C	1963	Casillio, P.	9	8		20	8		8	30	12	30	4	6		30	10							P. Casillio
SOC.SERV	2036	Williams, S.	9	8					1	00	4	00	3							35	12		.30	Sam Williams
V.A.	1845	Kelly, A.	9	9		20	8		9	00	5	00	8	28						25				A. Kelly
VNA	2306	Garcia, M.	9	10		40	15		8	30	12	30	4											M Garcia
SOC.SERV	1495	Garcia, M.	9	10		20	8		12	30	4	30	4							45	15			M Garcia

Sample of a Weekly Time Sheet

DAILY AND WEEKLY SCHEDULING

As a beginning home health aide, you may have some difficulty in scheduling your activities. The authors have prepared a time checklist which they recommend be used until you have established a pattern of work. It provides a reminder of what is expected. An individual notebook, detailing the procedures done and the time required for each, can be kept instead of a checklist.

You should become accustomed to making a working schedule and putting it into practice. Post conferences with your instructor may be quite helpful in recognizing areas in which you can make adjustments leading to greater efficiency and ease of accomplishing goals. The need for personal flexibility should be stressed. You should be flexible in order to meet client needs and still maintain the home within reasonable bounds.

As each procedure is completed, note the time required. At the end of the day make a note of undone tasks, and see if the time spent could have been used more effectively.

Daily Checklist

Duties	Completed	Time Required
A.M. Client Care	_____	_____
Client Unit—Bedroom/Bath	_____	_____
Breakfast Made/Served	_____	_____
Kitchen Clean Up	_____	_____
Shopping	_____	_____
House Cleaned	_____	_____
Lunch Made/Served	_____	_____
Aide's Lunch Period	_____	_____
Kitchen Clean Up	_____	_____
Laundry/Ironing	_____	_____
Major Job—Clean Oven	_____	_____
Refrigerator		
Mop Floor		
Vacuum		
Other Client Care	_____	_____
List Procedures		
_____	_____	_____
_____	_____	_____
_____	_____	_____
P.M. Client Care	_____	_____

Observations by home health aide _____

_____

_____

appendix d   child growth and development

CHARACTERISTICS	NEEDS

BIRTH TO 1 MONTH

At birth the infant is helpless, with uncontrolled and uncoordinated movements.
Undifferentiated crying.
Sucking, swallowing and rooting reflexes present at birth.
No tears when crying.
Self and social concept very limited.
Bowel movements three or four times daily.
Interested primarily in eating.
Returns to sleep toward end of feeding.

Physical care (to be fed, positioned, kept warm and dry).
To sleep as desired.
To develop a basic attitude of trust.
Love and affection (holding, fondling, caressing, pleasant vocal tones).

1 TO 2 MONTHS

Raises head from prone position.
Tears appear.
Cries to be picked up.
Cries at loud noises.
Almost continuous arm and leg movement when awake.
Reaching movements lying on back.
Meaningless vowel sounds.
Interested in rattle.
Fascinated by light or moving object.

"Chuckling" and smiles from adults.
Protection from extreme and unnecessary frustration.
Physical care as above.
Love and affection as above.
A safe rattle.
DPT immunization.
Poliomyelitis immunization.

3 TO 4 MONTHS

Sleeps 8 to 12 hours without awakening.
Remains awake after eating.
Interested in solids.
Two to four naps per day.
One to two bowel movements per day.
Grasps at objects. Makes sounds.
A beginning concept of communications.
Mimics facial expressions.
Holds head erect when supported in sitting position.
Back is becoming straight.
Self contained period.
Coos and chuckles, laughs and smiles.
Enjoys other people.
Saliva appears. Drooling.
Follows objects with eyes.

Mother or mother-figure as child recognizes mother.
A high chair.
A schedule that is more or less stable.
Experience with spoon feeding.
To learn small frustration such as slight delay in feeding.
To hear certain sounds repeated in specific situations so child can form associations.
To reason vocally when played with.
To be permitted to splash in bath.
Physical care.
To have more attention, play and love.
Play with adult other than mother.
To learn to swallow saliva.
To have bright objects to focus upon.

5 TO 8 MONTHS

Back straight.

Sits with no support (6 months).

Controls head when leaning forward in sitting position (5 months).

Rolls from supine to prone position (5 months).

"Crows" with pleasure (5 months).

Can support own weight for short periods (7 months).

Plays with feet and puts them in own mouth.

Afraid of strangers.

Manipulates and chews small objects.

Recognizes self in a mirror.

Night sleeping continuous.

Two or three naps per day.

One bowel movement per day.

Frequent voidings.

Cup feedings begun.

Increased motor ability.

Verbalizes with people and toys.

Can grunt, growl and gurgle.

"Mama" and "Dada" are spoken.

Affection for family appears.

Stretches arms to loved adults.

Own room.

Attention.

To respond to more than one person at a time.

To suck the thumb to relieve tension.

A toothbrush after four teeth appear.

Biscuits or toast to bite on.

To assign different demands on each parent.

Small soft rubber or cloth toys.

To eat with family schedule.

Introduction to first solid foods.

More play during bath.

To learn the meaning of "no" (to learn to tolerate frustration).

Physical care and love.

To suck for pleasure.

Immunization: third diphtheria pertussis tetanus, and third oral poliomyelitis by 5 months.

9 TO 12 MONTHS

Can sit up indefinitely.

Preference for right or left hand appears.

Crawls at 9 months.

Can maintain balance turning from side to side and can lower self from standing to sitting by holding on to stable objects.

Cries when scolded (9 months).

Walks holding on to furniture for support (10 months).

Can bring hands together (10 months).

Imitates adult inflection on a specific word (10 months).

Listens and responds to own name (10 months).

Stands alone at 11–12 months.

Speaks single words (9–11 months).

Walks holding onto hand for support.

Can pick up small objects with fingers.

Can bend, grasp, and manipulate objects.

Security and limits.

Physical care and love.

To hear tonal reprimand.

To hear tonal praise.

Play pen.

To listen to adults converse.

To hear own name.

To learn the meaning of "no."

Mother's security when confronted with anything new or different.

Tuberculin test at 11 months of age.

Measles vaccine at 12 months of age.

Play with adults in give-and-take manner.

To be included at table in high chair with family.

9 TO 12 MONTHS (continued)

Shy with a stranger.

Upset by changes in household.

Is an observer.

Can sit from standing position without assistance.

Happy and busy.

Handles genitals although true masturbation
is not evident.

Beginning concept of give-and-take.

Plays spontaneously.

Eats three meals per day and one afternoon
treat.

One nap per day.

Handles cup well.

Food dislikes may become evident.

13 TO 18 MONTHS

Early walking characterized by wide stance and
short steps up on toes.

Can make actual markings with crayon.

Explores in and out of house.

Ceaseless activity.

Assertive and independent.

At 15 months throws objects.

Holds a cup.

Turns pages in a book.

Concept of adult activities and of self as a person.

Anger and temper tantrums.

Negativism begins.

Ritualistic behavior begins.

Afraid of noises, especially noisy machinery.

Decrease in appetite.

Urination better controlled.

Bowel movements may be less regular.

Can respond to need to go to the toilet.

May resist bathing.

Handles cup well.

Interested in dressing and undressing.

Pulls toys.

Can use four or five words.

Still spills when handling spoon.

Uses jargon which will develop into sentences.

Security and love.

Supervised and regulated independence.

To explore drawers and closets.

Pull and push toys.

Adult supervision.

Pots and pans to play with.

To move objects about.

To do things for self within reason. (Assists
in self-determination.)

To have a place for things.

To know own belongings.

To imitate adults.

To be controlled so as not to be destructive.

To be permitted to feed self with supervision.

To sleep with favorite toy or blanket.

Toilet training unless resistant.

To be asked to indicate need.

To be bathed.

To have teeth brushed.

To be permitted to participate in both dressing
and undressing.

To name objects in a picture book.

To hear conversations.

18 TO 21 MONTHS

Can walk backward and sideways.
Can unlace and remove shoes.
Neater self-feeding.
Spontaneous scribbling.
Hand preference obvious.
Turns pages in a book.
Can build a tower of three to four blocks.
Understands simple directions.
Can use 10 words.
Independence alternating with sudden dependence.
Temper tantrums, negativism and ritualistic behavior continue.
Imitates adult activities seen in the home.
Uses two- or three-word phrases or sentences.
Fairly steady gait.
Walks upstairs holding rail, but needs help walking downstairs.
Holds spoon well; drinks from a glass; handles cup well.
Obeys simple commands.
Tries to put on simple garments.
Runs, but falls are frequent.
Begins to use pronouns.
May be toilet trained during day.

Toilet training to continue.
To participate in dressing and undressing.
To feed self with supervision.
Toys: crayon and paper, blocks, broom, telephone, picture book, pots and pans.
To have mother admire accomplishments.
To be held and reassured as child indicates.
To be bathed.
To assist with handwashing and brushing of teeth.
To be permitted to feed self.
To be given simple errands about the house.
To put on own mittens and cap and assist in dressing and undressing.
To be cuddled and reassured as indicated by child.
Repeated correction to get pronouns correct.
To have bathroom wishes respected.
To have harmful objects out of reach.

24 MONTHS

Crude jumping from low heights.
Walks up and down stairs without assistance.
Makes short sentences.
Toilet trained during day.
Dressing ability improved.
Increased sense of individuality.
"Me" and "mine" dominate.
Cannot share possessions.
Gives name when asked.
Points to objects named in picture books.
Does not know how to play with children (hugs or pushes).
Thumbsucking and temper tantrums decrease.
Negativism, ritualism, and dawdling increase.
Cannot wait for things.

To express desires and to be heard.
To be permitted to dress and undress with limitations.
Opportunity to please others.
Toys to hoard.
Praise for correct recognition.
Adult supervision when around other children.
To have the company of other children.
To learn to tolerate delays.

30 MONTHS

Walking is automatic.

Increased finger control; can imitate both vertical and circular line acceptably.

Can build an eight block tower.

Likes bathing.

Can undress easily.

Cannot play cooperatively.

Rigid, ritualistic and perfectionistic.

Changes in routine will produce fear reactions.

Curiosity about physical differences between sexes.

Appetite fluctuations.

Can feed self but may demand an adult to do so.

Bedtime rituals can become excessive.

Sleep may be restless.

Cannot make choices.

Bowel training is established but bowel movements are irregular.

Bladder control may not be quite established.

Can use words that refer to past, present, and future.

To be permitted to play in the tub.

To be permitted to undress.

Supervised play experience with children of the same age.

Reassurance when fear reactions appear.

To begin to learn correct terminology for genitals.

Routine meals.

To be permitted some testing of limits.

To be permitted some rituals.

To take toys to bed.

To be protected from having to make choices.

To experiment with verbalization.

3 YEARS

Less negative and more easily cared for than the toddler.

Understands words better.

Interested in new activities so learning from experience is rapid.

Rides a tricycle, using the pedals.

Walks backward.

Walks downstairs alone; walks upstairs alternating feet.

Jumps from a low step.

Can pour fluid from a pitcher.

Begins to use scissors.

Tries to draw pictures.

Undresses self; can unbutton buttons.

Helps to dress self.

Goes to the toilet.

Washes hands.

May be able to brush teeth.

Feeds self well.

Help in taking turns and sharing in group play.

Encouragement to eat appropriate foods.

Help in coping with fears, real or imagined.

Positive reinforcement/approval for acceptable behaviors and accomplishments.

Reinforcement of gender identification.

Simple explanations in response to sexual curiosity.

Opportunity to practice and develop abilities.

Positive role model for acceptable behavior.

Careful supervision as a result of increased independence.

3 YEARS (continued)
Has a vocabulary of about 900 words.
Plays simple games with others.
Talks in sentences.
Begins to understand taking turns.

4 YEARS

Can climb and jump well.
Can lace shoes.
Can brush teeth.
Uses scissors successfully to cut out pictures.
Has a vocabulary of about 1500 words.
Exaggerates, boasts, and tattles on others.
Talks with an imaginary companion.
Tends to be selfish and impatient.
Takes pride in accomplishments.
Aggressive physically as well as verbally.
Cooperative in group activities.
Longer attention span.
Can dress and undress self.
High level of energy and motivation.

Help in developing positive social behaviors.
Assistance in dealing with fears.
Encouragement to "work through" unresolved conflicts.
Help and reinforcement in acquiring a sense of right and wrong.
Opportunity to exhibit abilities and independence appropriately.
Help in recognizing and observing limits.

5 YEARS

Very energetic and restless.
Wishes constant activity.
Fatigue may be indicated by a display of crossness.
Self-centered and has growing desire to make own decisions.
Interference with play or possessions is resented.
Beginning sense of property rights.
Increased growth in social relationships with less grabbing, pushing, crying.
Verbally critical but shares more.
Cooperative play is much enjoyed.
Plays with the same age, younger, or older, but likes to be "bigger than."
Shows off but at times may be shy.
Can recognize the skills of others.
Interests of boys and girls are similar; they play together.

Security within the family is a primary need.
Companionship of other children is important.
There is pleasure in initiating and playing simple games with several other children.
There must be a wide variety of activities to develop the muscles of arms and shoulders, the trunk, and the legs and feet.
Climbing and hanging activities are essential.
Kiddie-cars, wagons, scooters, tricycles and boats are enjoyed.
Pounding nails and building blocks are desirable.
Additional play may be with sand, toys, dolls, etc.
Adults should deal rationally with the child if child exhibits an overinterest in the sex organs. Cleanliness, loose clothing, supervision of toilet habits and substitution of other interests are needed.

5 YEARS (continued)

Boys are more quarrelsome than girls.

Both locomotor and manipulative play are enjoyed.

The use of imagination in play is seen.

Laughter is a frequent form of communication.

Those who do not communicate readily through speech may be unable to achieve close relationships with other children.

Toilet habits, getting a drink, etc. are well established.

The child should sleep about 12 hours or longer per day; sleep is a prime essential in building sturdy health.

An afternoon nap of one to two hours is needed.

Development of liking for all types of food is a necessity, but should be accomplished without stress or strain.

Regularity of mealtime is important.

The child should have opportunities to do things for self.

The child likes to "help." This takes longer for the adult, but is valuable for the child's development.

appendix e   obstructed airway procedures

A. CONSCIOUS ADULT
1. Victim may be using the universal signal of choking—holding the throat with one hand.
2. Ask the victim if he/she is choking.
3. Determine if the airway obstruction is complete. If the victim can speak or cough, do not interfere. The victim may be able to expel the obstruction through his/her own efforts.
4. If the obstruction is complete and the airway is blocked, perform subdiaphragmatic abdominal thrusts (Heimlich maneuver).
   a. Stand behind the victim.
   b. Place your arms around the victim's waist.
   c. With one hand, form a fist and grasp the fist with the other hand.
   d. Place the thumb side of the fist in the middle of the victim's abdomen slightly above the navel.
   e. Press fist into the abdomen, using quick inward and upward thrusts to push air from the lungs into the airway to remove any blockage.
5. A chest thrust may be performed on women in late pregnancy and on obese people.
   a. Stand behind the victim.
   b. Place your arms around the victim's chest under the armpits.
   c. Make a fist, grasp the fist with the other hand, and place the thumb side of the fist on the middle of the breastbone.
   d. Press the fist into the chest, using quick backward thrusts.
B. CONSCIOUS ADULT BECOMES UNCONSCIOUS
1. If repeated efforts to dislodge the obstruction fail and the victim becomes unconscious, turn the victim on his/her back while supporting head and neck, if necessary.
2. Call for help; call for emergency medical services or summon a bystander who will call for help.
3. Tilt the head back by pushing down on the forehead with one hand and lift the chin forward with the other hand. This is the open airway position.
4. Open the mouth and check for obstruction. Perform a finger sweep deeply into the mouth to try to remove obstruction.
5. With the head tilted back and the chin lifted in position for an open airway, pinch the nostrils between the thumb and forefinger of the hand on the victim's forehead, and place your mouth over the victim's mouth, making a tight seal. Give two breaths, inhaling deeply for each breath.
6. Watch the victim's chest to see if it rises as the lungs expand.
7. If there is no sign that rescue breathing is having any effect and the airway is still blocked, perform subdiaphragmatic abdominal thrusts.
   a. Straddle the victim's thighs.
   b. Place the heel of one hand on the midline of the victim's abdomen slightly above the navel.
   c. Place the second hand on top of the first hand.
   d. Press upward on the abdomen with quick thrusts (6–10 thrusts).
   e. Open the mouth to check for a dislodged obstruction; perform a finger sweep deep in the mouth along the cheek to remove any obstruction.
   f. Place the head in the open airway position with the head tilted back and the lower jaw lifted forward.

g. Pinch the nostrils closed and give breaths by sealing your mouth over the victim's mouth.

h. Watch for any movement of the chest, indicating that the airway is cleared.

i. In rapid sequence, repeat abdominal thrusts, finger sweep, and breaths until the airway is opened.

C. UNCONSCIOUS ADULT

1. Gently shake the shoulder to try to arouse victim. Shout "Are you OK?"

2. Call "Help!" to alert bystanders. Send someone to call emergency medical services.

3. If the victim is not on his/her back, turn the body as a unit, supporting the head and neck, if necessary.

4. Place the head in the open airway position—with one hand push down on the forehead to tilt the head back, and, with the other hand, lift the lower jaw forward.

5. Place your ear over the victim's mouth and listen for breath sounds, watch for chest movement, and feel for breaths on your cheek.

6. Give breaths by pinching the nostrils shut with the fingers of the hand on the victim's forehead. Seal your mouth over the victim's mouth. Give breaths, inhaling deeply before each breath.

7. If the airway is still obstructed, give 6–10 subdiaphragmatic abdominal thrusts following the steps listed in B. 7.

D. CONSCIOUS INFANT (LESS THAN ONE YEAR OF AGE)

1. Perform the procedure only if you are sure the breathing difficulty is caused by an obstruction and coughing is not effective in removing the obstruction. In all other situations, get the infant to advanced life support services immediately.

2. Place the infant face down, straddling your forearm (support the infant on your thigh) and support the head and neck with your hand.

3. Give four forceful back blows between the infant's shoulder blades using the heel of one hand.

4. Turn the infant over while supporting the head and neck.

5. Support the infant on your lap with the head lower than the trunk.

6. Using your forefinger and middle finger, give four chest thrusts in the middle of the sternum.

7. Alternate four back blows and four chest thrusts until the airway is cleared or the infant becomes unconscious.

E. CONSCIOUS INFANT BECOMES UNCONSCIOUS (LESS THAN ONE YEAR OF AGE)

1. Call for help. If someone comes, tell him to call for emergency medical services.

2. Place the infant on his/her back on a firm surface, supporting the head and neck during turning, if necessary.

3. Place the head in the open airway position—tilt the head back with one hand on the forehead and use the other hand to lift the lower jaw.

4. Look into the mouth. If you can see an obstruction, remove it. Do not perform a finger sweep.

5. Make sure the head is in the open airway position and give two gentle breaths by covering the nose and mouth of the infant with your mouth.

6. Turn the infant on his/her stomach, supporting the head and neck, and give four back blows.

7. Turn the infant on his/her back, supporting the head and neck, and give four chest thrusts.

8. Position the head in the open airway

position and check the mouth for obstruction. Remove the obstruction if it can be seen.

9. Maintain the open airway head position and give two gentle breaths as in step 5.

10. Repeat steps 6–9 until the airway is cleared.

11. When the obstruction is removed, check for breathing and pulse.

12. If there is no pulse, give two breaths and start CPR.

13. If there is a pulse, open the airway and check for breathing.

14. If there is no breathing, give breaths at the rate of one every three seconds (20 breaths per minute).

F. UNCONSCIOUS INFANT (LESS THAN ONE YEAR OF AGE)

1. Ensure that the infant is unconscious by gently shaking the shoulder.

2. Call for help to alert any bystanders to an emergency.

3. Turn the infant on his/her back on a firm surface, supporting the head and neck if necessary.

4. Place the head in the open airway position—place one hand on the forehead and press down to tilt the head back (do not tilt the head too far back); use the other hand to lift the lower jaw upward.

5. Place an ear over the infant's mouth and listen for breathing, watch the chest for movement indicating breathing, and feel for any breath with your ear.

6. Give two gentle breaths by sealing your mouth over the infant's nose and mouth.

7. Check that the head is in proper open airway position and repeat step 6.

8. Call for, or have someone else call, emergency medical service.

9. Turn the infant on his/her stomach, supporting the head and neck, and straddle the infant over your forearm resting on your thigh.

10. Give four back blows between the shoulder blades using the heel of one hand.

11. Turn the infant on his/her back, supporting the head and neck, and place the infant on your lap with the head lower than the trunk.

12. Using your forefinger and middle finger, give four chest thrusts in the middle of the sternum.

13. Lift the lower jaw forward and look into the mouth. If an obstruction can be seen, remove it.

14. Place the head in the open airway position and give two breaths with your mouth sealed over the nose and mouth of the infant.

15. Repeat steps 9–13, until the airway is cleared.

16. Remove any obstruction and check for pulse.

17. If there is no pulse, give two breaths and start CPR.

18. If there is a pulse, open the airway and check for breathing.

19. If there is no breathing, give breaths at the rate of one every three seconds (20 breaths per minute).

G. CHILD (ONE TO EIGHT YEARS OF AGE)

1. The procedure for clearing an obstructed airway is the same as that for adults with the following exception.

2. Do not perform the finger sweeps.

3. Tilt the head back and lift the lower jaw to open the airway.

4. Look into the airway. Use a finger to remove the obstruction only if it can be seen.

appendix f   cardiopulmonary resuscitation

A. CPR ON ADULTS (ONE RESCUER)

1. Try to get the victim to respond: gently shake the shoulder and shout "Are you OK?"
2. Call for help to summon anyone nearby.
3. If the victim is not on his/her back, turn the victim as a unit if necessary. Support the head and neck. Positioning should not take more than 4–10 seconds.
4. Open the airway as follows:

    a. Kneel beside the victim's shoulder.
    b. Place one hand on the victim's forehead and push down.
    c. Lift the lower jaw up with the other hand so the head is tilted backward.
    d. The mouth is partially open.
    e. Maintain the airway while you place your ear over the victim's mouth. For 3–5 seconds, listen for sounds of breathing, observe the chest for movement, and feel for breath on your cheek.

5. While keeping the head tilted back, pinch the nostrils shut between the thumb and forefinger of the hand on the victim's forehead.
6. Open your mouth, take a deep breath, and seal your mouth over the victim's mouth.
7. Breathe twice into the victim's mouth at the rate of 1 to 1½ seconds for each breath. Inhale deeply before each breath.
8. While maintaining the head tilt, check for pulse for 5–10 seconds as follows:
    a. Locate the carotid pulse using two or three fingers.
    b. Place your fingers on the victim's Adam's apple and slide them down the side of the throat to rest on the groove next to the muscle.
9. Send someone to call emergency medical services to summon help and provide information about the victim.
10. A cycle consists of two breaths and 15 chest compressions.
11. Perform chest compressions as follows:
    a. Position yourself at the victim's shoulder.
    b. Locate the proper hand position by using the forefinger and middle finger of one hand to trace the lower margin of the rib cage up to the lower end of the sternum. Place the middle finger at this point.
    c. Place the heel of the hand closest to the victim's head next to the index finger of the hand on the victim's chest.
    d. Place the other hand on top of this hand.
    e. Your shoulders should be directly over your hands with your arms straight and locked so your weight is transmitted straight down to the victim's chest.
    f. Keeping your fingers off the victim's ribs, begin compressions. Between each compression, the weight is released so the chest returns to its normal position, but the hands are not removed from the chest.
    g. Compressions are applied at the rate of 80–100 per minute. Establish a rhythm by counting "one-and-two-and-three-and-four-and. . . ."
    h. With each compression, the sternum is depressed 1½ to 2 inches.

12. After 15 compressions, give two breaths.
    a. Place the head in the open airway position.
    b. Pinch the nostrils closed, inhale deeply, and seal your mouth over the victim's mouth.
    c. Give breaths at the rate of one every 1 to 1½ seconds.
13. After four complete cycles of breaths and compressions, check for the carotid pulse for five seconds.
14. If there is a pulse but no breathing, give breaths at the rate of one breath every five seconds (12 per minute).
15. If there is no pulse, continue the cycles.

B. CPR ON ADULTS (TWO RESCUERS)
1. When a second rescuer appears who is certified in CPR, the first rescuer ends a cycle with two breaths.
2. The second rescuer checks the pulse for five seconds.
3. If there is no pulse, the second rescuer starts one-person CPR with two breaths.
4. The first rescuer assists by watching for the chest to rise during breaths and by checking for a pulse.

C. CPR ON A CHILD (ONE TO EIGHT YEARS OF AGE) (ONE PERSON)
1. Try to get the child to respond: gently shake the shoulder and shout ''Are you OK?''
2. Call for help to summon someone nearby.
3. If the child is not on his/her back, turn the child, supporting the head and neck. Positioning should not take more than 4–10 seconds.
4. Open the airway as follows:
    a. Kneel beside the child's shoulder.
    b. Place one hand on the child's forehead and push down.
    c. Lift the lower jaw up with your other hand so the head is tilted backward.
    d. The mouth is partially open.
    e. Maintain the airway while you place your ear over the victim's mouth. For 3–5 seconds, listen for sounds of breathing, observe the chest for movement, and feel for breath on your cheek.
5. While keeping the head tilted back, pinch the nostrils shut between the thumb and forefinger of the hand on the child's forehead.
6. Open your mouth, take a deep breath, and seal your mouth over the child's mouth.
7. Breathe twice into the child's mouth at the rate of 1 to 1½ seconds for each breath. Inhale deeply before each breath.
8. While maintaining the head tilt, check for a pulse for 5–10 seconds as follows:
    a. Locate the carotid pulse using two or three fingers.
    b. Place your fingers on the child's Adam's apple and slide them down the side of the throat to rest on the groove next to the muscle.
9. Send someone to call emergency medical services to summon help and provide information about the victim.
10. A cycle consists of one breath and five chest compressions.
11. Perform chest compressions as follows:
    a. Position yourself at the victim's shoulder.
    b. Locate the proper hand position by using the forefinger and middle finger of one hand to trace the lower margin of the rib cage up to the

lower end of the sternum. Place the middle finger at this point.

c. Place the heel of one hand only (the hand closest to child's head) next to the index finger of the first hand on the child's chest. Remove the first hand.

d. Your shoulders should be directly over your hands with your arms straight and locked so your weight is transmitted straight down to the child's chest.

e. Keeping your fingers off the child's ribs, begin compressions. Between each compression, your weight is released so the child's chest returns to its normal position, but your hand is not removed from the chest.

f. Compressions are applied at the rate of 80–100 per minute. Establish a rhythm by counting ''one - and - two - and - three - and - four - and. . . .''

g. With each compression, the chest (sternum) is depressed 1 to 1½ inches.

12. After five compressions, give one breath.

a. Place the child's head in the open airway position.

b. Pinch the nostrils closed, inhale deeply, and seal your mouth over the child's mouth.

c. Give breaths at the rate of one every 1 to 1½ seconds.

13. After ten complete cycles of breaths and compressions, check for the carotid pulse for five seconds.

14. If there is no pulse, give one breath and continue CPR.

15. If there is a pulse, check for breathing. If there is no breathing, give one breath every four seconds (15 breaths per minute).

D. CPR ON A CHILD (ONE TO EIGHT YEARS OF AGE) (TWO RESCUERS)

1. When a second rescuer appears who is certified in CPR, the first rescuer ends a cycle with one breath.

2. The second rescuer checks the carotid pulse for five seconds.

3. If there is no pulse, the second rescuer starts one-person CPR with one breath.

4. The first rescuer assists by watching for the chest to rise during breaths and by checking for the pulse.

E. CPR ON AN INFANT (ONE RESCUER)

1. Try to get the infant to respond: gently shake his/her shoulder.

2. Call for help to summon anyone nearby.

3. If the infant is not on his/her back, turn the infant on the back on a firm surface, supporting the head and neck.

4. Open the airway as follows:

a. Place one hand on the infant's forehead and push down to tilt the head back. Do not tilt the head too far back.

b. Lift the lower jaw up with your other hand.

c. The mouth is partially open.

5. While keeping the head tilted back, place your mouth over the nose and mouth of the infant. Give two gentle breaths at the rate of 1 to 1½ seconds per breath.

6. While keeping the infant's head tilted back to maintain an open airway, feel for the pulse.

7. For an infant, feel for the brachial pulse on the inside of the upper arm using your forefinger and middle finger.

8. Send someone to call emergency medical services.

9. A cycle consists of one breath for every five chest compressions.
10. Perform chest compressions as follows:
   a. Find the proper location for your fingers for compressions.
   b. Visualize a line between the infant's nipples.
   c. At the middle of this line, place two fingers one finger's width below that line.
   d. Compress the chest ½ to 1 inch at the rate of at least 100 times per minute.
   e. After five compressions, give one breath.
11. Complete ten cycles of breaths and compressions.
12. Check the brachial pulse.
13. If there is no pulse, give one breath and continue chest compressions.
14. Check for a pulse every few minutes.
15. If a pulse is present, check for breathing.
16. If there is no breathing, give one breath every three seconds (20 breaths per minute).

appendix g   living will declaration

The Society for the Right to Die makes available legally recognized documents forms to residents of those states that have enacted right-to-die laws. For use in states which have not yet enacted right-to-die laws, the Society supplies Living Will Declaration forms.

Society for the Right to Die
250 West 57th Street/New York. NY 10107

Living Will Declaration

INSTRUCTIONS
Consult this column for help and guidance.

To My Family, Doctors, and All Those Concerned with My Care

This declaration sets forth your directions regarding medical treatment.

I, _____. being of sound mind. make this statement as a directive to be followed if I become unable to participate in decisions regarding my medical care.

If I should be in an incurable or irreversible mental or physical condition with no reasonable expectation of recovery. I direct my attending physician to withhold or withdraw treatment that merely prolongs my dying. I further direct that treatment be limited to measures to keep me comfortable and to relieve pain.

You have the right to refuse treatment you do not want, and you may request the care you do want.

These directions express my legal right to refuse treatment. Therefore I expect my family. doctors, and everyone concerned with my care to regard themselves as legally and morally bound to act in accord with my wishes. and in so doing to be free of any legal liability for having followed my directions.

You may list specific treatment you do not want. For example:

   Cardiac resuscitation
   Mechanical respiration
   Artificial feeding/fluids by tubes

Otherwise, your general statement, top right, will stand for your wishes.

I especially do not want: _____
_____
_____
_____
_____

You may want to add instructions for care you do want—for example, pain medication; or that you prefer to die at home if possible.

Other instructions/comments: _____
_____
_____

If you want, you can name someone to see that your wishes are carried out, but you do not have to do this.

Proxy Designation Clause: Should I become unable to communicate my instructions as stated above. I designate the following person to act in my behalf:

Name_____
Address_____

If the person I have named above is unable to act in my behalf. I authorize the following person to do so:

Name_____
Address_____

Sign and date here in the presence of two adult witnesses, who should also sign.

Signed:_____ _____Date:_____

Witness:_____Witness:_____

Keep the signed original with your personal papers at home. Give signed copies to doctors. family. and proxy. Review your Declaration from time to time; initial and date it to show it still expresses your intent.

Reprinted by permission of the Society for the Right to Die, 250 West 57 Street, New York, NY 10107.

glossary

abbreviations—shortened forms of written words.

abortion—interruption of pregnancy before delivery date; may be natural or medically induced by the physician.

abuse—mistreatment; physical and/or mental cruelty. Abused wives are victims of beatings by their husbands. Abused children suffer physical maltreatment by one or both parents.

accelerated—speeded up; rapid.

acidosis—a condition in which the balance of acids and bases in the body is disturbed because of loss of salts, sodium and potassium or the accumulation of acids.

acute illness—a change from normal body functioning to a sudden pathological condition requiring immediate care.

addiction—a dependency on a drug or substance such as alcohol, cocaine, methadone, or cigarettes that block normal habits and body functions of everyday living.

adjustment—changes a person makes in behavior in order to deal with a situation.

adolescence—the period of physical and emotional development from early teens to young adulthood (usually between the ages of 13 to 18).

Age of Information—the general classification of today's society which relies heavily on computer sciences, micro chips, rapid transmittal of information via television, radio and telephone.

agitator—the spindle in a washing machine which rotates and forces the dirt out of clothes by forcing water and soap through the fabrics.

agrarian—a time in society during which life revolved around farming and rural population.

AIDS (anti-immune deficiency syndrome)—a crippling and fatal disease. It was first diagnosed in 1981. The disease breaks down the body's natural immune system so that its victims are vulnerable to almost any infection.

airborne—transmitted through the air. Sneezing and coughing are examples of pathogens being transmitted through the air.

A/K—above the knee amputation.

Al-Anon—a support group for the spouses of alcoholics. The group meets regularly to learn how to work and live with a family member who is an alcoholic.

Alateen—a support group for children of alcoholic parent(s). The children meet with a counselor and learn to recognize shared problems and how to deal with them on a daily basis.

Alcoholics Anonymous—a support group that provides help for the alcoholic based on getting through one day at a time without taking an alcoholic drink.

alcoholism—an addiction to alcohol leading to physical and social breakdown; generally considered to be an illness caused by the body's inability to metabolize alcohol.

allergy—a heightened sensitivity to a substance such as food, pollen, or dust that causes a physical reaction such as sneezing, runny nose, hives, etc. Allergies can often be relieved by a series of injections or avoidance of the substance bringing on an attack.

Alzheimer's disease—a progressive, degenerative illness causing loss of memory and mental incapacity.

ambulation—walking.

amputation—the surgical procedure in which a limb or part of a limb is removed.

aneurysm—localized enlargement of a blood vessel, may be due to a congenital defect of weakness of the vessel's wall.

angina pectoris—a severe pain in the chest that may radiate to the left arm and into the jaw. It is usually caused by an insufficient blood supply to the heart.

anticoagulant—a drug that delays or prevents the formation of blood clots within the circulatory system. Anticoagulants are not effective in dissolving clots that have already formed.

antiseptic—a product or technique preventing the growth of microorganisms or stopping and slowing the growth of pathogens.

anuria—no urinary output as a result of kidney failure.

anxiety—an unpleasant emotional or psychological state of constant fear or apprehension.

aphasia—impaired or lost ability to communicate through speech due to dysfunction of brain centers. There can be a loss of verbal understanding, word blindness, inability to understand the meaning of spoken or written words, or speaking in meaningless phrases.

apnea—absence of breathing or respirations.

apoplexy (stroke)—another term for a cerebral vascular accident.

arteriosclerosis—a condition in which the arteries become hard and lose the elasticity needed for good blood circulation.

arthritis—inflammation of the joints causing pain, swelling and enlargement of the joints. Usually associated with aging but can attack young people as well.

articulates—utter intelligible sounds; speaks.

ascites—the collection of fluid in the abdomen or peritoneal cavity, characterized by a swollen abdomen that feels hard to the touch.

asepsis—techniques to rid the environment of microorganisms and provide a sterile area.

asthma—a disorder of the respiratory system. Symptoms may include labored breathing, wheezing, coughing. There may be a secretion of fluid from the bronchials. Condition may be caused by pollutants, infection, emotional stress, and allergies.

atherosclerosis—fatty tissue (lipid) collected within or beneath the surface of blood vessels causing impaired circulation. Common cause of arterial occlusion (blocking).

attention span—increasing your ability and time to study with comprehension of the assigned reading material.

auditory—relating to hearing.

automatic speech—continuous repetition of phrases or words with no meaning.

axillary—the triangular space at the underside of the shoulder between the upper part of the arm and the side of the chest commonly called the armpit.

bacteria—one-celled microorganisms that are round, rod-shaped or spiral in form. They can cause infections in the body or in the environment.

Basic Four—the four food groups making up good nutritional standards for humans. The Basic Four food groups are the Fruits and Vegetables Food Group, The Dairy Food Group, the Breads and Cereals Food Group, and the Meats and Meat Substitute Food Group.

behavior—how an individual responds to a given situation.

benign tumor—a noncancerous growth that is usually covered or encased in a capsule.

bile—a yellowish green product of the liver which is manufactured and stored in the gallbladder. Bile is used by the body to metabolize fat in the small intestine.

biopsy—the surgical technique in which a sample of tissue is removed from an area where cellular change is suspected and examined under the microscope for signs of cancer.

B/K—below the knee amputation.

bland diet—food prepared with no spices featuring easily digested items that are soothing to the digestive tract.

blood lancet—small pointed surgical instrument used to pierce the skin to obtain a blood sample.

blood pressure—the force exerted by the blood on the walls of the blood vessels.

body language—a form of communication using gestures and facial expressions instead of words.

body mechanics—the techniques used to get the most effective and least taxing body movements. Bending the knees when lifting to avoid unnecessary strain to the back and legs is an example of good body mechanics.

bony prominences—areas of the body where bones protrude, e.g., the elbows, wrists, knees, pelvic bones, spinal column. Such bones have little natural padding and are areas where decubitus ulcers can easily form.

brachial—relating to the arm; commonly referred to when taking the blood pressure and checking the brachial artery or taking the brachial pulse.

bradycardia—an extremely slow heartbeat.

brooding—an emotional response to depression characterized by sadness and lack of communication.

bulk—roughage foods needed by the body to prevent constipation and to keep the stool soft. High-bulk foods are fruits, green leafy vegetables, potatoes, and whole-grain cereals.

cancer—a disease characterized by rapid growth of abnormal cells that form a tumor; it often spreads to other sites.

capillaries—the tiny vessels joining arteries and veins within the circulatory system.

carcinogen—a substance or agent which produces cancer; may be related to environment or heredity.

cardiac—anything related to the heart and the disorders associated with the heart.

cardinal sign—those signs which quickly indicate the status of a person's life functions. Cardinal signs include pulse, temperature, respirations, and blood pressure; these signs are often referred to as vital signs.

cardiopulmonary resuscitation—the restoring of respirations and heart beat by artificial means. It is performed by an individual following standard procedures which include establishing a clear airway for the victim, breathing into the victim's mouth, and compressing the victim's chest in order to restore breathing.

carotid—pertaining to the main arteries at the side of the neck which provide the main supply of blood to the neck and head area.

catheter—plastic or rubber tube inserted in the body to release or introduce fluids, e.g., dyes are introduced during heart catheterization, urine is released by use of the Foley catheter.

cerebral infarction—the condition in which a portion of the brain dies when an artery becomes blocked and blood is prevented from reaching that part of the brain.

cerebral vascular accident—a disorder of the blood vessels of the brain due to a blockage caused by an embolus or hemorrhage.

certified—meeting a specified standard. One who has special training in a particular subject as required by state law is said to be certified.

cesarean section—surgical abdominal delivery of a fetus; performed when normal birth canal delivery would be dangerous to the mother or fetus.

challenge—an invitation to participate in a competition.

chemotherapy—a treatment for cancer in which chemicals are used to destroy or slow the growth of cancerous cells.

cheyne–stokes respirations—term used to describe respirations: periods of apnea followed by periods dyspnea.

chronic illness—a long-term condition.

civilized—meeting standards of refinement; the act of being polite.

clinical—relating to a clinic; procedures such as bedmaking, bathing, oral care, etc.

cognitive—relates to thinking.

colon—the large intestine which is divided in three parts—the ascending, transverse, and descending.

colostomy—the removal of the diseased area of the gastrointestinal tract and making an external opening on the abdomen called a stoma. In some cases this may be a temporary solution and at a later date the intestine can be reattached to the bowel. Other colostomies may be permanent.

collateral circulation—when small blood vessels take over the circulation from near-by damaged or scarred blood vessels. These vessels enlarge themselves in order to carry the blood to the body parts.

coma—a state of unconsciousness in which there is little or no eye movement, diminished response to external stimuli and the inability to talk or communicate.

communication—the sending and receiving of messages; may be verbal or nonverbal.

compensation—making up for a weakness by becoming very good in some other area.

complication—the worsening of a body condition due to added factors.

components—the separate parts of a machine or a procedure which make up the whole.

conception—occurs when a female egg is fertilized by the male sperm; a zygote is formed and cell growth and multiplication takes place and a fetus develops.

confident—self-assured; ability to perform in an efficient manner.

confidentiality—keeping a client's personal affairs private. A home health aide must not give out information about the client except to the nursing supervisor or doctor.

confined—restricted to a certain location or area.

consultation—the exchange of views on a particular subject; a conference between physicians about a patient and the patient's treatment.

contagious—a condition that is transmitted to others easily; a communicable disease.

contaminated—that which is dirty and contains pathogens which may lead to infection.

congestive heart failure—a condition in which the heart cannot pump enough blood to the body. This can start as an acute problem which leads to a chronic condition with slow deterioration and the possibility of complications to other body systems.

consciousness—a normal state of awareness and responsiveness during the waking period.

constipation—infrequent or difficult bowel movements where the feces are unusually hard.

constrictive—something that is tight or narrowed.

contracture—a permanent shortening of muscle tissue causing deformity or distortion.

convenience foods—prepared foods that are ready to serve or require only cooking. These foods are often more expensive and may not be as tasty as foods prepared from fresh products.

conversion reaction—a defense mechanism whereby suppressed emotion takes the form of a physical symptom.

convulsion—abnormal, involuntary series of violent muscle contractions; often associated with epilepsy.

coronary occlusion—a condition in which a blood vessel in the heart muscle closes or is blocked by a blood clot.

crisis—an unstable, critical period that can alter ones life, either for better or for worse.

crisis intervention center—specialized units often run by volunteers who give information on how to deal with a specific problem. Drug hot lines, alcohol information centers, abortion clinics, Planned Parenthood, and poison control centers could all be considered crisis intervention centers.

critical—a dangerous time; relates to a crisis period in an illness.

culture—the learned behavior patterns of a race, nation or people; the life-style standards in society.

custom—common practice among a group of individuals or within a family or community; the ordinary or usual manner of acting.

cyanosis—lack of oxygen in the blood causing the client to appear bluish; indicates improper heart/lung function.

cyanotic—a bluish skin tone due to some problem of the respiratory system preventing proper inspiration and exhalation; the result of lack of oxygen to the blood cells.

cystitis—inflammation of the bladder.

debilitating—causing weakness.

decubitus ulcer—bedsore; breakdown of the skin covering a bony area. Reddening of the skin is the first sign; ulceration can occur within a period of 18 to 24 hours.

defense mechanism—a technique used by an individual to protect the self from unpleasantness, shame, anxiety or loss of self-esteem.

degenerative—a disease or condition causing tissues or organs to weaken and become abnormal. May be a progressive degeneration in which the condition becomes worse and worse with time.

delicatessen—a specialty store selling cheeses, coldcuts, sodas, sandwiches, and convenience foods.

denial—refusal to accept an unpleasant fact.

depression—a mental state characterized by loss of hope, feelings of rejection, generalized sadness and, in severe cases, the inability to function.

dermis—the inner layer of skin.

diabetes—a chronic disorder related to metabolism. It is caused by the inadequate functioning of the islets of Langerhans in the pancreas which produce insulin. Insulin is needed for the proper metabolism of sugars in the body.

diabetic complications—the results of untreated or improperly treated diabetes which can lead to blindness, gangrene, heart and kidney failure.

diabetic diet—a measured and low- or no-sugar diet for diabetics.

diagnosis—the identification of a disease or condition.

diarrhea—a condition in which stools are watery and frequent.

diastolic—measurement of blood pressure when the heart is relaxing.

dietary—relating to the diet or food eaten by an individual. Certain religious groups have dietary laws which prohibit the eating of certain foods.

diet modification—special diet changes required for a particular set of conditions, e.g., low-fat diet, liquid diet, diabetic diet.

digitalis—a therapeutic drug used to slow down the heart beat and to increase the force of the heart muscle contractions thus enabling the heart to pump more blood.

disinfectant—a chemical substance used to kill bacteria.

disinfected—use of a medication or germ-fighting agent to destroy microorganisms.

disorganized—confused and unable to follow and plan a step-by-step practical course of action.

disoriented—confused or mixed up; loss of the sense of time, place or identity.

displacement—taking one's own anger or frustration out on someone else, e.g., yelling at a child because you are angry with another person and afraid to yell at that person.

dispute—disagreement leading to argument.

distended—to become bloated or swollen. A distended abdomen becomes hard to the touch and bulges out.

diuretic—a drug used to reduce fluid accumulation in the body. Persons taking a diuretic urinate frequently.

diversion—a change or distraction to help a person relax. Soft music, television, or talking can be diversions to keep the client from thinking about the illness.

doffing—removing of the prosthesis.

donning—application of the prosthesis.

DPT—a combination immunization given to infants to prevent diphtheria, pertussis (whooping cough), and tetanus.

ductless gland—that part of the endocrine system that releases hormones directly into the blood and lymph systems.

dyslexia—a learning disability which prevents a person from reading or understanding the written word.

dysphasia—speech difficulty resulting from a brain lesion.

dyspnea—difficult or labored respiration.

-ectomy—a suffix which indicates removal of.

edema—the swelling of legs and/or arms or other body parts when water is being retained unnaturally.

efficient—performance of tasks without wasted time and effort and doing them well.

embalming—the process of removing blood and fluid from a dead body and replacing the fluids with a chemical preservative to keep the body from decomposing before burial.

embolism—obstruction of a blood vessel by a blood clot or foreign matter.

emergency—a sudden, unexpected happening usually related to a danger.

emotion—basic feelings common to all such as love, fear, anger, sorrow and anxiety.

emotional impact—how one is affected by a situation or individual and how one responds to that situation or individual.

emotional support—the depth of understanding for the emotional needs of others and the way in which a person successfully meets those needs.

empathy—the ability to observe and share the feelings of others in a supportive manner.

emphysema—an abnormal condition of the lung tissue in which the lungs lose their normal spongy and elastic character making for a poor exchange of gases needed for normal respirations. The condition may be acute or chronic.

empty calories—foods high in carbohydrates and fats and low in proteins, minerals and vitamins; ''junk'' food.

endocrine—a body system made up of ductless glands which secrete hormones directly into the blood and lymph system.

environment—the sum total of the conditions surrounding an individual.

enzymes—proteins produced by the body that break down organic matter (food) within the body; necessary for digestion and metabolism.

epidermis—the outer layer of the skin.

epilepsy—an illness related to brain dysfunction that may or may not bring on convulsions. Heredity seems to play some part in the transmission of this illness; it may also result from a head injury. Medication can control the condition in many cases.

epiglottis—thin irregular shaped structure located at the rear of the tongue and covers the larynx (voice box) when a person swallows. It prevents food or liquids from entering the airway.

ethics—a code of behavior. Medical ethics is the standard of professional conduct by health team members.

euphoria—a state of high feeling.

evacuation—to empty or remove the contents from.

evaluation—a determination of how well a given duty or demonstration of skill is performed.

exhale—to breath out.

experience—knowledge, skill, or practice derived from the direct participation in events; being part of an event.

extended care facility—a nursing home, residence, or hospital wing that is licensed by the state to provide long-term care.

external stimulus—a message or impulse sent to the nervous system from outside the body that causes a mental or physical response.

extinguish—to cause to stop burning; to quench.

familiar—that which is well known.

family unit—a group of people, usually related, who may or may not live under the same roof.

fanfold—to fold in pleats.

fantasizing—daydreaming; engaging in imagination that is not real.

femur—bone in thigh, going from the hip to the knee.

fermented—rotted.

fertilization—uniting of the female ova and the male sperm which starts a new being.

fibula—secondary and smaller bone in the lower leg, next to the shin bone.

finances—related to the money earned, spent, or saved by an individual, family, or organization.

first aid—the immediate help given in case of accident or injury.

fixed income—usually refers to the sum total of money coming in to a retired, elderly, or disabled person on a regular monthly basis.

flexible—the ability to adapt to new situations or conditions; pliant.

foot drop—a condition in which the muscles of the foot are out of alignment; may be due to injury or paralysis.

fracture—a break in a bone requiring an X ray to determine the type and treatment.

fraternal twins—result from the fertilization of two female eggs by two separate male sperms. The two embryos are encased in separate amniotic sacs and have separate placentas. Fraternal twins may or may not be of the same sex.

frustration—a sense of insecurity and dissatisfaction due to unfulfilled needs and/or unresolved problems.

gait—term used for walking style.

gait deviations—any abnormalities found in a walking style.

gambling—betting on the outcome of an event; may be an addictive behavior pattern among certain individuals.

gamma globulin—an immune factor of blood plasma which can be manufactured and injected into the body to prevent or diminish the effects of diseases such as measles, polio, chicken pox, hepatitis, etc.

gangrene—the formation of large areas of dead tissue which can become a serious complication.

gas gangrene—a complication of diabetes which causes the skin to decay requiring surgical removal of a limb or body part.

gestation period—the time required from conception until birth. In humans the gestation period is nine months.

gesture—body, hand, muscle movements; in body language, gestures are used to communicate without words.

glucose—a form of sugar required by the body.

glucose tolerance test—a procedure used to measure the metabolism of carbohydrates in the body; usually refers to blood and/or urine tests to diagnose and treat diabetes.

goiter—a thyroid disorder causing unnatural enlargement of the thyroid gland which is visible as a lump at the front of the neck.

gonorrhea—a venereal disease which develops within 48 hours after sexual contact with an infected person. Painful burning sensation during urination among males; females have urinary burning and vaginal discomfort. Complications can lead to reproductive disorders, liver involvement and blindness (more common among women). Immediate treatment is required.

hazard—that which is dangerous or could cause a serious accident.

heat exhaustion—an acute response to exposure to high temperatures; often associated with an overexposure to hot sunlight.

Heimlich maneuver—technique for removing a food particle or foreign object that has become lodged in the trachea thereby preventing flow of air to the lungs. To administer the Heimlich maneuver, wrap your arms around the victim's waist from behind; make a fist with your one hand and place it against the victim's abdomen between the navel and the rib cage; grasp your fist with your other hand and press into the victim's abdomen with a quick upward thrust. Repeat if necessary.

hemiplegia—a weakness or paralysis confined to one side of the body.

hemophilia—a blood disease usually found only among males; the blood clotting factor is missing and even small injuries can cause severe blood loss that may require transfusion.

hepatitis—inflammation of the liver.

herbs—plants having an aroma that may be used in medicines or as a seasoning for foods to enhance taste.

heredity—the passing of physical and mental traits from parents to their offspring, e.g., height, weight, general appearance, skin color, talents, and intelligence.

herpes—a sexually transmitted virus for which there is no known cure.

high-bulk diet—diet including foods that are high in fiber in order to stimulate bowel action.

home health aides—individuals who are specially trained to provide safe and proper physical care to sick persons; members of the health team who are supervised by nurses.

hormones—products of body glands which assist in healthy body function.

homosexual—a person who feels sexual attraction to members of the same sex.

hygiene—the study of health and the observance of health rules.

hypertension—high blood pressure.

hypotension—low blood pressure.

hysterectomy—a major surgical technique in which the uterus is removed. In the case of a panhysterectomy, all the female reproductive organs are removed.

identical twins—result from the fertilization of one female egg by one male sperm. The fertilized egg divides into two embryos encased in separate amniotic sacs that share one placenta. Identical twins are always of the same sex.

ileostomy—the surgical removal of a diseased portion of the small intestine and the preparation of an external abdominal stoma (usually permanent) from which a liquid stool is expelled.

illiterate—the inability to read due to lack of education or a learning disability.

immobilize—to hold rigidly in one position.

immunity—the ability to resist a particular disease.

immunization—injections and/or oral vaccines given to prevent the onset of communicable diseases.

impacted—tightly wedged. In reference to the stool, impaction is a condition in which the feces become hardened and lodged in the lower colon or rectum.

incinerator—a furnace for burning trash and garbage.

incontinence—the loss of voluntary control of the bladder muscles causing uncontrolled voiding.

incubation period—the time between entry of germs into the body and the appearance of the first signs of the disease.

Industrial Society—refers to that period of time when technology and industry became the basis of economic development and the farming society decreased in importance.

infection—invasion of pathogenic organisms causing inflammation, discomfort, or illness. Infections may be caused by viruses, bacteria, fungi, or animal parasites.

infraction—violation of a rule or law.

inhale—to breathe in; that part of the breathing and respiration cycle in which oxygen is drawn into the lungs.

injection—the forcing of a fluid into a blood vessel or body cavity or under the skin.

instinct—an inborn trait.

insulin—a hormone produced by the islets of Langerhans in the pancreas which is essential for the maintenance of proper blood sugar levels. Insulin can be medically prepared from animal pancreas for use in diabetes.

insulin shock—a condition in which there is too much insulin in the body resulting in abnormally low blood sugar. The condition is characterized by nervousness, dizziness, perspiration, headache, blurred vision. Immediate treatment such as eating candy or sugar or drinking orange juice is necessary.

interaction—the reciprocating actions between two people or between members of a group.

interfere—to concern oneself in the affairs of others; meddle.

intergenerational conflict—the problems occurring among individuals of differing ages living together who all have needs and desires which may cause disagreements, anger, or unhappiness.

intermittent positive pressure breathing (I.P.P.B.)—clients suffering from pulmonary disease such as emphysema breathe through a mask connected to a machine which produces intermittent positive air pressure. Increasing the air pressure inflates the lungs; when the pressure is released, the client exhales. This helps the client to breathe easier.

internal stimulus—a message or impulse from within the body that is transmitted through the nervous system and causes a mental or physical response.

interpersonal relationships—behaviors among individuals related to communication and getting along in a satisfactory manner.

intrafamily—the relationships among members of a specific family or group of individuals living together as a family.

involuntary—body responses not subject to control that occur naturally and automatically.

irrigation—the use of a fluid to cleanse an area.

—separating the client from others in the family to prevent the spread of pathogens.

-itis—a suffix which means inflammation.

jaundice—a condition in which there is a yellowish color to the skin, mucous membranes, and eyes. It is associated with liver failure when excessive amounts of bilirubin enter the blood.

jejunostomy—surgical opening of the jejunum.

Judaism—the religious practices of Jews, including dietary laws, attending services on Saturday, following the teachings of the Old Testament.

juvenile diabetes—a form of diabetes occurring among persons under the age of 25; generally a condition that is hard to keep under control requiring careful medical attention.

kosher—dietary law practiced by some Jewish people. Rules include how animals are killed, what kinds of foods may be used, and keeping separate pots, pans and dishes when preparing milk and meat products or special holiday meals.

laryngectomy—the surgical removal of the larynx (voice box) because of disease. Laryngectomy patients can be taught to speak through an artificial airway by gulping air through the external stoma into the esophagus.

larynx—the voice box.

legal—having to do with the law and or laws.

lesion—a well-defined abnormal change in tissue due to disease or injury. Examples of lesions are crusts, scales, scars, ulcers, chancres, raised and reddened areas, pimples, pus.

lethargy—a state of unnatural tiredness, feelings of exhaustion and sleepiness.

liability—something for which a person has a responsibility or duty.

ligaments—the tough elastic fibers that hold the bones in place.

listening—hearing with thoughtful attention.

lobectomy—partial removal of a lung.

localized—pertaining to a specific area.

low-birth-weight baby—a full-term infant weighing less than five pounds.

low-residue diet—diet in which only foods low in bulk are allowed; used to lessen bowel activity.

low-sodium diet—diet containing foods with low salt content; no extra salt is to be added.

LPN—licensed practical nurse; a person who has met state educational mandates, passed a state examination, and is licensed to practice in the state.

malignant—uncontrolled growth that is resistant to treatment and has a tendency to spread to surrounding areas; often said of cancerous growths.

malnutrition—a condition resulting from poor diet that lacks needed nutrients to maintain health; early signs include muscle weakness.

mammography—X rays of the female breasts used to determine if a tumor is present in the breasts.

mandible—lower jaw bone.

manipulation—a behavior that uses insidious means to control others to one's own advantage.

mastectomy—the surgical removal of the female breast(s); may be total or partial.

masturbate—self-stimulation of the genitalia.

maxilla—upper jaw bone.

Meals-On-Wheels—prepared meals which are delivered to homebound clients or to senior citizens centers to help assure the disadvantaged, handicapped, ill, or aged have at least one meal a day that is nutritionally sound.

measles—a highly contagious viral disease characterized by the eruption of distinct red circular spots; other symptoms are fever, general malaise, sneezing, nasal congestion, and brassy cough. Children should be immunized to prevent the disease.

mechanical life support—machines used to keep the heart and lungs working when they do not function naturally, e.g., heart-lung machines or oxygen.

medical asepsis—procedures used to stop the spread of pathogens from person to person or place to place.

Medic Alert ID—a bracelet or necklace worn by individuals with specific medical problems such as allergies, diabetes, or hemophilia. In an emergency, the ID may provide information necessary to save the person's life.

medical terminology—those words that specifically relate to a medical condition or describe medical procedures.

menopause—cessation of the monthly menstrual cycle. It normally occurs during a woman's middle years (late forties to late fifties). Following menopause, reproductive ability ceases.

mental—relating to the mind; the nonphysical health condition of an individual.

metabolic rate—the speed and efficiency of the body systems in using the nutrients in the blood after digestion has taken place; related to growth, energy and waste elimination.

metastasize—to spread; refers to the uncontrolled spread of cancer cells throughout the body from the original cancer site.

microorganism—organism that is not visible with the naked eye such as bacterium or protozoan; some microorganisms cause serious illnesses.

midwife—a specially educated person who cares for pregnant women and can deliver babies. In most states, it is required that a physician be available as backup in case of an emergency.

mildew—a fuzzy, grayish fungus growth that appears in damp, dark areas.

misconduct—improper behavior; mismanagement of responsibilities.

mobile—that which moves about. Pathogens are mobile and may be carried through the air. Families who move from place to place because of job changes are called mobile families.

multiple sclerosis—a progressive disease involving the nerves of the brain and spinal cord. It may start slowly and become worse throughout life or there may be periods of remission when the condition seems to stay about the same. Signs and symptoms are tremors and inability to coordinate muscles.

muscular dystrophy—a progressive degenerative disease of the muscles surrounding the skeleton; characterized by loss of strength, physical disability and deformity.

myocardial infarction—an acute coronary occlusion commonly called a heart attack.

myth—a story that is unverifiable.

neuropathy—having mainly to do with diabetic clients, but is any disease of the nerves.

nitro-patch—a patch containing nitroglycerin; when placed on the chest nitroglycerin is released and absorbed into the body through the skin. The nitro-patch is a replacement for the nitroglycerin tablet which is taken sublingually.

nonverbal—a way of communicating without words using gestures, facial expressions or other body language.

nutrient—the usable products derived from the food eaten after the food has been acted on by the digestive juices. Nutrients are absorbed through the walls of the small intestine and carried through the body.

nutrition—the sum of those processes using food for growth, development and body maintenance.

oath—a solomn promise to do what one has said will be done.

occult blood—hidden blood, must be seen by a microscope, sometimes a stool is sent to the lab for occult blood testing.

offensive—causing displeasure.

oliguria—lowered urinary output.

optimal health—highest point an individual can achieve mentally and physically as adapted from Abraham Maslow's hierarchy of needs.

optimist—one who expects a positive outcome to a situation.

oral hygiene—care given to the oral cavity to prevent diseases of that area and to keep bad odors from forming.

osteoporosis—loss of bone density and strength; the bones become increasingly porous and brittle which may lead to malformations such as a dowager's hump or hip fractures. Postmenopausal women are at high risk. An adequate intake of calcium helps to prevent the disease.

-otomy—suffix meaning to cut into.

otosclerosis—chronic, progressive deafness, especially to low tones.

outsider—one who is not part of an organized group.

ovulation—that time of the month when the ovum (egg) produced in the female reproductive system's ovary is released and enters the fallopian tube where it may be fertilized.

oxygen—the colorless, tasteless, odorless gaseous element in the atmosphere which is essential to breathing.

Pap smear—a medical technique whereby a sample of the vaginal cells are tested for cancer; recommended for women annually to detect early signs of cancer.

paralysis—loss of sensation in a body part making it difficult or impossible to move that part of the body.

paraplegic—paralysis of the lower body involving both legs.

patella—knee cap.

patella tendon—tendon found below knee cap.

pathogens—microorganisms causing disease or infection in the body.

peer pressure—the attitudes and behavior patterns within a particular group which all group members are expected to follow. (A peer is an equal; one of same age group, rank, social status.)

perishable—likely to spoil or decay.

peristalsis—the progressive, wavelike movements that occur involuntarily to move food through the digestive system.

permanent press—fabric with combination of natural and man-made threads that require little or no ironing.

persistent—constantly repeated; permanent, or stubborn in a course of action.

personal reference—a person, other than a member of the individual's family, who can give a prospective employer a recommendation concerning the character and ability of an individual seeking employment.

pessimist—one who expects a negative or bad outcome to a situation or who looks on the gloomy side of life.

phantom pain—a sensation of pain felt in an amputated part. It is caused by the nerve endings that have not had time to heal from the surgery.

phobia—an abnormal fear.

pilferage—to repeatedly steal in small amounts or value.

pistoning—stump slipping up and down in the prosthesis.

pitch—the high or low tone of voice with which one speaks. Pitch is related to the sound wave frequency that causes variations in sounds from high to low.

pneumonectomy—surgical removal of the entire lung.

pneumonia—an acute inflammation of the lungs caused by bacteria, viruses or fungi; characterized by high fever, chills, headache, cough and chest pains.

poliomyelitis—an inflammation of the spinal cord's gray matter which can cause paralysis and respiratory problems; a communicable disease that has been almost wiped out as a result of vaccines.

polyester—a man-made fabric.

practice—repeatedly going over a procedure until one does it well; the clientele of a doctor or medical practice.

prefix—series of letters placed at the beginning of a word that produces a derivative word.

premature—an infant born before full term (37 weeks gestation is considered full term among humans).

prescription—usually refers to medication ordered by the doctor to be used following specific instructions and in controlled dosages.

preventative health measures—use of inoculations, special diets, or other techniques to avoid illness before it starts.

priority—decision as to what items or tasks should be done first based on their importance.

privilege—a special benefit or opportunity offered to a person or group.

procedure—the steps taken to accomplish a particular task; a course or plan of action.

produce—fresh fruits and vegetables.

professional—one who is skilled or experienced in a particular area of training or learning.

prognosis—the probable outcome of an illness.

progressive degenerative disease—disease which grows worse as time goes on, often resulting in greater and greater physical loss to a particular part of the body.

projection—a defense mechanism whereby an individual blames someone else for his or her own failure.

prolonged—that which lasts over a long period of time.

prosthesis—artificial replacement for a body part.

protozoa—tiny, one-celled microscopic animals.

psychology—the study or science concerned with mental processes and behavior of an individual; the study concerned with mental health.

psychosocial—relating to both psychological and social problems/happenings in the life of an individual.

puberty—the time period following childhood when the body matures and reproduction becomes possible.

pulse—the measurement of the number of heartbeats per minute.

quadraplegic—paralysis of four extremities—arms and legs.

radical mastectomy—the surgical removal of the entire breast including the underlying muscles and lymph glands under the arm. It is performed in the hope of stopping further spread of cancer cells.

rales—bubbling sound from the lungs when fluid or mucus is trapped in the air passages.

range of motion exercises—the exercises designed to prevent contractures and loss of motion and function in the joints; usually planned by a physical therapist.

rationalization—a defense mechanism whereby a person gives excuses to account for personal failings.

reality orientation—techniques used to keep confused clients in touch with reality.

recreation—a pleasurable activity following a period of work; distraction from normal activity in an effort to have fun or enjoy a change of pace.

rectum—the last segment of the digestive system from which feces are expelled.

registry service—an agency that employees certified individuals to give home health care.

rehabilitation—the restoring of physical and/or mental abilities following an accident or illness. Some patients can be fully restored to normal functioning; others are brought up to the best possible level through exercise and retraining.

reinforcement—the act of supporting another individual by words and actions. Reinforcement may be either positive or negative.

remedies—the methods and medications used to cure or make well.

remission—a period in an illness when the symptoms cease or become less severe.

residue—that which is left over. In nutrition, high or low reside refers to the amount of bulk and fiber food in the diet. These foods are usually low in vitamins.

respiration—the sum total of the processes by which the body exchanges oxygen and carbon dioxide in the respiratory system.

respirations—one of the vital signs in which the breaths of the person are counted. Illness can cause the respirations to fluctuate or become abnormal.

rigidity—stiffness or inability to bend; associated with the pain and joint stiffness caused by arthritis.

RN—registered nurse; an individual who has attended nursing school or college, taken and passed state examinations, and is licensed to practice in the state.

root word—the main part of a compound word that has a prefix or suffix.

sanitary—of or relating to health and cleanliness.

satiety—the feeling of satisfaction or fullness after eating.

schedule—a plan to organize work so that everything that needs to be done can be completed within a certain time.

security—the feeling of being comfortable or safe in a given situation.

seizure—a sudden attack; a convulsion.

self-esteem—value one places on one's self as a person functioning in society.

self-scheduling—the individual plan of action that allows one to determine priorities and to work as his/her own pace in order to accomplish set goals.

self-understanding—the awareness of one's own behavior and feelings in any given situation.

semicoma—the third level of unconsciousness in which it is difficult to rouse the patient or get the patient to respond.

senescence—the period of old age; the process of growing old.

senile—pertaining to old age.

senile dementia—a group of mental disorders afflicting some aging individuals.

sensitive—being aware of the physical and emotional needs of others.

sensory deficits—lack or lessening of ability to receive stimuli in a particular sense (loss of hearing, weak eyes, weakened taste buds, inability to feel heat or cold, etc.)

septum—divider, as seen in the division of the heart. The septum divides right side from left side.

Seventh Day Adventist—a religious sect observing the Sabbath on Saturday and following a set of standards of daily living that may be different from other religious groups.

shrinking—decreased, as in swelling.

sibling rivalry—the normal jealousy and competition found between brothers and sisters in the family setting.

sickle cell anemia—a hereditary and chronic blood anemia in which the red blood cells are shaped in a crescent formation and look like a sickle. This disease occurs mainly in Blacks.

sign—in medicine, a change in the patient that can be observed or measured.

single-parent family—a family group headed by a mother or a father in which there is no other adult providing emotional and/or financial support.

skin breakdown—any cut or scaping of the skin due to pressure or positioning too long in the same position.

social service agency—a governmental body which provides assistance in solving problems such as housing, living conditions, clothing or food stamps for those unable to find jobs or support themselves.

soft diet—diet in which soft, easily digested foods are ordered for clients recovering from surgery or who have ulcers; this diet causes little upset to the digestive system.

somnolence—a state of drowsiness and lethargy; the desire to sleep.

spasticity—increased tension in the muscles causing irregular movements of the body part involved.

special children—the term used to refer to children with handicaps who need extra assistance.

specialist—one who has studied in a concentrated area and has specialized in one particular field of knowledge.

sperm—the male germ cell ejaculated during intercourse that fertilizes the ovum and starts the cycle of reproduction.

sphygmomanometer—the instrument used to measure blood pressure.

stabilized—under control and on an even course.

staple items—those foodstuffs normally kept in most homes which are used in many ways and are the basis for preparing meals, e.g., flour, sugar, spices, herbs, canned goods.

sterile—free of pathogens.

stimuli—messages sent from the five body senses to the brain so that a response can be made. Internal stimuli start within the body; external stimuli come from outside the body.

stoic—not affected by or showing emotions.

stoma—the surgically formed opening between a body cavity or passage and the body's surface.

stressful—a situation that is filled with pressure and causes anxiety and signs of discomfort.

stump—term used for the remaining portion of the amputated limb.

subcutaneous—under the skin.

sublingually—under the tongue.

suffix—series of letters placed at the end of a word that produces a derivative word.

suicide—the act of taking one's own life.

supervisor—one who is in charge of other people.

sympathetic—having concerns or sharing the feelings of others; being sensitive to the needs of others.

symptom—those changes reported by the patient such as feeling pain which may not be visible.

syphilis—an infectious, chronic venereal disease characterized by open lesions which can spread to the entire body and affect the nervous system.

system—a group of structures or organs related to each other that work together to perform certain functions.

systolic—measurement of blood pressure when the heart is contracting.

tachycardia—a very rapid heartbeat.

technique—the way a particular task or procedure is done following acceptable guidelines.

technological—related to scientific advances that increase productivity of machines and eliminates manual operations.

temperament—the usual mood of an individual.

temporal—temples; that part of the face and head near and above the ears.

terminal asepsis—the careful cleaning of an area after a sick person has been removed from the room to destroy any pathogens that may be in the room.

theory—the practical and necessary information one must learn about a particular topic or subject.

thrombus—a blood clot that obstructs a part of the circulatory system.

TIA—transient ischemic attack.

tibia—prominent bone in the lower leg (shin).

tone—related to voice pitch but includes the quality and length of sound when speaking.

topical—pertaining to a particular area; local.

trachea—the main tube running from the throat to the lungs to bring air in and out of the body; the windpipe.

tracheostomy—a surgical procedure to create an opening in the trachea; an emergency operation in cases where the trachea is obstructed and the person cannot breathe.

tremors—a spastic condition of the muscles in which a body part develops an uncontrollable shaking.

unconscious—a state of unawareness with four possible levels—somnolence, stupor, semicoma, and coma.

underestimate—placing too low a value on a condition or situation; to assess as being less than actual.

upward mobility—moving upward.

urgent—requiring immediate attention.

vaccine—a manufactured product administered to develop a resistance to an infectious disease.

vasoconstriction—narrowing of the blood vessel.

vasodilation—widening of the blood vessel.

vegetarian—one who does not eat meat or meat products.

venereal disease—a group of diseases usually transmitted by sexual contact with one having that disease.

verbal—communication through the use of words.

virus—microorganism that lives and grows by feeding on living cells; the cause of many infections.

vocational—related to the job or profession in which one is employed.

voluntary movements—actions controlled by the brain after messages are sent by the senses through the nervous system; the body chooses the appropriate action.

wellness—free of illness; a state of well-being free of psychological or physiological symptoms.

withdrawal—removing one's self physically or mentally from an uncomfortable or frightening situation.

index